CHILDREN, FAMILIES, AND HIV/AIDS

Children, Families, and HIV/AIDS

PSYCHOSOCIAL AND THERAPEUTIC ISSUES

Editors

Nancy Boyd-Franklin, PhD
Gloria L. Steiner, EdD
Mary G. Boland, MSN, RN

Foreword by James Oleske, MD, MPH

THE GUILFORD PRESS
New York   London

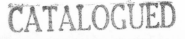

©1995 The Guilford Press
A Division of Guilford Publications, Inc.
72 Spring Street, New York, NY 10012

Printed in the United States of America

This book is printed on acid-free paper.

Last digit is print number: 9 8 7 6 5 4 3 2

Library of Congress Cataloging-in-Publication Data

Children, families, and HIV/AIDS: psychosocial and therapeutic
    issues / editors, Nancy Boyd-Franklin, Gloria L. Steiner,
    Mary G. Boland.
        p.   cm.
    Includes bibliographical references and index.
    ISBN 0-89862-147-X (hard)   ISBN 0-89862-502-5
(pbk.)
        1. AIDS (Disease) in children—Social aspects.   2. AIDS
    (Disease) in children—Psychological aspects.   3. AIDS
    (Disease) in children—Patients—Family relationships.
    4. AIDS (Disease) in children—Patients—Services for.
    I. Boyd-Franklin, Nancy.   II. Steiner, Gloria L.   III.
Boland,
    Mary G.
    RJ387.A25C48   1995
    362.1'98929792—dc20   93-34761
                                                            CIP

To the children and families
who are living with HIV/AIDS

Royalties from the sale this book will be donated
to the Starfish Foundation for Children with AIDS, Inc.,
to provide an emergency fund for children and families
living with HIV/AIDS.

Contributors

Julia del C. Alemán, MSW, *Assistant Director of Social Work/Pediatrics, Newark Beth Israel Medical Center, Newark, NJ*

Jacqueline A. Bartlett, MD, *Director of Consultation/Liaison, Department of Psychiatry, University of Medicine and Dentistry of New Jersey/New Jersey Medical School, Newark*

Mary G. Boland, MSN, RN, *Associate in Pediatrics, University of Medicine and Dentistry of New Jersey/New Jersey Medical School, Newark; Director, AIDS Program, Children's Hospital of New Jersey, Newark*

Nancy Boyd-Franklin, PhD, *Professor of Psychology, Graduate School of Applied and Professional Psychology, Rutgers University, Piscataway, NJ; Consultant, National Pediatric HIV Resource Center, Children's Hospital of New Jersey, Newark*

Patricia M. Brady, EdD, *private practice, Kendall Park, NJ*

Lynn Czarniecki, MSN, RN, *Clinical Nurse Specialist, AIDS Program, Children's Hospital of New Jersey, Newark*

Elizabeth W. Drelich, MSW, *Social Worker, AIDS Program, Children's Hospital of New Jersey, Newark*

Haftan Eckholdt, PhD, *Director of Information Technology, Department of Psychiatry, University of Medicine and Dentistry of New Jersey/New Jersey Medical School, Newark*

Katherine A. Gomez, RN, MA, *Psychology Clinician, Department of Child Psychiatry, Children's Hospital of New Jersey, Newark*

Heidi J. Haiken, MSW, MPH, ACSW, *Social Work Services Coordinator, AIDS Program, Children's Hospital of New Jersey, Newark*

Jennis Hanna, PhD, *Assistant Supervising Psychologist, AIDS Program, Children's Hospital of New Jersey, Newark*

David C. Harvey, MSW, LCSW, *Executive Director, AIDS Policy Center for Children, Youth, & Families, Washington, DC*

Michèle M. Jean-Gilles, MA, *Research Associate, Department of Psychiatry, Center for Family Studies, University of Miami School of Medicine, Miami, FL*

Steven E. Keller, PhD, *Professor, Department of Psychiatry, University of Medicine and Dentistry of New Jersey/New Jersey Medical School, Newark*

Patricia Kloser, MD, FACP, *Associate Professor of Clinical Medicine and Associate Professor of Preventive Medicine, University of Medicine and Dentistry of New Jersey/New Jersey Medical School, Newark; Medical Director, AIDS Services, University Hospital, Newark, NJ*

Theresa Kreibick, PsyD, *Pscyhology Resident, Newington Children's Hospital, Newington, CT, and Charter Oak Terrace/Rice Heights Health Center, Hartford, CT*

Mary Ellen La Brie, RNC, *Research Nurse, AIDS Clinical Trials Unit, University of Medicine and Dentistry of New Jersey/New Jersey Medical School, Newark*

Olivia R. Lewis, MA, *Staff Clinician, Child and Adolescent Unit, Community Mental Health Center, University of Medicine and Dentistry of New Jersey, Newark, NJ*

Sandra Lewis, PhD, *Assistant Professor of Clinical Psychiatry and Pediatrics/Psychologist Educator, National Pediatric HIV & Family Resource Center, University of Medicine and Dentistry of New Jersey/New Jersey Medical School, Newark*

Mark Mintz, MD, *Head, Division of Pediatric Neurology, Cooper Hospital University Medical Center, Robert Wood Johnson Medical School, Camden, NJ*

Bradley C. Norford, PhD, *Supervising Psychologist, Devereux Foundation, Glenmoore, PA*

James M. Oleske, MD, MPH, *Francois Xavier Bagnoud Professor of Pediatrics and Director, Division of Allergy, Immunology, and Infectious Diseases, University of Medicine and Dentistry of New Jersey/New Jersey Medical School; Medical Director, Children's Hospital AIDS Program, United Hospital Medical Center, Newark*

Sylvia W. Pollock, PhD, *Supervising Psychologist, Newark Beth Israel Medical Center, Community Mental Health Center, Newark, NJ*

Ann Silver Pozen, PsyD, *Adjunct Faculty, Center for Psychological Studies, Nova University, Fort Lauderdale, FL*

Steven J. Schleifer, MD, *Professor and Chairman, Department of Psychiatry, University of Medicine and Dentistry of New Jersey/New Jersey Medical School, Newark*

Elena Schwolsky-Fitch, RN, *Nurse, Early Intervention Program, Children's Hospital of New Jersey, Newark*

Laurie N. Sherwen, PhD, FAAN, *Director, Masters of Science Degree Program in Nursing, College of Allied Health Science, Thomas Jefferson University, Philadelphia, PA*

Hazel Staloff, JD, *private practice, New York, NY*

Gloria L. Steiner, EdD, *Clinical Associate Professor and Director of Psychology Training, Division of Child and Adolescent Psychiatry, University of Medicine and Dentistry of New Jersey/New Jersey Medical School, Newark; Consultant, Natinal Pediatric HIV Resource Center, Children's Hospital of New Jersey, Newark*

Cheryl L. Thompson, PhD, *Associate Professor, Department of Professional Psychology and Family Therapy, Seton Hall University, South Orange, NJ*

Marge Iurato Torrance, PsyD, *private practice, Princeton, NJ*

Susan Tross, PhD, *private practice, New York, NY*

Acknowledgments

We would like to express our special thanks to our families: Dr. Anderson J. Franklin; Jay, Deidre, Remi, and Tunde Franklin; Regina Boyd; Dr. Charles Steiner; Charles Steiner Jr.; Susan S. Sher; Dr. Jeanne L. Steiner; and grandchildren Graham, Evan, Hannah, and Jesse; and Jaime, Jenny, and Julie de Jesus.

In addition, we would like to give our deepest thanks to Hazel Staloff, our editor and coordinator of word processing services for our many authors. Our editors at Guilford have all been wonderful, including: Suzanne Little, who guided us through the early phases; Marie Sprayberry, who copyedited the book with precision; and Anna Brackett, who helped us to bring the book to completion. Thanks also to Jim Oleske for his encouragement and support.

Finally, we would like to express our appreciation to all of the staff of the Children's Hospital AIDS Program, the Family Place, and the National Pediatric and Family HIV Resource Center for their help and support throughout this process.

Foreword

In my role as a health care provider for children and families living with HIV/AIDS, I have witnessed and experienced many paradoxes inherent in their situation. Many HIV-infected individuals not only live with this most frightening and painful disease, but also endure prejudice, scorn, and rejection by their birth families. Yet these same individuals are often offered compassion and love by a "family" defined by those who provide care and support rather than by blood relationship. I have seen these hopelessly ill and dying individuals giving hope and encouragement to others. I have witnessed the strength and courage of individuals ravaged by AIDS as they overcome attitudes of prejudice and ignorance and convert them into understanding. I have held the hand of a weakened child with AIDS and gained strength; I have received comfort while trying to give comfort. All too often I have watched as a mother seeks the best possible medical care for her infected infant, while sacrificing her own health through a refusal to accept care for herself. Unfortunately, I have been told by many of my health care colleagues that my patients are expendable. They share with the rest of society misunderstanding, fear, and contempt, although their professional oaths have pledged them to understanding, enlightenment, and compassion. I have also been enriched by colleagues who have quietly led by example, giving to families and patients living with HIV/AIDS the full measure of their expertise with kindness, gentleness, and concern. I have seen the worst in people during this epidemic of HIV/AIDS but I have also seen the best.

By choosing to deal with the psychological and social problems encountered by families caring for HIV-infected children, the editors of this book have begun to extend the horizon of care to include the most important environment—the family. Classical medical diagnosis, treatment, and care must be provided by clinicians who recognize and respect the specific family structures and culture of their patients. This textbook provides critical information for all care providers faced with patients, clients, and family who are struggling to maintain both their individual and collective self-esteem and health.

James Oleske, MD, MPH

Preface

Over 240,000 lives have been lost to acquired immune deficiency syndrome (AIDS) in the United States over the past 13 years, and it is estimated that an additional 1 million people continue to live with human immunodeficiency virus (HIV) infection. HIV/AIDS is a worldwide problem that is striking women and children in developing nations with particular virulence. The secondary effects of HIV on the individual lives of affected people, the economic loss it causes, and its societal impact are only now being recognized. As we prepare to enter the 21st century, HIV/AIDS can no longer be viewed as strictly a health problem or a medical illness. Our nation must begin to focus on the psychosocial and psychotherapeutic aspects of the disease, and to view these within a behavioral, cultural, and social context. The response, to date, has ranged from ignorance and fear to stigmatization and isolation.

Working since the mid-1980s in a city and community wounded deeply by HIV/AIDS, we have seen firsthand the devastation of this illness. Confronted daily by the challenges of this epidemic, we began by directing our energy toward assuring that the basic medical services were available to those infected with HIV. While we worked to accomplish this, the mental health implications became evident as we recognized the enormity of the epidemic and its potential impact on women and families. By focusing this book on the psychological and psychosocial issues of children and their families, we hope to share our experience with others.

It is our goal that this book serve as a resource to psychologists, family counselors, counselors, physicians, nurses, social workers, teachers, and other service providers working with children, youths, and families whose lives have been affected by HIV infection, either through infection itself or through the loss of a parent, relative, friend, or coworker to AIDS. The contributors describe clinical interventions on several levels, a variety of which can decrease many of the devastating repercussions of this disease. Many treatment modalities are discussed, including family, individual, and group therapy. These multisystems interventions have the goal of family preservation, despite the tragedy of HIV in families affected by substance abuse, poverty, social isolation, and illness in multiple family members.

We have chosen to define "family" in the broadest and most generous sense as consisting of those adults, youths, and other children whose relationship is of major emotional and psychological significance to a child. This definition includes those with legal and biological relationship, as well as foster and adoptive parents, and older caretaking siblings. The family may have members from multiple systems, including the foster family, the biological parent(s), extended family members, volunteers, and members of HIV/AIDS agencies. Often, the staff of the treatment program becomes a supportive part of the extended family; such relationships last many years and increase in intensity as the family faces the advanced stages of AIDS in its members.

We see and understand the world through a family-centered lens. Our model is a "frontline" one. It has evolved from our interventions in the inner city with families coping with multiple problems and multiple systems as well as the diagnosis of HIV. Many of these families must also contend with poverty, homelessness, racism, classism, and the intrusion that often comes from such bureaucratic agencies as child protective services, welfare, courts, police, schools, and hospitals.

We are privileged to have the opportunity to witness the courage of these children and the strength of their caregivers and families, who, drawing on a wellspring of inner resources, must suffer through the pain of illness, death, and loss. We are especially inspired by the grandmothers we see, who, after suffering through the death of their own adult children, choose to serve as primary caretakers of their HIV-infected and affected grandchildren. It is to these children and families that we have dedicated this book.

Nancy Boyd-Franklin, PhD
Gloria L. Steiner, EdD
Mary G. Boland, MSN, RN

Contents

SECTION IV
THERAPEUTIC APPROACHES WITH HIV-INFECTED CHILDREN AND THEIR FAMILIES

SECTION V
SERVICE DELIVERERS AND SYSTEMS ISSUES

SECTION VI
RESEARCH AND PUBLIC POLICY

Section I

INTRODUCTION

1

. . . .

Rationale and Overview of the Book

. . . .

Gloria L. Steiner, EdD
Nancy Boyd-Franklin, PhD
Mary G. Boland, MSN, RN

In our work with various agencies, providing effective medical, health care, psychosocial, and mental health services to children and their families with human immunodeficiency virus (HIV) or acquired immune deficiency syndrome (AIDS), has been foremost in our minds. More recently, we have also been involved in training numerous health care providers, mental health workers, and social service providers in all disciplines—physicians, nurses, social workers, psychologists, and psychiatrists—from all over the world. This book introduces the Multisystems HIV/AIDS Model for the provision of effective service delivery and care to HIV/AIDS children and families. The model is family-focused, culturally sensitive, and systems-coordinated.

To demonstrate the need for a new treatment approach to HIV/AIDS families, we explore the medical and psychological realities of this illness in the first part of this chapter. The second section of the chapter presents the Multisystems HIV/AIDS Model and its three-part treatment approach. The third part of the chapter provides an overview of the book to orient the reader to our conceptual framework.

MEDICAL AND PSYCHOLOGICAL REALITIES

Psychosocial Stressors: Attitudes toward HIV/AIDS

Any service provider intending to work with HIV-infected children and families must first understand the societal attitudes, beliefs, and biases about HIV/AIDS that these children and families confront daily.

Stigma and Fears of Contagion

The common response to this disease is often "AIDS phobia"—a stigmatization that has profoundly affected the lives of HIV-infected children and their families, and is linked to homophobia, judgments about sexual promiscuity or drug abuse, and (most notably) fear. Fear of contagion persists despite evidence that AIDS can be acquired only through sexual transmission or exposure to contaminated blood products. Some families, schools, day care centers, doctors, nurses, teachers, and social workers still perceive a risk in normal daily contact and respond apprehensively toward an HIV-infected child. Indeed, some school systems have barred HIV-infected children; families have become homeless when landlords refuse to rent apartments to them; parents have lost employment; and children are rejected by their peers.

Shame, Guilt, and Anger

The stigma associated with HIV infection causes many families to experience intense shame, guilt, and anger. Mothers and fathers who are themselves HIV-infected and who have become infected through unprotected sex, prostitution, drug use, and/or needle sharing often feel tremendous guilt. Mothers who acquire the virus through heterosexual transmission often experience complicated feelings of guilt and anger toward both themselves and their partners when confronted with a diagnosis of HIV in their newborn children.

Guilt can also be manifested in the grandparental generation when an adult child has died of AIDS contracted through drug use or prostitution. The raising of infected or noninfected grandchildren who have been orphaned may provide a "second chance" at parenting for grandparents who may feel that they have failed their own children. However, a caretaker can easily become overwhelmed with the responsibility of raising many children.

Anger is a common emotion in families coping with HIV/AIDS. The infected individuals may have a sense of "Why me?" Families may feel rage toward a member for abusing drugs, and may find it difficult to forgive a family member who has stolen from them or been manipulative or abusive in the past.

There is also a tendency among health and mental health care providers to blame parents, particularly drug abusers, for "causing" their children's illness. Clinical and medical staff members may need to discuss their feelings of anger, so that they do not impose them on already deeply burdened parents and family members.

Secrecy and Social Isolation

Too often, many HIV-infected children and their families live in a "conspiracy of silence" (Septimus, quoted in Anderson, 1990) because of the stigma and shame associated with AIDS, as well as related issues and risk factors (homosexuality, bisexuality, drug abuse, prostitution, and promiscuity). For many reasons, HIV/AIDS is often a well-kept secret. An HIV/AIDS diagnosis may also expose an individual's drug use, homosexuality, or prostitution to his or her family for the first time. Many such families fear that they will be rejected in their communities if the secret becomes known.

One disturbing consequence of the "conspiracy of silence" is that families may withdraw, become socially isolated, and become "emotionally cut off" (Bowen, 1976) from their traditional support systems. These family members are at particularly high risk for mental health problems, such as depression and suicide, and for withdrawal from or poor compliance with medical care.

Impact of the HIV Diagnosis

Denial

The diagnosis of HIV infection in a child threatens the integrity of the family in a unique way. It may cause the mother to be tested and to discover that she is seropositive; further testing may involve the father and other siblings. On hearing the diagnosis, a parent unable to take in the information may resort to denial or disbelief. It is particularly difficult for adult family members to cope with their feelings about the death of a child.

Denial takes different forms. Some families attempt to withdraw or run away from medical facilities. In an individual or family where alcohol or other substance abuse exists, the emotional trauma upon hearing the child's diagnosis may trigger a binge or relapse. The oblivion provided by "getting high" allows the denial to persist.

Denial is also viewed as serving an adaptive role in chronic illness. Some denial helps the family to return to routine functioning. But denial can also thwart acceptance and impede growth. An important function for any clinician working with an HIV-infected child and family is helping family members to establish a balance between the need to face the realities of the child's condition, and the need to put the illness aside and continue "living." The nature and extent of denial also serve a diagnostic function and help the clinician to determine the nature of the clinical intervention (Pollock & Boland, 1990).

The profound emotional shock following the initial denial may be expressed in a variety of ways, from hysteria to anger. Anger is usually directed at those believed to be responsible: a lover, multiple partners, or oneself. Sometimes the anger is displaced or directed against others, such as doctors, other medical caretakers, or the government. Many alternate between anger at others and at themselves, particularly if the mode of transmission is stigmatized by the public, such as injection drug use or bisexuality.

These critical feeling states may remain, or even be followed by depression and withdrawal. Shame and guilt over the implicating past behavior may result in feelings of low self-worth and withdrawal, which often jeopardize compliance with needed medical treatment. These shifting stages of affect and thought are often accompanied by clinical signs of anxiety, depression, regression, isolation, and dependency. With the help of family, friends, and other social supports, the individual may be able to transcend feelings of hopelessness and helplessness to reach a stage of acceptance. The person may even be able to establish a new identity in which he or she participates in life, engages in activities, and can take action to help others in a similar predicament.

Death and Dying/Life and Living[1]

Many of these children and families must cope with multiple deaths and losses, and thus have little time either to prepare for death or to mourn past losses. Thus, bereavement is a major psychosocial and mental health stressor in their lives.

There is a paradox, however, because as HIV-infected children are living longer, the families must learn to cope with issues related to death and dying while simultaneously attempting to provide some degree of "normality" for these children and other family members. Service providers have looked to the literature on other chronic pediatric illnesses, particularly those that are ultimately terminal. The

[1]Thanks to Heidi Haiken and Lyn Czarniecki for the use of this title.

chronic illness model as a framework for dealing with these complex issues is discussed next.

HIV/AIDS as a Chronic Illness

The marked increase in the number of cases of HIV/AIDS in children intensifies the challenge and strain on the health care delivery system. In the early stages of the epidemic, children infected with HIV/AIDS rarely survived infancy. However, with the introduction of prophylaxis for opportunistic infections and the use of antiviral agents such as zidovudine, pediatric HIV/AIDS patients are now living longer. With this reality, the psychosocial issues for all members of the family have intensified. Now HIV/AIDS can be seen as a chronic disease, similar to other childhood chronic and/or terminal illnesses such as pediatric cancers, leukemia or diabetes (Boland, 1989).

Similarities to Other Chronic Illnesses

The many similarities between pediatric HIV/AIDS and other childhood illnesses provide the foundation for mental health interventions. It is a well-documented fact that most pediatric chronic illnesses have psychological sequelae (Adams-Greenly, Shiminski-Maher, McGowan, & Meyers, 1986; Breslau, 1985; Garralda, Jameson, Reynolds, & Postlethwaite, 1988; Perrin, Ramsey, & Sandler, 1987; Stein & Jessop, 1985). Research in the 1950s and 1960s focused on the presence of a specific illness as an overriding factor in determining the psychological adjustment of the child. Inconsistencies in results led to the conclusion that the relationship between illness and psychological functioning is neither simple nor linear. Thus, elements in all chronic illnesses—the handicapping potential of the illness, the child's sense of being different, and the chronicity (Stein & Jessop, 1982)—determine the possible outcomes in terms of adjustment. With any chronic illness there may be periods of "normality," but there are also often crises, when familial, psychological, medical, economic, and social resources are heavily taxed. In general, a chronic illness interferes with a child's ability to engage in developmentally appropriate activities. Normal development can be compromised both by the illness itself and by necessary medical interventions.

Even in the best of circumstances, managing chronic illness in a child places enormous and continual strain on family functioning (Stein & Jessop, 1982). Often the parents of a chronically ill child are the only consistent links in the child's health care system. They know the most about the child's symptoms, treatment, and responses (Boland

& Czarniecki, 1991). The family reorients its existence around the child's constant need for care, with the concomitant financial, social, and emotional strains.

Differences from Other Chronic Illnesses

A number of critical features distinguish HIV/AIDS from other chronic childhood illnesses: the need for secrecy; the association with high-risk or undesirable behaviors; and fear of social isolation. In addition, HIV/AIDS has had a major impact on the family system, often dramatically altering the needs and roles of different family members. In most childhood chronic illnesses, the primary caretaker (usually the mother) is likely to be both emotionally and physically available. In childhood HIV/AIDS, however, one or both parents are likely to be infected themselves and unable to care for the child. When parents become more disabled or symptomatic, or die from this disease, other members of the immediate or extended family must assume child care responsibilities.

The stress inherent in a diagnosis of HIV/AIDS places new challenges on the relationship between patients and various health care providers, highlighting the need for more cultural sensitivity in the administration of treatment. And finally, the complexity of the illness and the probability of several illnesses in a single family underscores the need within the larger health care system for coordinated systems of care. For this reason, we have come to view HIV/AIDS as a multisystems problem.

CONCEPTUAL FRAMEWORK: THE MULTISYSTEMS HIV/AIDS MODEL

To treat pediatric HIV/AIDS, health and mental health practitioners must go beyond a child-focused approach. The Multisystems HIV/AIDS Model provides a framework for addressing the different levels of intervention, including the child, the family, the service providers, and the myriad institutions (medical, mental health, and social services) that may become involved in the provision of care. The components of the Multisystems HIV/AIDS Model are as follows:

1. HIV/AIDS is a multigenerational family disease.
2. There is a need for cultural sensitivity in treating this disease.
3. A multisystems approach is needed to coordinate care for HIV/AIDS families.

The first major reality is that HIV/AIDS is often a multigenerational family disease; deaths and losses occur across generations. The second is that many HIV/AIDS families come from cultures (African-American, Hispanic/Latino, and Haitian) with which health and mental health care providers may be unfamiliar. This model provides a culturally sensitive framework to help practitioners offer more effective medical and clinical interventions.

Finally, all families living with HIV/AIDS have had to learn to navigate the many systems of health care, including hospitals, clinics, subspecialties, emergency rooms, intensive care units (ICUs), visiting nurse service, insurance carriers, and so on. In addition to these systems, many families live in poverty in inner-city or rural areas. This exacerbates the problem of providing coordinated care, as such families may be working with additional institutions and agencies (child welfare agencies, courts, police, mental health services, schools, welfare departments, housing agencies, Supplemental Security Income [SSI], Medicaid, etc.).

HIV/AIDS: A Multigenerational Family Disease

For many inner-city patients, HIV has crossed generational boundaries and infected many individuals within each family. Often parents are infected through injecting drugs or through contact with sexual partners. As mothers become infected, the disease is transmitted prenatally, perinatally, or via breast feeding to children. By the time a diagnosis of HIV/AIDS has been made, one or more significant family members in the parental generation may have already died of AIDS. When this loss occurs, the burden of raising these children often falls to an older generation of extended family members (grandmothers, grandfathers, aunts, uncles).

In groups most seriously affected by HIV/AIDS—African-American, Latino, and Haitian families—complex extended families frequently exist, in which child rearing is shared. In some of these families, HIV/AIDS has taken its toll through multigenerational drug abuse, which may include needle sharing among brothers, sisters, mothers, fathers, cousins, and close friends. Many individuals within these families have survived multiple deaths and losses in all generations, which create a constant "emotional shock wave" (Bowen, 1976; Boyd-Franklin, 1989). They often do not have the opportunity to mourn one death sufficiently before another loss occurs.

The Multisystems HIV/AIDS Model expands our lens and our definition of "the patient" from the traditional pediatric emphasis on the child to a broader, more inclusive family focus. Death in the parental generation complicates the issue of caretaking, depletes family resources, and forces us to examine the devastating impact of multiple losses on family stability and support. These realities have forced practitioners from fields such as medicine, nursing, social work, family therapy and psychology to look not only at the *in*fected patients (i.e., the children, mothers, and fathers), but also at the extended family members who are *af*fected by this disease (i.e., the caretakers and the noninfected children).

Caregivers may be so impeded by their own lifestyles or illnesses, or the deaths of other loved ones, that they cannot be emotionally available to children. If they are advanced in age, they may also lack the physical strength and stamina for caretaking. Many grandparents, who have not resolved the mourning for their own adult children who have died, may be reluctant to form an attachment to grandchildren who also have a terminal illness. In addition, these caregivers are often burdened by financial hardship. In many states, extended family members receive little or no reimbursement for the care of a relative, and often services are available to other foster parents (e.g., respite care) that may not be available to them.

The second affected group of family members consists of the noninfected children whose parents have HIV/AIDS or whose siblings are infected. These survivors have been described as "the forgotten children" in these families. Since so much of the families' emotional, financial, and psychological resources have gone into caring for the infected family members, the "forgotten children," feeling neglected and abandoned, frequently become enraged. Their rage is often manifested in the forms of acting-out behavior and conduct disorders. When death occurs, these children also need an opportunity to mourn, to discuss their feelings of sadness, and to remember their deceased parent or sibling.

Our Multisystems HIV/AIDS Model has provided us with a conceptual framework that is family-focused and addresses the needs of both the *in*fected and the *af*fected members.

The Need for Cultural Sensitivity

A key component of the Multisystems HIV/AIDS Model is its emphasis on cultural sensitivity and competence. The high prevalence rate of HIV/AIDS among African-American, Latino, and Haitian families has created the necessity for health and mental health practitioners to learn about these cultures as they expand their understanding of the medical and psychological issues in HIV/AIDS. As stated above, all three of these cultures are characterized by complex extended families in which there may be multiple caretakers. Health and mental health practitioners may unknowingly make critical medical decisions without consulting extended family members, who often wield great power and have the ability to ensure adherence to prescribed medical treatment.

Cultural, spiritual, and/or religious beliefs about the care and course of illness can also influence the family members' responses to medical care. Some families will resist the use of medication, because it involves "giving drugs to children." Others will resist disclosure issues because of their own reluctance to discuss issues of death, particularly with children. In some Haitian families, one often encounters beliefs that illnesses are caused by "voodoo" practices. In Latino families that practice *espiritismo* or *santeria,* one may encounter a belief that spirits are responsible for illness causation as well as cure. Often families are very reluctant to share these beliefs with the hospital staff.

Understanding a family's spirituality can illuminate how family members perceive illness causality and how this affects their beliefs about illness, as well as their understanding of death and dying and their belief in a life after death. Moreover, these spiritual beliefs of different family members can be used to facilitate healing from the psychological pain of multiple deaths and losses.

Finally, cultural sensitivity is important to understanding the lack of trust with which some clients approach the health care and mental health care systems. Often, racism, discrimination, and years of experience with the intrusiveness of the welfare system have produced feelings of "healthy cultural paranoia" (Grier & Cobbs, 1968), which influence many African-American families' approach to clinics and hospitals. Many of these families are very reluctant to discuss "family secrets" with service providers until trust has been established. Lack of sensitivity to this issue is often demonstrated in the intrusive intake questions that families are inevitably asked when they first enter service agencies.

A Multisystems Approach: Coordinated Care for HIV/AIDS Families

The third component of the Multisystems HIV/AIDS Model goes beyond the multigenerational family issues to explore the impact of broader systems on the lives of HIV/AIDS children and families. Poverty and its attendant problems (homelessness, crime, unemployment, drugs, etc.) compel families to deal with a host of "systems." These include schools, courts, police, juvenile justice, drug and alcohol treatment programs, the welfare department, child protective services, and so on (Boyd-Franklin, 1989). HIV/AIDS brings an additional series of frequently intrusive systems into the lives of these children and their families, including hospitals, clinics (pediatrics, OB/GYN, infectious disease, immunology, the emergency room, the ICU, etc.), visiting nurse programs, Medicaid, SSI, medical transportation systems, and often social services and mental health services. Barth, Pietrzak, and Ramler (1993) have shown that a given child and family may have as many as 12 case managers. Families as well as service providers may be overwhelmed by duplicative services, mixed messages, overlapping case management, and conflicting treatment plans and goals. Paradoxically, this state of affairs often leads to the loss of services, as a family's needs fall into the bureaucratic abyss.

The multisystems approach we advocate offers a way to empower families and service deliverers by showing how care workers can provide effective case management and coordination of the many systems involved in family-focused care. The emphasis in this approach is on the concepts of empowerment and cooperation, so that service providers and family members can begin to understand and directly intervene in the many systems that affect their lives (Boyd-Franklin, 1989).

OVERVIEW OF THE BOOK

Given the current realities of the AIDS epidemic, this book offers a conceptual framework that orients the service provider to the medical, cultural, psychosocial, and mental health needs of HIV-infected infants, children, and adolescents; mothers and other relatives who are also infected with HIV/AIDS; and uninfected but nonetheless affected family members or other caretakers.

In Section II of this book, Chapter 2 provides an epidemiological perspective on the health care needs of HIV-infected children and their families. Among the devastating sequelae of HIV/AIDS in the pediatric population has been the neurological and neurodevelopmental symptomatology that many of these children develop; Chapter 3 addresses the neurological manifestations of the disease, and presents data from neurological examinations and neuropsychological testing to illustrate these issues. Research data, and clinical and pharmacological interventions, are also discussed. As HIV-infected children are living longer and becoming school aged, this chapter has major implications for their educational needs. Many such children present with learning disabilities and developmental delays that require interventions.

Section III of the book deals with the psychosocial context of HIV/AIDS. As AIDS has spread to inner-city areas in the 1980s and 1990s, health service providers and mental health clinicians have found themselves confronted with patients whose families come from cultural and racial groups about which they know very little. This paucity of cultural knowledge in this area often puts professionals at a distinct disadvantage in their attempts to provide services to these different groups. Chapter 4 provides an overview of this area and a cultural competence model to help clinicians understand and work with the rich diversity among African-American, Latino, and Haitian families—the three cultural groups most affected by HIV/AIDS in women and children.

Professionals may also fail to consider the particular needs of adolescents, who represent less than 1% of those infected with HIV/AIDS (Centers for Disease Control, 1993). This is a very serious oversight, because this statistic represents an increase of 40% since 1990. Because many young adults who are currently HIV-infected were first infected during their adolescence, the needs of this age group, along with the task of prevention and educational strategies, must be addressed if the epidemic is to be curtailed. Chapter 5 discusses the current research and clinical material relevant to the treatment of adolescents.

Finally, in order to understand the full epidemiological scope of the issues in pediatric HIV/AIDS, the reader must be aware of the issues that affect women who are themselves infected with HIV. It is unfortunate that service providers who work with children often overlook the impact of the illness on women. Chapter 6 provides an understanding of the medical, psychosocial, and cultural issues for women who have HIV or AIDS.

Section IV is entitled "Therapeutic Approaches with HIV-Infected Children and Their Families." Utilizing our view of HIV/AIDS as a multigenerational family disease, this section provides in-depth chapters written by service providers that describe actual clinical interventions in a number of therapeutic treatment modalities: family therapy, bereavement counseling, individual therapy, hypnotherapy, children's group therapy, and a multiple-family group approach.

Chapter 7 applies a family systems lens to the treatment of this multigenerational disease, and discusses the other family systems approaches to families living with AIDS. Once again, the concept of clinical empowerment is drawn upon in mobilizing families. Because of the realities of the health care needs of HIV/AIDS patients, much of the family therapy must also incorporate a crisis intervention model.

In our emphasis on the family system, it is essential that we not overlook the needs of the child. Chapter 8 explores the special dynamics of children who are living with HIV, as the complex issues involved in the development of a therapeutic relationship within the context of ongoing death-and-dying/life-and-living issues.

Chapter 9 presents trailblazing work on hypnotherapy with HIV-infected children. Many of these techniques have greatly improved the quality of life and medical care of these children by providing non-pharmacological approaches to pain management for the children and their families.

In Chapter 10, the emphasis is upon creating a safe, therapeutic family environment where HIV-infected children can explore their concerns about their illness, their pain and losses, and their joy in living in spite of their illness. Often they do not have the opportunity to discuss these issues openly at home. Chapter 11 focuses on empowering the caretakers of HIV-infected children—mothers, fathers, grandmothers, grandfathers, other relatives, or foster or adoptive parents—to cope with complex issues: social isolation; the need to advocate for the children they care for; death, loss, and ongoing grief; guilt and suicidal feelings; and the burden of secrecy. The emphasis in both of these group approaches is upon empowering children and family members to create support systems for themselves. Often such a group becomes a true network or "family of choice," which continues long after the group has ended.

Chapter 12 discusses issues of bereavement and mourning for the surviving family members of persons with AIDS, within the conceptual framework of a multigenerational family disease. The paradoxical challenge for service providers, as well as for the families, is learning how to cope with the enormity of death and dying while remaining focused on the issues of life and living.

Within Section V, "Service Deliverers and Systems Issues," Chapter 13 discusses the larger multisystems issues affecting case management coordination and continuity-of-care issues for HIV-infected children and their families. Consistent with the focus throughout this book, Chapter 13 places these children and their families within their own societal context, which involves racism, poverty, AIDS phobia, and stigma. Many of these families live in substandard conditions (e.g., inadequate housing, poor nutrition) and must contend on a daily basis with homelessness, poverty, crime, violence, drug abuse, and victimization. Given that many of these families must contend with a host of complex and bureaucratic systems (e.g., hospitals, mental health centers, schools, child protective agencies, etc.), Chapter 13 introduces the conceptual framework of the multisystems approach (Boyd-Franklin, 1989), which can guide both families and clinicians in finding ways to coordinate services and provide continuity of care.

Until this point, this book has focused primarily on the needs of the children and their families. Chapter 14 explores the psychosocial issues presented by professional caretakers—nurses, doctors, social workers, and psychologists—with particular stress on the fact that AIDS patients elicit many different and complex responses from both health and mental health service providers. Fear of contagion, discomfort with open discussions of sexual behavior, feelings of professional inadequacy and helplessness, overidentification, and the complex issues of multiple losses may be triggered by ongoing work with dying patients and their families. The chapter discusses the need for support systems, including groups for clinicians, as well as administrative support for these dedicated service providers.

As children with HIV continue to live longer, school systems must be helped to address their needs. Chapter 15 is devoted to HIV/AIDS education, prevention, and outreach in the schools. Schools are an important component of a multisystems family approach and a focus of major policy implications.

The AIDS epidemic has presented service providers with a range of ethical and moral dilemmas, as well as complex legal problems. Chapters 16 and 17 discuss these issues and provide a framework for those who are working directly with HIV/AIDS families.

The sixth and last section encompasses research and public policy concerns. Chapter 18 discusses the current research and provides directions for future work. Chapter 19 discusses the public policy implications of the many issues discussed in this book. This chapter is written with "front-line" clinicians in mind, and discusses their role as public policy makers and advocates for HIV-infected children and their families. It also explores the political issues involved in HIV/AIDS public policy as well as mental health policy issues, including initiatives by federal agencies and decisions about service delivery, research, clinical trials, prevention strategies, risk assessment, and the development of counseling services. The chapter places particular emphasis on directions for the future in HIV/AIDS treatment, education, and prevention strategies.

REFERENCES

Adams-Greenly, M., Shiminski-Maher, T., McGowan, N., & Meyers, P. A. (1986). A group program for helping siblings of children with cancer. *Journal of Psychosocial Oncology, 4*(4), 55–67.

Anderson, G. (1990). *Courage to care: Responding to the crisis of children with AIDS.* Washington, DC: Child Welfare League of America.

Barth, R., Pietrzak, J., & Ramler, M. (1993). *Families living with drugs and HIV: Intervention and treatment strategies.* New York: Guilford Press.

Boland, M. (1989). *Generations in jeopardy: Responding to HIV infection in children, women and adolescents in New Jersey.* Newark, NJ: New Jersey Department of Health.

Bowen, M. (1976). Theory in the practice of psychotherapy. In P. J. Guerin (Ed.), *Family therapy: Theory and practice* (pp. 42–90). New York: Gardner Press.

Boyd-Franklin, N. (1989). *Black families in therapy: A multisystems approach.* New York: Guilford Press.

Breslau, N. (1985). Psychiatric disorders in children with physical disabilities. *Journal of the American Academy of Child Psychiatry, 24,* 87–94.

Boland, M., & Czarniecki, L. (1991). Starting life with HIV. *Registered Nurse, 54*(1), 54–58.

Centers for Disease Control. (1993, July). *HIV/AIDS surveillance report.* Atlanta: Author.

Garralda, M. E., Jameson, R. A., Reynolds, J. M., & Postlethwaite, R. J. (1988). Psychiatric adjustment in children with chronic renal failure. *Journal of Child Clinical Psychology and Psychiatry, 29*(1), 79–90.

Grier, W., & Cobbs, P. (1968). *Black rage.* New York: Basic Books.

Perrin, E., Ramsey, B., & Sandler, H. (1987). Competent kids: Children and adolescents with a chronic illness. *Child: Care, Health and Development, 13,* 13–32.

Pollock, S. W., & Boland, M. G. (1990). Children and HIV infection. *New Jersey Psychologist, 40*(3), 17–21.

Stein, R. E., & Jessop, D. J. (1982). A noncategorical approach to chronic childhood illness. *Public Health Reports, 97,* 354–362.

Stein, R. E., & Jessop, D. J. (1985). Delivery of care to inner city children with chronic conditions. In N. Hobbs & H. Perrin (Eds.), *Issues in the care of children with chronic illness* (pp. 382–401). San Francisco: Jossey-Bass.

SECTION II

THE EPIDEMIOLOGICAL AND MEDICAL CONTEXT

2

. . . .

The Health Care Needs of Infants and Children

An Epidemiological Perspective

. . . .

Mary G. Boland, MSN, RN
James Oleske, MD, MPH

Delivery of services to HIV-infected youngsters is a particularly complex and multifaceted process. First, many clinical settings lack access to the sophisticated technology capable of making the diagnosis in young infants. Since the screening tests for HIV infection currently in clinical use detect HIV antibodies rather than the virus itself, virtually all infants born to infected mothers initially test positive for HIV. However, only about 25% of these infants will themselves develop HIV infection (Sanchez & Paya, 1992). The remainder will seroconvert, eventually showing signs neither of HIV antibody nor of HIV infection. Second, it is also not yet known at what stages of pregnancy or delivery infants can become infected. Although virus has been detected in the tissues of fetuses as early as 13 weeks after conception, most infants born to HIV-infected mothers have negative studies for the virus at birth.

Third, progress in the development of antiretroviral and prophylactic drugs for infected children has increased their lifespans substantially. As a result, it has created a demand for health and social services for such children over an extended period of time and in an increasing variety of settings, including long-term care facilities, day care centers, and schools.

Finally, many of these families—especially when one or both parents have developed HIV-related illness—find it difficult to provide their infected children with proper attention or adequate care. A large portion of these infected parents may also be chemically dependent; they are thus doubly hindered, both psychologically and physically, in their capacity to meet their children's health needs. Minimal prenatal care, inadequate nutrition, substandard housing, and lack of access to badly needed medical treatment are often causes, as well as consequences, of the injection drug abuse that is found in many of these HIV-afflicted families (Novello, 1991). In some cases foster care may be necessary. By contrast, some infected mothers dedicate themselves to the care of their ailing children and neglect to seek necessary services for themselves. All of these factors complicate the delivery of care to HIV-infected children.

We begin this chapter with a brief look at HIV/AIDS among children and adolescents with hemophilia, because youngsters with coagulation disorders who received contaminated blood products made up a large proportion of pediatric HIV cases in the early stages of the epidemic. We then present epidemiological data that indicate the prevalence of HIV/AIDS in infants and children at present. We also review current knowledge on methods of diagnosis, symptoms, and disease course, and the impact of this knowledge on treatment and service needs for HIV-infected children.

HIV/AIDS AMONG CHILDREN WITH HEMOPHILIA

The recognition in the early 1980s that AIDS was caused by a viral agent, and the subsequent widespread availability of the enzyme-linked immunosorbent assay (ELISA) test for HIV antibody, led to the realization that not only blood but blood products could transmit HIV. HIV-contaminated blood and blood products have resulted in significant infection of the estimated 20,000 persons with hemophilia in the United States. Several studies showed that 70% of hemophiliacs intensively treated with factor VIII concentrates were seropositive in 1984 (Eyster, 1994). Since 1985, screening of all blood for HIV antibodies and modifications in the manufacturing process have prevented further transmission to hemophiliacs and others who are dependent on blood products to treat coagulation disorders. Although HIV infection is most common among those with severe hemophilia who received multiple infusions of infected factor, infection has also been identified in those with mild and moderate disease who received infected factor.

Those children with hemophilia who were infected early in the epidemic are now in the age range from late childhood to young adulthood. Early optimism that those infected with HIV would not progress to AIDS has been dampened over time by the progression to AIDS of increasing numbers of persons. The symptoms seen are similar to those of adults, including opportunistic infections and neurological manifestations. Management is similar to that of other children and adolescents, but is complicated by management of the underlying coagulation disorder.

Approximately 50–60% of persons with hemophilia receive their care through the national network of comprehensive hemophilia treatment centers. At these centers, multidisciplinary staffs provide comprehensive care similar to that advocated for other children with HIV infection. Praised for their success in erasing mortality and decreasing morbidity and disability from hemophilia, the staffs have struggled to cope with the emergence of HIV and the new needs of patients and families they have known for years. Regional and national workshops have been held to address the addition of HIV counseling and testing to the care provided at the centers, since denial was at first a prevalent coping mechanism for professionals and patients alike. Because many infected hemophiliacs are adolescents, intensive efforts have been made to develop not only educational strategies but interventions that will have an impact on behavior. The teams have developed training materials and increased their skill in education to prevent sexual transmission. As a result of screening of the blood supply since 1985, new HIV infections among hemophiliac children have declined significantly. Since the majority of HIV-infected children are currently infected perinatally through their mothers, whose risk factors were either heterosexual transmission or injection drug use, they are the major focus of this chapter and this book.

THE PREVALENCE OF HIV/AIDS
IN INFANTS AND CHILDREN

As of June 1994, 5,734 cases of pediatric AIDS (AIDS in children from birth to 13 years of age) had been reported in the United States (Centers for Disease Control and Prevention [CDC], 1994a) representing approximately 2% of all reported AIDS cases. Because AIDS is the most severe manifestation of HIV infection, this statistic accounts for only a fraction of the total number of HIV-infected infants and children.

The prevalence of pediatric HIV infection in the United States can best be estimated using the results of national surveys of HIV infection in childbearing women conducted between 1988 and 1992. These results—based on anonymous HIV antibody screening of heelstick samples from all newborns in such states as Minnesota, Florida, New Jersey, and New York during intervals of several months—suggest that approximately 1.5 newborns per 1,000 in the United States are born to HIV-infected women. According to statistics of seroprevalence rates by location, an estimated 7,000 HIV-infected women will give birth annually in the United States (CDC, 1993). In conjunction with an estimated mother—infant transmission rate of 25–30%, these numbers translate to approximately 2,000 HIV-infected infants born annually in the United States. The estimated total number of HIV-infected infants and children in the United States is currently between 10,000 and 20,000.

The risk of being born with HIV infection in the United States varies significantly by race and ethnicity. Of children under 13 years reported with AIDS, Black children represent 50% of cases, Hispanic 25%, and White 21%. The numbers of Black and Hispanic children are disproportionate to their representations of 15% and 13%, respectively, in the U.S. population (CDC, 1994a).

As noted above, many of the earliest cases of pediatric HIV infection in the United States resulted from the presence of the virus in blood product transfusions used for children with hemophilia. Since universal screening of blood and treatment of blood products in the United States began in 1985, this vector of transmission has been all but eliminated. By the end of 1993, infection through blood and blood products accounted for approximately 10% of all reported pediatric HIV cases in the United States, while mother—infant transmission accounted for 89% (CDC, 1994a).

Transmission from mother to infant ("vertical transmission") can occur both prenatally and at the time of delivery. Studies done with fetal tissue suggest that prenatal transmission of HIV can occur as early as the eighth week of gestation (Lewis, Reynolds-Kohler, Fox, & Nelson, 1990). The fact that infants can present with symptoms in the first months of life suggests prenatal infection. Serial serological evaluation of infants has documented the appearance of HIV-specific immunoglobulin antibodies (IgM, IgG3, and IgG1) in some who lacked HIV-specific IgM antibodies at birth, thereby providing evidence for HIV transmission at about the time of delivery (Gabiano et al., 1992). This mode of transmission is also suggested by the documented perinatal transmission of other blood-borne viruses, such as hepatitis B virus. However, it is still unclear exactly when in relation to gestation and delivery the majority of transmissions occur, and whether the timing of transmission correlates with the severity of disease. Why some infants become infected and others do not is not yet known; ongoing research is investigating whether there are maternal factors that can predict the likelihood of perinatal transmission. The recent report that the administration of zidovudine (formerly known as azidothymidine, or AZT) decreased perinatal transmission by two-thirds has been greeted with tremendous enthusiasm by the medical community (CDC, 1994b). A selected group of "well" HIV-infected pregnant women who enrolled in AIDS Clinical Trials Group Protocol 076 received zidovudine during pregnancy, labor and delivery and their infants received the drug for the first six weeks of life. The double-blind study was stopped in early 1994 and recommendations to prevent perinatal transmission in this group of women have been published. Despite the documented benefits, there are many unknowns regarding long-term effects of the drug on the non-infected infants and gaps in knowledge regarding the benefit to women whose clinical condition does not correspond to the group enrolled in the study.

Postpartum transmission of HIV infection from mother to newborn via breast feeding has been reported and documented in women who acquired HIV infection after delivery through sexual relations and blood transfusion (Oxtaby, 1994). The documented cases may be accounted for by the significant HIV antigenemia and presumed increased infectivity in the first 3–6 months after acquisition of HIV infection.

Whether breast feeding is a significant mode of transmission in women who are already HIV-infected during pregnancy and clinically stable is unclear. The risk–benefit ratio from breast feeding in HIV-infected women is influenced by the availability of sterile formula. It is currently recommended that in the United States and other developed countries, breast feeding be discouraged for women who are HIV-infected.

DIAGNOSIS AND CLASSIFICATION OF HIV IN INFANTS

HIV-exposed infants can be identified at birth if testing is available to pregnant women. The recent advances in antiretroviral therapy and the efficacy of early prophylaxis of opportunistic infections cannot be translated into improved duration and quality of life unless HIV-infected infants and children are diagnosed early, before the onset of clinical symptoms. For this reason, public health officials increasingly recommend voluntary, confidential testing for all pregnant women and those contemplating pregnancy, particularly when there has been a history of high-risk activity. Such testing should always be accom-

panied by culturally sensitive counseling, both before tests are conducted and when the results are given. At a minimum, pretest counseling should clarify that the test is for HIV infection, how HIV infection
is related to AIDS, why the test is desirable, and what its possible outcomes and consequences are. Techniques to prevent HIV transmission
can also be discussed at counseling sessions. When an infant is to be
tested, the consent of a parent or guardian (or a child protective agency, where appropriate) should be obtained prior to the test. Test results
should be given only in person and, in the case of an infant, to the
caregiver, and their implications need to be explored with care.

Because infants retain maternal HIV antibodies for as long as 18
months after birth, the standard ELISA and Western blot tests used to
diagnose HIV in older children and adults yield indeterminate results
for infants. In a child younger than 18 months, a diagnosis of HIV infection can be established by a positive p24 antigen test or polymerase chain reaction (PCR) if HIV is cultured from blood or tissues. In
an infant born to an HIV-infected mother, clinical symptoms consistent with HIV, and evidence of dysfunction or the appearance of an
AIDS-defining illness, are sufficient to permit a clinical diagnosis. Because of the toxicities associated with antiretroviral treatments, these
interventions should be given only to truly infected infants and children, and not to children in whom possible infection is merely suspected. For those children in whom the tests detect HIV infection, such
early intervention can be of substantial benefit.

The CDC issued a revised classification scheme for pediatric HIV
infection in 1994. The original system, issued in 1987, was developed
for epidemiological purposes. It was not helpful to clinicians and did
not reflect the emerging knowledge regarding disease progression. The
indeterminate status has been removed and the new system addresses
only those children who have been diagnosed with HIV infection based
on described criteria. The new system classifies infected children into
mutually exclusive categories based on infection status, clinical condition, and immunological status (CDC, 1994c). It is anticipated that
it will better reflect the stage of disease and be of help for both epidemiological and clinical purposes.

Asymptomatic Infection

Illness contracted by asymptomatic HIV-infected children rarely requires hospitalization, and in the vast majority of cases treatment can
be given on an outpatient basis. The major goal of care for asymptomatic children is management of HIV infection to prevent infections
and opportunistic illnesses, through both supportive care and
prophylaxis. Prophylaxis is intended to prevent primary or recurrent

infection in children known to be HIV-infected or in HIV-exposed infants who have decreased lymphocyte counts. Although studies of prophylaxis for *Pneumocystis carinii* pneumonia (PCP) have not yet been conducted on children, results in adults have shown trimetho-prim-sulfamethoxazole (Bactrim, Septra) to be effective in both preventing the onset of PCP and reducing its morbidity and mortality. The combination has also been shown to be effective in preventing recurrent otitis media and other infections in children. Prophylaxis to prevent primary and recurrent PCP infection in infants and children is now recommended, as PCP is the major cause of morbidity and mortality for children with AIDS (CDC, 1991). Researchers are increasingly devoting efforts to develop prophylaxis regimens for other opportunistic infections in children with immunocompromise secondary to HIV.

Symptomatic Infection

In children, as in adults, HIV affects organ systems throughout the body. A common abnormality found in HIV-infected children is generalized lymphadenopathy, and many children with this condition also develop splenomegaly. Hepatomegaly also occurs, frequently late in a child's first year. Skin conditions are common (especially *Candida* and seborrheic rash), resulting from either unidentifiable chronic infection or circulating immune complexes. *Candida esophagitis* also occurs frequently, interfering with nutrition by making it painful for a child to swallow. Other symptoms include a failure to thrive related to anemia, recurrent diarrhea, and gastrointestinal problems. Unusual enteric pathogens have been found in infected children, including cryptosporidium, persistent adenovirus infection, and cytomegalovirus enteritis.

HIV-infected children have a high incidence of lower respiratory tract infections, especially PCP and bacterial pneumonia. Lymphoid interstitial pneumonitis may affect as many as half of all HIV-infected children. Sinusitis and chronic otitis media are also found.

Neurological disorders can be subtle in their initial manifestations, but longitudinal studies have identified such problems in up to 90% of HIV-infected children (Burns, 1992). Infants with HIV infection appear to be particularly susceptible to encephalopathy, which is manifested in developmental delays, a deterioration of motor skills and intellectual abilities, and abnormal behaviors (see Chapter 3). Malignancies and susceptibility to unusual bacterial infections, such as sepsis, pneumonia, meningitis, abscesses, and cellulitis, are often among the early symptoms of pediatric HIV infection.

Symptoms can be divided into three categories: nonspecific findings, findings related to immunodeficiency, and end organ abnormalities. Nonspecific findings are those that are seen in other illness and do not by themselves indicate HIV. Included are symptoms such as lymphadenopathy, hepatomegaly, and fever. Findings related to immunodeficiency include opportunistic infections and malignancies; these occur as a direct consequence of the HIV-induced immunosuppression. These symptoms can be controlled by ongoing treatment, but may be life-threatening if treatment is delayed or interrupted. Finally, as children are being treated successfully for early manifestations of HIV, abnormalities of organ systems have been identified. The etiology is unclear, but major organ systems such as the heart, lungs, gastrointestinal tract, kidneys, and endocrine system can be threatened. Treatment for these manifestations is based on the symptoms and is usually supportive in nature.

DISEASE COURSE

The chronic nature of pediatric HIV infection is being increasingly recognized with advances in treatments and prolonged survival of children. Although there are a significant percentage of children who develop disease early in life and have a very poor prognosis, with survival of only a few years, the survival of the group as a whole is much longer. In one large prospective study, it was determined that the cumulative proportion surviving at the age of 9 years was 49.5%, with a median survival of 96.3 months (Tovo et al., 1992). Of 202 living HIV-infected children currently being followed at the Children's Hospital AIDS Program (CHAP) in Newark, New Jersey, 96 are over 6 years old and 56 are over 9 years of age (Grubman et al., in press) Management of chronically ill children with HIV is often complicated by the premature deaths of their mothers, their primary caretakers. At CHAP, 76% of the children older than 9 years who were infected by mother–infant transmission have been orphaned as a result of maternal death. In 1991, an estimated 13% of children in the United States whose mothers died of all causes were children of women who died of HIV-related diseases. It is estimated that by 1995, over 45,000 children and adolescents will be orphaned as a result of maternal death secondary to AIDS, with the vast majority from poor communities of color (Michaels & Levine, 1992).

Ongoing studies attempting to trace the natural history of maternally transmitted HIV infection in children indicate that the disease does not follow any single course. The age at onset of symptoms and type of symptoms both vary in children. A small number of children may be asymptomatic for long periods of time; others present with acute symptoms that can be treated successfully. Thus, many children with HIV live lives similar to those of other children with chronic illness. The course for each child is individual and can rarely be predicted even by an experienced HIV health care provider. Medical management of pediatric HIV disease is very complex, and each child should be treated on the basis of individual symptoms, needs, and response to therapy. Evidence based on the experiences of the past 10 years suggests that infected children who receive care in programs with expertise in pediatric HIV have a better quality of life.

TREATMENT

Strategies to prevent or delay the onset of serious illness in HIV-infected children include attempts to block the action of specific infectious agents, to block replication of HIV, and to strengthen the immune system. For many of the conditions affecting HIV-infected children, investigational therapies offer the only hope for curative treatment. Because HIV causes damage to many body systems, therapy must reach multiple sites. Moreover, because of the integration of proviral sequences into target cells, treatment needs to be continued potentially for the life of the child. It is unlikely that any one drug will be effective over the long term. Therapy must include multiple agents used in combination to minimize side effects or toxicity while providing benefit.

CONCLUSIONS

The epidemiological data on pediatric HIV/AIDS make it clear that in the United States there has been a disproportionate impact upon the poor and people of color, particularly those with histories of injection drug use. The health care needs of this population have traditionally been underserved, and previous contact with public agencies may dispose them toward distrust and discourage them from seeking timely medical care. Often one of the first relationships of trust that affected families develop is with the health care providers who treat their children. Health care professionals should attempt to establish partnerships with these families, rather than reinforcing the more traditional role of passivity and dependence.

Mothers are typically the strongest advocates for their children, but this advocacy may be hindered by the fact that the mothers of HIV-infected children are often single-parent heads of poor households. As stated previously, symptomatic HIV infection or drug use may interfere with a mother's ability to care properly for her child; more often, however, mothers are assertive in seeking care for their children while neglecting their own care needs. The general shortage of openings in drug treatment programs is especially severe for women who are HIV-infected or pregnant or who have children. All of these socioeconomic conditions have to be addressed in designing effective health care systems for families with HIV infection.

On the other hand, ongoing advances in medical technology that enable health professionals to identify HIV infection in infants and to treat infected children with antiretroviral and prophylactic therapies will continue to improve the prognosis for HIV-infected children. Already there has been a shift in the management of HIV infection to a chronic illness model. As the life expectancy for infected children increases, the quality of their lives assumes greater importance. It has become realistic to expect that many infected children will be able to participate in the normal growth processes and activities of childhood. Thoughtfully designed and competently administered systems of care will assist HIV-infected children to live for many years.

REFERENCES

Burns, D. (1992). The neuropathology of pediatric acquired immunodeficiency syndrome. *Journal of Child Neurology, 7*, 332–346.

Centers for Disease Control (CDC). (1991, March 15). Guidelines for prophylaxis against *Pneumocystis carinii* pneumonia for children infected with human immunodeficiency virus. *Morbidity and Mortality Weekly Report, 40*(RR-2), 1–11.

Centers for Disease Control (CDC). (1993). *HIV Serosurveillance Summary, 3,* 15–18.

Centers for Disease Control and Prevention (CDC). (1994a, June). *HIV/AIDS Surveillance Report, 6*(1), 11.

Centers for Disease Control and Prevention (CDC). (1994b, August 5). Recommendations for the use of zidovudine to reduce perinatal transmission of human immunodeficiency virus. *Morbidity and Mortality Weekly Report, 43*(RR-11), 1–20.

Centers for Disease Control and Prevention (CDC). (1994c, September). 1994 Revised classification system for human immunodeficiency virus (HIV) infection in children less than 13 years of age. *Morbidity and Mortality Weekly Report, 43*(RR-12), 1–5.

Eyster, M. E. (1994). Continuing issues regarding transfusion and coagulation factor acquired HIV infection in children. In P. Pizzo & C. Wilfert (Eds.), *Pediatric AIDS: The challenge of HIV infection in infants, children and adolescents* (2nd ed., pp. 51–69). Baltimore: Williams & Wilkins.

Gabiano, C., Tovo, P. A., de Martino, M., Galli, L., Capello, N., et al. (1992). Mother-to-child transmission of human immunodeficiency virus type 1: Risk of infection and correlates of transmission. *Pediatrics, 90,* 369–374.

Grubman, S., Gross, E., Lerner-Weiss, N., Hernanley, M., McSherry, G., et al. (in press). Older children and adolescents living with perinatally acquired HIV infection. *Pediatrics.*

Lewis, S., Reynolds-Kohler C., Fox, H., & Nelson, J. (1990). HIV-1 introphoblastic and villous Hofbauer cells and haematologic precursors in eight-week fetuses. *Lancet, i,* 565–568.

Michaels, D., & Levine, C. (1992). Estimates of the number of motherless youth orphaned by AIDS in the United States. *Journal of the American Medical Association, 268,* 3456–3461.

Novello, A. (1991). *Family centered comprehensive care for children with HIV infection.* Bethesda, MD: U.S. Public Health Service.

Oxtaby, M. (1994). Vertically transmitted HIV infection in the United States. In P. Pizzo & C. Wilfert (Eds.), *Pediatric AIDS: The challenge of HIV infection in infants, children and adolescents* (2nd ed., pp. 3–20). Baltimore: Williams & Wilkins.

Sanchez, E., & Paya, J. (1992, July). *Estimating HIV vertical transmission: A meta-analytic approach.* Paper presented at the VIII International Conference on AIDS/III STD World Congress, Amsterdam.

Tovo, P., de Martino, M., Baiano, G., Capello, N., Palomba, E., et al. (1992). Prognostic factors and survival in children with perinatal HIV-1 infection. *Lancet, 339,* 1249–1253.

3

. . . .

Neurological and Neurodevelopmental Functioning in Pediatric HIV Infection

. . . .

Jennis Hanna, PhD
Mark Mintz, MD

Although relatively little published research documents the effects of HIV infection on neuropsychological functioning, there is increasing recognition that neurological involvement is a common feature of pediatric HIV/AIDS. Impairments in attention and concentration, expressive behavior, motor coordination, and language have all been noted. The incidence of neurodevelopmental abnormalities in pediatric AIDS patients has been estimated at 40–90%. Younger children may show delays in achieving developmental milestones; older children may show deteriorating cognitive skills. The central nervous system (CNS) is a key target of HIV infection, which can result in debilitating neurological disease.

This chapter describes the impact of HIV infection on the neurodevelopmental functioning of pediatric patients, including its effect on the CNS. Findings from both psychological and neurological assessments are presented in case study data. Results of treatment with antiretroviral agents, and implications for communities and school systems, are also discussed.

CLINICAL MANIFESTATIONS

An unfortunate consequence of HIV type I infection is the virus's ability to access and infect the CNS. It may remain clinically silent for an extended period of time, as demonstrated by the case study material in this chapter. Once HIV establishes residence in the brain, however, it can create substantial and often devastating neurological complications (Epstein, Sharer, Oleske, et al., 1986). The mechanism by which the virus operates and wreaks severe devastation in the brain is not fully known (Mintz & Epstein, 1992). The most severe manifestation of CNS HIV infection is a progressive neurological deterioration, or "progressive encephalopathy" (PE), which occurs in up to 50% of pediatric patients with AIDS. This is characterized by a failure to attain, a plateau in, or a loss of developmental milestones (see Figure 3.1); an impairment of brain growth (see Figures 3.2, 3.3, and 3.4);

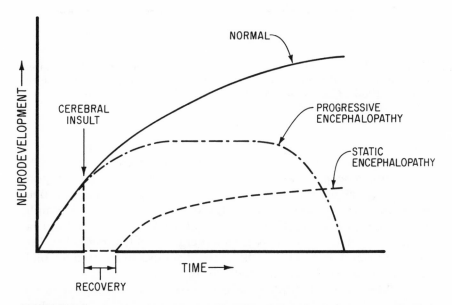

FIGURE 3.1. Comparison of the curves of neurodevelopment in an acquired cerebral insult (i.e., static encephalopathy; dashed line) and a neurodegenerative process (i.e., progressive encephalopathy; dotted/dashed line), as compared to normal neurodevelopment (solid line). Since the slope of the developmental curve of static encephalopathy is often not as steep as the normal developmental curve, children with static encephalopathies can sometimes be mistakenly classified as having progressive encephalopathies. Adapted from Rapin & Johnson (1987). Copyright 1987 by Appleton & Lange. Adapted by permission.

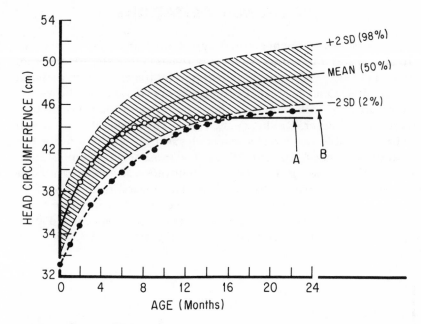

FIGURE 3.2. Serial head circumference measurements for (A) acquired microcephaly, and (B) microcephaly vera ("true" microcephaly). Adapted from Nellhaus (1968). Copyright 1968 by the American Academy of Pediatrics. Adapted by permission of *Pediatrics.*

and progressive motor dysfunction. The natural course of an HIV-related PE can be quite variable. Although there may be observed spontaneous "honeymoon periods" characterized by plateaus or improvements, the overall course is most frequently a relentless, downhill, stepwise deterioration (Belman, Diamond, Dickson, et al., 1988; Diamond, 1989; Mintz, Epstein, & Koenigsberger, 1989; Mintz, 1992; Ultmann, Diamond, Ruff, et al., 1987). The diagnosis of PE carries a high morbidity rate (Scott, Hutto, Makuch, et al., 1989).

Children with HIV infection may also manifest nonprogressive neurological deficits or "static encephalopathies," of which cerebral palsy is one subtype. The majority of static encephalopathies are not necessarily related to infection of the CNS by HIV (Kairam, 1989; Mintz, 1992). Among the other factors that may be implicated are genetic syndromes (e.g., Down's syndrome); metabolic disorders (e.g., untreated phenylketonuria); birth factors (e.g., prematurity, low birth weight); toxins (e.g., lead poisoning, gestational drug exposure); and influence of the environment (e.g., poor nutrition, poor stimulation). Head trauma or exacerbation of systemic diseases related to HIV infection may

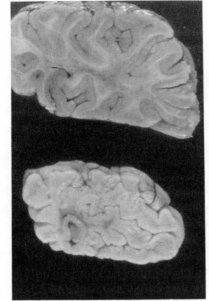

FIGURE 3.3. Postmortem brain specimens: (A) a 6-month-old non-HIV-infected infant; (B) a 7-month-old infant with AIDS. Reprinted from Epstein, Sharer, & Goudsmit (1988). Copyright 1988 by Little, Brown and Company. Reprinted by permission.

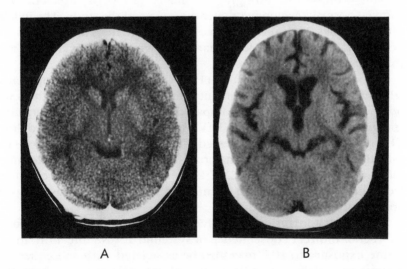

FIGURE 3.4. CT scans: (A) head of a normal child; (B) head of an HIV-infected child with neurological disease. Note the "atrophic" appearance of B, characterized by enlargement of fluid-containing spaces (dark areas) secondary to loss of brain tissue volume.

also be implicated in subsequent developmental delays and learning disabilities. When one or more of these conditions coexist with HIV, as they often may, attributing the consequent developmental delay solely to the direct effects of HIV infection may be inaccurate.

Research has been conducted specifically to clarify the impact of HIV infection on early childhood development. The results suggest that HIV may be implicated in some cases where children present with both HIV infection and developmental aberrances. A study by Hittleman (1992) compared the developmental status of serologically HIV-positive (HIV+) and HIV-negative (HIV–) babies born to two groups of women. One group was in treatment for drug abuse; the other group had no history of drug use. Both groups of women had members who were infected and uninfected with HIV. They came from the same racial, ethnic, and socioeconomic groups within one urban neighborhood. This sample allowed the author to compare the effects of HIV infection on the infants, independently of the influence of maternal drug use. Hittleman found that the HIV-infected babies, as compared to the HIV– sample, showed clear lags in development by 18 months of age, regardless of the history of maternal drug use.

A similar study was completed by Cohen, Morgan, Rivera, et al. (1991). Again, the HIV+ babies demonstrated significant developmental and neurological abnormalities as compared to the HIV– and indeterminant groups. Interestingly, a ''small'' group of infected babies showed normal development over the course of the study. The indeterminant babies scored somewhat better than the HIV+ babies, but demonstrated more problems than those who were never exposed to the virus, the HIV– babies.

Koch, Jeremy, Lewis, et al. (1989) measured the development of HIV-infected and uninfected infants born to HIV-infected mothers who injected drugs. These were compared to scores obtained from a control group of children born to HIV– mothers who also injected drugs. This modest-sized study suggested that despite lack of direct fetal HIV infection, mere exposure to maternal HIV infection might be detrimental to the developing fetal CNS. Early developmental lags characterized both the infected and uninfected infants as contrasted to the control group.

Thus, HIV infection may adversely affect neurodevelopment, as a direct or indirect consequence of systemic or CNS infection. Intrauterine exposure to HIV may also be associated with subsequent developmental delays even in those infants who are not themselves infected. The consequent developmental delays occur separately from other handicapping factors, and thus do not seem to be solely the consequence of maternal drug use or other environmental influences.

ASSESSMENT

Psychological assessment has become an integral component in the evaluation and treatment of neurological deterioration in HIV-infected patients. Results from psychological evaluations are used by the medical team as a guide to assessing the efficacy of antiretroviral treatment. In addition, parents or caretakers can use feedback regarding cognitive abilities to help them establish realistic expectations for behavior, self-help skills, achievement, and so on, when the child's deteriorating health is an issue. Finally, when areas of deficit are identified, a program of rehabilitative therapies can be implemented.

Thus far, standard psychological testing batteries have typically been used in clinical trials and other studies of the neurodevelopmental effects of HIV infection. An adequate battery is thought to consist of a measure of cognitive development, such as the Bayley Scales of Infant Development (Bayley, 1969), the fourth edition of the Stanford–Binet Intelligence Scale (Thorndike, Hagen, & Sattler, 1986), the Kaufman Assessment Battery for Children (Kaufman & Kaufman, 1983), the McCarthy Scales of Children's Abilities (McCarthy, 1972), or a test from the Wechsler series such as the Wechsler Intelligence Scale for Children—Third Edition (WISC-III: Wechsler, 1991); a measure of achievement, such as the Wide Range Achievement Test—Revised (WRAT-R; Jastak, Jastak & Wilkinson, 1984) or the Peabody Individual Achievement Test—Revised (Markwardt, 1989); a language scale, such as the Peabody Picture Vocabulary Test—Revised (Dunn & Dunn, 1981) or the Expressive One-Word Picture Vocabulary Test (Gardner, 1979); a measure of graphomotor skills, such as the Beery Developmental Test of Visual–Motor Integration (VMI; Beery, 1982); and a measure of behavioral and emotional functioning (i.e., projective tests and/or behavior checklists). A comprehensive battery may include a standardized measure of gross motor skills as well (the Bayley Scales and the McCarthy Scales offer such a measure), or a supplemental test such as the Peabody Developmental Motor Scales (Folio & Fewell, 1983) may be incorporated. Though specific neuropsychological measures have been recommended, the value of these measures with a pediatric population has yet to be determined. Thus far, no relationship has been shown to exist between particular subtest scores and neurodevelopmental deficits. Similarly, no cluster of subtests has been identified that serves as a marker for CNS involvement in HIV-infected children.

A baseline assessment immediately upon diagnosis of HIV infection is preferable. This allows a clinician to gather information on the neurodevelopmental functioning of the patient, presumably before the disease has progressed. However, at some institutions this may not always be feasible, because of large numbers of newly diagnosed patients. Alternatively, testing prior to institution of antiretroviral agents, such as zidovudine (formerly known as azidothymidine or AZT) or dideoxyinosine (ddI) is essential, so that periodic re-evaluations can be compared to baseline measures to provide consistent monitoring of the patients' status (O'Donnell, Mintz, Maha, et al., 1991). In most cases, 6-month testing intervals are sufficient to show significant change. One can expect patients to maintain their previous level of functioning or, more optimistically, to improve somewhat. Any plateau or decline in test scores is cause for alarm. However, practice effects tend to obscure findings somewhat; it is not always clear whether significantly improved test scores represent a positive response to treatment or just overexposure to test material. In essence, though, the patients form their own control group, since all have the same opportunity for practice. Therefore, practice effects become less of an issue, as they are controlled across the population.

In addition to the problem presented by the practice effect, researchers have found other limitations with existing test batteries. For example, problems arise when attempting to compare children of different ages and developmental stages, since psychological tests do not all yield comparable information. Also, Watkins, Brouwers, and Huntzinger (1992) emphasize the need for "interactional" evaluations, taking into account the effect the child's environment has on his or her developmental functioning. Qualitative aspects of behavior worthy of investigation are cited (p. 135). Researchers that agree there is a need for standardized and reliable measures of psychological and neurological functioning—measures that can accurately quantify change over time (Stover, Pequenat, Huffman, et al., 1990).

The clinical neurological assessment of children with HIV infection is essential. Furthermore, correlation with the results of psychometric testing is pertinent and allows for a more pragmatic interpretation of results. A complete neurological evaluation is desirable, but one essential aspect is a serial assessment of head circumference growth (see Figure 3.2). In the child over 2 years of age, an inordinate amount of time may be necessary to reflect a loss of velocity in head growth; therefore, in such children, serial neuroimaging studies can be utilized to assess for a loss of brain volume ("atrophy") (see Figure 3.4). The neurological evaluation should also include an appraisal of gross and fine motor function, and an evaluation of ambulation and gait. A baseline neuroimaging study (computed tomography [CT] or magnetic resonance imaging [MRI]) with serial follow-up studies should be considered (see Figure 3.4) and is mandatory if a mass lesion is suspected. Obtaining cerebrospinal fluid (CSF) to analyze for evidence of the virus (p24 antigen or HIV culture) can be useful as an adjunct in defining HIV-associated neurological disease or in determining the efficacy of antiretroviral treatment (Epstein, Goudsmit, Paul, et al., 1987; Ho, Rota, Schooley, et al., 1985). However, obtaining CSF is essential if there is an acute opportunistic bacterial or other infection of the CNS (and if lumbar puncture is not contraindicated).

CASE STUDIES

The findings reported in this section of the chapter are based on initial assessments of approximately 100 HIV-infected children aged 4 months to 15 years. These 100 patients were selected from a larger clinic population in a nonrandom fashion and were seen for psychometric testing prior to institution of antiretroviral treatment. Most of these children were infected via mother–infant transmission, though a small number (fewer than 10%) were infected via blood transfusion or sexual abuse. Although all were symptomatic and some had AIDS, there was considerable variation in the extent of neurological involvement. This was the key feature distinguishing these patients. Case study data will be presented for each of the three classifications: normal, static encephalopathy, and PE. Each study is based on an actual case, but names and other identifying information have been changed to protect confidentiality.

Normal

The majority of the selected cohort could be classified as cognitively normal, since at any given time most (approximately 80%) functioned within the average range of intelligence, and, more importantly, demonstrated no evidence of neurological involvement. These patients generally had histories of normal health and development during infancy. Consistent with others' observations, they demonstrated years of normal cognitive functioning. However, in some there were episodic health problems that, in retrospect, could have been HIV-related. For example, histories of repeated otitis media, unexplained fevers, or failure to thrive were common. However, some children were found to be HIV-infected only because they were screened following the diagnosis of an HIV-infected parent or sibling. These children were never symptomatic. Others were only diagnosed after they developed symptoms of an opportunistic infection characteristic of HIV.

On observation, these children might present as somewhat smaller and thinner than others their age. Otherwise, they showed no distinguishing characteristics. No phenotype has been identified that typifies HIV-infected children, despite early claims to the contrary (Marion,

Wiznia, Hutcheon, et al., 1986; Nicholas, 1988). Unfortunately, school achievement problems are common among such children, in spite of adequate cognitive ability. In fact, nearly 50% require special services (remedial assistance or special class placement) in public school (Haiken, Hernandez, Mintz, et al., 1991). In addition, they are at risk for more significant future learning problems as their neurological status deteriorates.

Case 1

Eleven-year-old Angela and her two younger siblings lived with their maternal grandparents in a middle-class suburb. The mother had died several years previously of what was probably AIDS, though it had not been diagnosed at the time. The father was not a reliable parent, as he continued to inject drugs and use alcohol. His whereabouts and health status were not known.

Angela was an honor student and involved in many school activities. She had been exceptionally healthy until an acute illness progressed to *Pneumocystis carinii* pneumonia (PCP), causing her to be placed on a ventilator for 2 weeks. She subsequently lost weight and was in fragile health for several weeks. At that time, she was found to be HIV-infected. When subsequently seen for a psychological evaluation, she was found to be functioning in the "bright average" range of intelligence: she earned a Verbal IQ (VIQ) of 120, a Performance IQ (PIQ) of 111, and a Full Scale IQ (FSIQ) of 118 on the WISC-R. Academically, she scored above grade level. A sensitive child, Angela understood the implications of her diagnosis and demonstrated a reactive depression at the time she was seen.

Within 2 months she regained her health and was able to return home. Angela was prescribed zidovudine and tolerated the medication well. After discussing the issue, the family decided to disclose the diagnosis to the school. This resulted in initial anger, fear, and rejection of the family by the community. These attitudes were gradually modified through intensive educational services provided to the community by Angela's case management team. Angela and her siblings (both of whom tested negative for HIV) were able to remain in school and resume their normal activities.

When Angela was seen 6 months later, she was in very good health. She had been seen for weekly group therapy for HIV-infected children, which alleviated her depression somewhat. On psychological re-evaluation, she functioned in the "superior" range (VIQ = 124; PIQ = 120; FSIQ = 125) and performed significantly above grade level on measures of achievement.

Static Encephalopathy

The second subgroup of our sample included children who demonstrated developmental delays, learning problems, and/or attentional deficits; however, their deficits were considered to be static, not progressive, in nature. Although their deficits did not worsen over time, improvements might occur at such a slow rate that the children might give the appearance of a progressive deterioration. In addition, their birth or medical histories were often indicative of multiple potential sources of cerebral insult in addition to HIV infection. Therefore, observed deficits were attributed to a variety of sources. Neurologically, these children presented with developmental delay, but not developmental regression; nonprogressive motor deficits; microcephaly that often paralleled a normal head circumference growth curve; and, on occasion, a concomitant seizure disorder. On psychometric assessment, cognitive status might vary from impaired to near-average. However, special educational services are often required to help remediate the observed delays.

Case 2

Two-year-old Leah had been observed at a pediatric HIV clinic since her early infancy. She was born prematurely to a young woman who died of an AIDS-related illness within weeks of her daughter's birth. Leah herself was diagnosed, by culture, as HIV-infected at 3 months of age. She demonstrated failure to thrive in the neonatal period and was treated for a septic episode. She had also been treated for multiple ear infections. An early CT scan suggested "mild cerebral atrophy" attributed, by the neurologist, to the prematurity of Leah's birth and not to HIV infection.

Leah had been seen for multiple developmental evaluations with the Bayley Scales. Though she initially demonstrated "low average" developmental skills, these gradually declined to the "borderline" range. Close analysis of her responses suggested not a loss of skills but, instead, poor progress in the acquisition of new skills. Specifically, Leah did not acquire expressive language skills at an appropriate rate. A referral for an audiological evaluation revealed a mild hearing loss. She was subsequently enrolled in speech therapy as well as an infant stimulation program.

Leah had been cared for by her maternal grandmother since the child's birth. The grandmother initially struggled with caring for a newborn while also grieving for her lost daughter. Involvement in a support group was helpful during that period. However, she continued to adjust to the reality of Leah's diagnosis.

Progressive Encephalopathy

A minority of our sample demonstrated progressive neurological manifestations at intake, and we expect that as many as 50% will eventually demonstrate signs of PE. The diagnosis of an HIV-associated PE is analogous to the AIDS–dementia complex reported in adults (Michaels, Sharer, & Epstein, 1988; Mintz, 1994). It often accompanies severe systemic immunodeficiency and disease (Mintz, 1992; Mintz, Epstein, & Koenigsberger, 1989). Onset may be abrupt and startling; global and rapid regression in cognitive skills, accompanied by changes in affect and behavior, is typical. In severe cases, children may no longer be able to feed, dress, and toilet themselves. They lose academic skills and are suddenly unable to function in their classroom setting. Often, they are aware of these dramatic changes in their own skills and behavior, and this awareness causes distress and depression. In addition, the parents or caretakers report that these children can be very irritable and difficult to console.

Diagnosis of a PE in childhood depends predominantly on clinical criteria. In a child with HIV infection, one of the three following persistent findings, present over at least a 2-month period in a child neurologically normal at baseline, is sufficient to classify a child as possessing an HIV-associated PE of childhood: impaired brain growth (acquired microcephaly or progressive loss of cerebral parenchymal volume on serial neuroimaging studies—see Figures 3.2 and 3.4); symmetrical and progressive motor dysfunction (manifested by two or more of the following: paresis, tone abnormalities, pathological reflexes, gait disturbance); or the failure to attain, a plateau in, or a loss of neurodevelopmental milestones (Working Group, 1993). Care must be taken to be sure that these findings are not a result of a known etiology (Sharer & Mintz, 1993) or malignancy (Mintz, Epstein, & Koenigsberger, 1989). Laboratory findings of the virus within the CSF is supportive but not diagnostic. The diagnosis of PE can be quite problematic under 1 year, and especially under 6 months, of age (Mintz, 1992).

When assessing for HIV-associated PE, one should be aware of other potential neurological complications seen in this population, some of which can mimic or confound the diagnosis of HIV-associated PE. Such complications include, but are not limited to, stroke syndromes (Park, Belman, Dickson, et al., 1988), primary CNS lymphoma (Epstein, DiCarlo, Joshi, et al., 1988), opportunistic and other infections of the CNS (Sharer & Mintz, 1993), seizure disorders (Mintz, Epstein, & Koenigsberger, 1989), nutritional deficiencies (Mintz & Epstein, 1992), myelopathies (Mintz & Epstein, 1992; Sharer & Mintz, 1993; Dickson, Belman, Kim, et al., 1989), and neuromuscular disorders (Dalakas & Pezeshkpour, 1988; Koch, Wesley, Lewis, et al., 1989;

Parry, 1988; Simpson, 1992). Appropriate investigations and interventions should ensue when such problems are suspected.

Psychometric testing in children with PE reveals a decline in IQ scores and loss of previously acquired skills. Changes in affect and attention/concentration are also often demonstrated. These children pose a special dilemma for schools, as their rapidly changing mental state requires flexible and creative responses from the school administrations.

Case 3

Jason was 4 years old when he was found to be HIV-infected. He and his three older siblings were all tested after it was learned that their mother was HIV+. Jason's medical history included a hospitalization at 6 months of age for failure to thrive, and again at 1 year for pneumonia. He was treated for repeated episodes of asthma and otitis media as well. However, his early development had been relatively normal. A psychological evaluation completed at the time of his diagnosis revealed a Stanford–Binet IQ of 96 (Form L-M; Terman & Merrill, 1973). However, he was noted to have lags in graphomotor skills, and his preacademic skills were somewhat delayed. Nevertheless, he was enrolled in a regular class in his private school system, where he made satisfactory progress over the years.

Jason's health gradually deteriorated: he was treated for thrush, herpes zoster, further otitis media, and asthma. Lymphadenopathy (swollen glands) and hepatomegaly (enlarged liver) were observed; lymphocytic interstitial pneumonitis was documented on chest X-ray. Jason gradually lost weight. He was offered antiretroviral treatment, but the family declined. Serial neurological evaluations suggested normal functioning, however. And Jason continued to function in the "average" range cognitively, as indicated by an assessment with the McCarthy Scales at 6 years.

However, Jason demonstrated a sudden and dramatic deterioration in behavior and development at 7 years of age. Jason's mother called to schedule an emergency appointment for her son, as she feared he was "losing his mind." Over the course of the previous few weeks, she had observed the following changes in Jason: He was no longer able to dress himself independently; he had become enuretic; he was afraid to climb stairs, so she had to carry him to level surfaces, where she observed that he tended to stumble when he walked. He seemed fully aware of these changes in behavior, and was profusely apologetic but also fearful. However, he was less aware of his decreased attention span and failing memory. The quality of Jason's school work also plummeted dramatically. The school was at a loss to help Jason.

Jason was seen for neurological and psychological evaluations. His CT scan indicated loss of cerebral parenchymal volume ("atrophy"). On cognitive assessment, this previously "average" child functioned in the "impaired" range: He earned a VIQ of 70, a PIQ of 68, and an FSIQ of 68 on the WISC-R. Subtest scaled scores varied dramatically from 1 to 9. Jason had obvious tremors of the hands and frequently dropped blocks, puzzle pieces, and the like. He also had difficulty controlling pencil pressure and broke three pencil leads when completing the Beery VMI. On this test, he scored at the 5½-year level (see Figure 3.5A). He was unable to perform academic

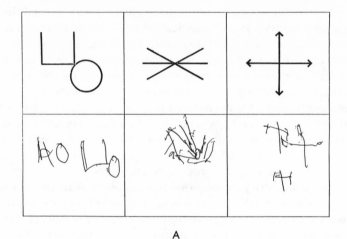

A

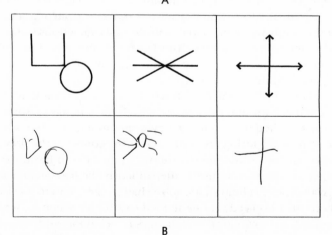

B

FIGURE 3.5. Comparison of graphomotor samples (Beery VMI) taken from child with PE (A) before treatment with zidovudine, and (B) 6 months after treatment was initiated.

tasks above the first-grade level on the WRAT-R. More striking was the change in affect and attention span. Previously reserved, he was now very disinhibited. He greeted members of the medical staff with enthusiastic hugs and chatted continually in a tangential, sometimes incoherent monologue. Whatever thought came to mind was immediately verbalized—including dialogue from movies and lyrics from songs.

Jason's mother consented to antiretroviral treatment. He was removed from school and placed on home instruction. Jason made gradual improvements in all spheres over the next few months. For example, within weeks he regained self-help skills (dressing and toileting), and his balance and equilibrium returned. Soon he was able to climb stairs to walk more smoothly. His attention and concentration only gradually improved, however. Unfortunately, academic skills showed a further decline before a rebound was noted on follow-up assessment.

When evaluated 6 months later, Jason continued to demonstrate significant impairments: He earned a VIQ of 78, a PIQ of 60, and an FSIQ of 68. However, there was a qualitative improvement in his performance: His attention and concentration were much improved, and he was able to inhibit impulses successfully. He was also coherent and logical in his thinking and modulated his affect more successfully. His VMI drawings best capture the qualitative improvement in his skills (Figure 3.5B). Academically, Jason still functioned at a very delayed level: he performed at the first- to second-grade level on the WRAT-R subtests. When he returned to school, he was placed in a special education class.

MEDICAL TREATMENT

The treatment of children with HIV-associated neurological disease has been frustrating and difficult (Mintz & Epstein, 1992; Mintz, 1994). However, encouraging early results with antiretroviral therapy suggest that neurodevelopmental deficits have been especially sensitive to this form of treatment (Brouwers, Moss, Welters, et al., 1990; McKinney, Maha, Connor, et al., 1991; Mintz & Epstein, 1992; Pizzo, Eddy, Falloon, et al., 1988; O'Donnell et al., 1991). The advent of antiretroviral medications has increased our ability to ameliorate debilitating neurological conditions. Administration of zidovudine to children with HIV infection has been shown to improve cognitive functioning (Brouwers et al., 1990; McKinney et al., 1991; Pizzo et al., 1988). Others (Watkins et al., 1992) have noted that the rate and magnitude of change exceed what would be expected during recovery from either forms of brain injury. For example, of the 20 patients in our population who were seen for follow-up evaluations after 6 months' treatment with zidovudine, 80% showed a dramatic increase in IQ scores. On average, a 20-point gain was noted. It may be that practice effects accounted for some of the gain noted; however, in each case genuine improvement in skills was also observed. In addition, concomitant positive changes have been documented on neuroimaging studies (Mintz & Epstein, 1992; Mintz, 1992; Pizzo et al., 1988). Analogous results have been found in adult populations (Schmitt, Bigley, McKinnis, et al., 1988; Mintz, 1994), but not to the same degree as in pediatric populations. Therefore, antiretroviral therapy has evolved to become a standard of therapy for children with HIV-associated progressive neurological disease (Mintz & Epstein, 1992). In the asymptomatic child with HIV infection, it is not known at the present time whether antiretroviral therapy can "prevent" or delay the onset of neurological or neuropsychological deficits. Ongoing treatment trials may better define this question.

Unfortunately, in some of our children with PE who demonstrated an initial improvement on zidovudine, neurological decline resumed during long-term treatment (Mintz, Connor, Oleske, et al., 1990; Mintz & Epstein, 1992). Thus, the beneficial effect of zidovudine on neurological functioning is not sustained in all children. This suggests the possible formation of resistant CNS viral isolates (Larder, Darby, & Richman, 1989; Tudor-Williams, St. Clair, McKinney, et al., 1992). Alternatively, the regression may be secondary to noncompliance by patients on long-term therapy (Mintz & Epstein, 1992). Other possible mechanisms of zidovudine failure include the release of neurotoxic factors that are not amenable to antiretroviral treatment (Mintz, Rapaport, Oleske, et al., 1989; Rosenberg & Fauci, 1989) or a direct neurotoxic effect of zidovudine (Dalakas & Pezeshkpour, 1989). Still, antiretroviral therapy remains the standard of care for pediatric patients with symptomatic HIV infection, especially in those with progressive neurological disease. Most children with neurological disease initially respond to antiretroviral therapy, and in many the effect is sustained. However, since some children may become tolerant to the benefits of zidovudine, future long-term therapy of children with HIV-associated neurological disease will require alternative antiretroviral agents, combinations of these agents, and the development of novel treatments to augment antiretroviral therapy (Butler, Husson, Balis, et al., 1991; Mintz, 1992, 1994; Mintz & Epstein, 1992).

Because of the sensitivity of neurodevelopmental surrogate markers to antiretroviral therapy, psychometric testing has become an integral part of determining drug efficacy in clinical trials involving children. An optimal testing battery in terms of both sensitivity to change and practical considerations has yet to be formulated, and protocols to date have relied heavily on standardized and commonly used tests (discussed previously in this chapter). What will be important for the future is to determine which subtests are most sensitive to change with the introduction of antiretroviral therapy and can be correlated with the clinical neurological condition. A psychometric marker of impending neurological decline would be useful as a predictive measure. However, in the asymptomatic infant or child, no formal neuropsychological marker is presently available. Likewise, similar attempts in the asymptomatic HIV-infected adult population have failed to identify any specific neuropsychological or cognitive deficit (Miller, Selnes, McArthur, et al., 1990; Selnes, Miller, McArthur, et al., 1990).

Since symptomatic HIV infection may be amenable to early intervention with antiretroviral therapy, it is incumbent to include HIV infection as a potential differential diagnosis in a child with unexplained developmental delay or deteriorating school performance. In addition, a school-aged child with known HIV infection is at risk for impairment of cognitive functioning. Therefore, psychometric testing and child study team evaluation are useful to identify children at academic risk, so that appropriate educational interventions can be set in place (Crocker, 1992). Though specific remediation strategies have not yet been identified, it is clear that special education services are often warranted and that early educational intervention is helpful (Armstrong, Seidel, & Swales, 1993).

Other forms of intervention may also be necessary. For example, children with severe neurological manifestations of HIV infection are susceptible to spasticity, and most will require vigilant physical and occupational therapies (Hinds, 1991). In addition, dysfunction of language formation and speech production are common features; these may be based on central dysphasia or secondary to oromotor dysfunction. Speech therapy should be employed to facilitate optimal speech functioning and to assist in problems with swallowing (Pressman, 1992). Sign language can be mastered when expressive language is impaired.

Since the CNS is not a totally separate entity from other organ systems, general health and well-being will have a great impact on neurological functioning. Accordingly, treatment of systemic difficulties (such as pulmonary disease or systemic infection), vigorous nutritional support, and antimicrobial therapy (when clinically indicated) will allow a child to make better developmental progress. Conversely, the CNS influences many aspects of systemic functioning. Thus, neurological and psychological health can only benefit when the overall system is operating optimally.

Obviously, the HIV-infected child requires an array of developmental, social, medical, and other ancillary services that are best accomplished through a multidisciplinary team (Boland, 1989; Crocker, 1989; Woodruff, Driscoll, & Sterzin, 1992). The geometric progression of the HIV epidemic will disproportionately add to the rolls of developmentally and physically disabled children, and will greatly tax available special services and rehabilitation resources. Foresight and pragmatism by education boards, and by state and federal governmental systems, will be necessary in planning for the future, since the epidemic among children has shown no signs of receding (Crocker, 1992).

SUMMARY

The majority of the 100 pediatric patients described in this chapter demonstrated average cognitive and neurological functioning at intake. Many of them have been able to function for years in regular classroom settings, though delays in achievement are common. Others, described here as having static encephalopathy, demonstrated persistent but not progressive delays in development, which have required ongoing remedial and therapeutic interventions. Ultimately, as many as 50% will eventually demonstrate symptoms of PE, characterized by global and rapid regression in skills, affect, and attention. The onset of this CNS involvement often signals the end stage of the disease process.

Treatment with antiretroviral agents has been effective in ameliorating debilitating neurological conditions. Patients may regain lost skills, though most do not resume previous levels of functioning. Unfortunately, however, some patients on long-term therapy show a tolerance for the medication and an eventual decline in functioning. In the future, treatment with combinations of different antiretroviral agents and CNS-specific augmentative therapies may be utilized to enhance outcome.

Health care and public education systems will bear the brunt of treatment for pediatric HIV patients in the future, as this once-terminal illness evolves into a chronic illness. Schools will have to be flexible in meeting the rapidly changing needs of individual children whose health is in constant flux. Chapter 15 explores in more depth how the educational system is responding to this challenge.

REFERENCES

Armstrong, D., Seidel, J., & Swales, T. (1993). Pediatric HIV infection: A neuropsychological and educational challenge. *Journal of Learning Disabilities, 26*(2), 92–103.

Bayley, N. (1969). *Manual for the Bayley Scales of Infant Development.* New York: Psychological Corporation.

Beery, K. (1982). *Revised administration, scoring and teaching manual for the Developmental Test of Visual–Motor Integration.* Cleveland: Modern Curriculum Press.

Belman, A., Diamond, G., Dickson, D., et al. (1988). Pediatric acquired immunodeficiency syndrome: Neurologic syndromes. *American Journal of Diseases of Children, 142,* 29–35.

Boland, M. (1989). *Generations in jeopardy: Responding to HIV infection in children, women and adolescents in New Jersey.* Newark: New Jersey Department of Health.

Brouwers, P., Moss, H., Wolters, P., et al. (1990). Effects of continuous-infusion zidovudine therapy on neuropsychologic functioning in children with symptomatic human immunodeficiency virus infection. *Journal of Pediatrics, 117,* 980–985.

Butler, K., Husson, R., Balis, F., et al. (1991). Dideoxyinosine in children with symptomatic human immunodeficiency virus infection. *New England Journal of Medicine, 324,* 137–144.

Cohen, D., Morgan, R., Rivera, I., et al. (1991, February). *A population based prospective study of neurodevelopment in infants at risk for human immunodeficiency virus type-I (HIV-I) infection.* Paper presented at the 6th Annual National Pediatric AIDS Conference, Washington, DC.

Crocker, A. (1989). Developmental services for children with HIV infection. *Mental Retardation, 27,* 223–225.

Crocker, A. (1992). Policy guidelines of various organizations. In A. Crocker, H. Cohen, & T. Kastner (Eds.), *HIV infection and developmental disabilities* (pp. 241–245). Baltimore: Paul H. Brookes.

Dalakas, M., & Pezeshkpour, G. (1988). Neuromuscular diseases associated with human immunodeficiency virus infection. *Annals of Neurology, 23*(Suppl.), 38–48.

Dalakas, M., & Pezeshkpour, G. (1989). AZT-induced destructive inflammatory myopathy with abnormal mitochondria (DIM-Mi): Study of seven patients. *Neurology, 39*(Suppl.), 152.

Diamond, G. (1989). Developmental problems in children with HIV infection. *Mental Retardation, 27,* 213–217.

Dickson, D., Belman, A., Kim, T., et al. (1989). Spinal cord pathology in pediatric acquired immunodeficiency syndrome. *Neurology, 39,* 227–235.

Dunn, L., & Dunn. L. (1981). *Peabody Picture Vocabulary Test—Revised.* Circle Pines, MN: American Guidance Service.

Epstein, L., DiCarlo, F., Joshi, V., et al. (1988). Primary lymphoma of the central nervous system in children with acquired immunodeficiency syndrome. *Pediatrics, 82,* 355–363.

Epstein, L., Goudsmit, J., Paul, D., et al. (1987). Expression of human immunodeficiency virus in cerebrospinal fluid of children with progressive encephalopathy. *Annals of Neurology, 21,* 398–401.

Epstein, L., Sharer, L. R., & Goudsmit, J. (1988). Neurological and neuropathological features of HIV infection in children. *Annals of Neurology, 23*(Suppl.), S19–S23.

Epstein, L., Sharer, L., Oleske, J., et al. (1986). Neurologic manifestations of HIV infection in children. *Pediatrics, 78,* 678–687.

Gardner, M. (1990). *Expressive One-Word Picture Vocabulary Test—Revised.* Los Angeles: Western Psychological Services.

Haiken, H., Hernandez, M., Mintz, M., et al. (1991). School-aged HIV-infected children and access to education. *Pediatric AIDS and HIV Infection: Fetus to Adolescent, 2,* 74–79.

Hinds, M. (1981). Physical therapy in pediatric HIV infection. In J. Muchland (Ed.), *Rehabilitation for patients with HIV disease* (pp. 343–358). New York: McGraw-Hill.

Hittleman, J. (1992). Neurodevelopmental aspects of HIV infection. In P. Kozlowski, D. Snider, P. Vietz, & H. Wisniewski (Eds.), *Brain and behavior in pediatric HIV infection.* Basel: Karger.

Ho, D., Rota, T., Schooley, R., et al. (1985). Isolation of HTLV-III from cerebrospinal fluid and neural tissues of patients with neurologic syndromes related to the acquired immunodeficiency syndrome. *New England Journal of Medicine, 313,* 1493–1497.

Jastak, S., & Wilkinson, G. (1984). *Wide Range Achievement Test—Revised.* Wilmington, DE: Jastak Associates.

Kairam, R. (1989, September). *The encephalopathies of pediatric HIV infection.* Abstract presented at the 5th Annual National Pediatric AIDS Conference, Los Angeles, CA.

Kaufman, A., & Kaufman, N. (1983). *Kaufman Assessment Battery for Children.* Circle Pines, MN: American Guidance Service.

Koch, T., Jeremy, R., Lewis, E., et al. (1989, June). *Developmental abnormalities in uninfected infants born to HIV infected mothers.* Abstract presented at the International AIDS Conference, San Francisco.

Koch, T., Wesley, A., Lewis, E., et al. (1989, June). *AIDS-related peripheral neuropathy in children and young adult hemophiliacs.* Abstract presented at the International AIDS Conference, San Francisco, CA.

Larder, B., Darby, G., & Richman, D. (1989). HIV with reduced sensitivity to zidovudine (AZT) isolated during prolonged therapy. *Science, 243,* 1731–1734.

Marion, R., Wiznia, A., Hutcheon, R., et al. (1986). Human T-cell lymphotropic virus type III (HTLV-III) embryopathy. *American Journal of Diseases of Children, 140,* 638–640.

Markwardt, F. (1989). *Peabody Individual Achievement Test—Revised (PAT-R).* Circle Pines, MN: American Guidance Service.

McCarthy, D. (1972). *McCarthy Scales of Children's Abilities*. New York: Psychological Corporation.

McKinney, R., Maha, M., Connor, E., et al. (1991). Protocol 043 study group: A multi-center trial of oral zidovudine in children with advanced human immunodeficiency virus disease. *New England Journal of Medicine, 324*, 1018–1025.

Michaels, J., Sharer, L., & Epstein, L. (1988). Human immunodeficiency virus type-1 (HIV-1) infection of the nervous system: A review. *Immunodeficiency Review, 1*, 71–104.

Miller, E., Selnes, O., McArthur, J., et al. (1990). Neuropsychological performance in HIV-1 infected homosexual men: The Multicenter AIDS Cohort Study (MACS). *Neurology, 40*, 197–203.

Mintz, M. (1992). Neurologic abnormalities. In R. Yoger & E. Conner (Eds.), *Management of HIV infection in infants and children* (pp. 247–285). St. Louis: Mosby–Year Book.

Mintz, M. (1994). Clinical comparison of adult and pediatric neuroAIDS. *Advances in Neuroimmunology, 4*, 207–221.

Mintz, M., Connor, E., Oleske, J., et al. (1990, July). *Neurologic deterioration in children on long-term zidovudine therapy*. Abstract presented at the 9th AIDS Clinical Trials Group Meeting, Bethesda, MD.

Mintz, M., & Epstein, L. (1992). Neurologic manifestations of pediatric acquired immunodeficiency syndrome: Clinical features and therapeutic approaches. *Seminars in Neurology, 12*, 51–56.

Mintz, M., Epstein, L. G., & Koenigsberger, M. R. (1989). Neurological manifestations of acquired immunodeficiency syndrome (AIDS) in children. *International Pediatrics, 4*, 161–171.

Mintz, M., Rapaport, R., Oleske, J., et al. (1989). Elevated serum levels of tumor necrosis factor are associated with progressive encephalopathy in children with acquired immunodeficiency syndrome. *American Journal of Diseases of Children, 143*, 771–774.

Nellhaus, G. (1968). Composite international and interracial graphs. *Pediatrics, 41*, 106.

Nicholas, W. (1988). Controversy: Is there an HIV-related facial dysmorphism? *Pediatric Annals, 17*, 214–224.

O'Donnell, K., Mintz, M., Maha, M., et al. (1991). Neurodevelopmental (ND) effects of pediatric HIV infection and treatment with oral zidovudine [Abstract]. *Pediatric Research, 29*, 181A.

Park, Y., Belman, A., Dickson, D., et al. (1988). Stroke in pediatric acquired immunodeficiency syndrome [Abstract]. *Annals of Neurology, 24*, 359–360.

Parry, G. (1988). Peripheral neuropathies associated with human immunodeficiency virus infection. *Annals of Neurology, 23*(Suppl.), 49–53.

Pizzo, P., Eddy, J., Falloon, J., et al. (1988). Effect of continuous intravenous infusion of zidovudine (AZT) in children with symptomatic HIV infection. *New England Journal of Medicine, 319*, 889–896.

Pressman, H. (1992). Communication disorders and dysphagia in pediatric AIDS. *Journal of the American Speech#Hearing Association, 35,* 45–47.

Rapin, I., & Johnson, W. (1987). Progressive genetic metabolic diseases: General principles. In A. Rudolph (Ed.), *Pediatrics* (pp. 1719–1725). Norwalk, CT: Appleton & Lange.

Rosenberg, Z., & Fauci, A. (1989). The immunopathogenesis of HIV infection. In F. Dixon (Ed.), *Advances in immunology* (Vol. 47, pp. 377–431). San Diego, CA: Academic Press.

Schmitt, R., Bigley, J., McKinnis, R., et al. (1988). Neuropsychological outcome of zidovudine (AZT) treatment of patients with AIDS and AIDS-related complex. *New England Journal of Medicine, 319,* 1573–1578.

Scott, G., Hutto, C., Makuch, R., et al. (1989). Survival in children with perinatally acquired human immunodeficiency virus type I infection. *New England Journal of Medicine, 321,* 1791–1796.

Selnes, O., Miller, E., McArthur, J., et al. (1990). HIV-I infection: No evidence of cognitive decline during the asymptomatic stages. *Neurology, 40,* 204–208.

Sharer, L., & Mintz, M. (1993). Neuropathology of AIDS in children. In F. Scaravilli (Ed.), *AIDS: The pathology of the nervous system* (pp. 201–214). Berlin: Springer-Verlag.

Simpson, M. (1992). Neuromuscular complications of human immunodeficiency virus infection. *Seminars in Neurology, 12,* 34–42.

Stover, E. Pequenat, W., Huffman, L., et al. (1990). CNS aspects of HIV-I infection and AIDS in infants and children: A collaborative research agenda. *Pediatric AIDS and HIV Infection: Fetus to Adolescent, 1,* 109–120.

Terman, L., & Merrill, M. (1973). *Stanford–Binet Intelligence Scale: Manual for the third revision, Form L-M.* Boston: Houghton Mifflin.

Thorndike, R., Hagen, E., & Sattler, J. (1986). *Stanford–Binet Intelligence Scale* (4th ed.). Chicago: Riverside.

Tudor-Williams, G., St. Clair, M., McKinney, R., et al. (1992). HIV-I sensitivity to zidovudine and clinical outcome in children. *Lancet, 339,* 15–19.

Ultmann, M., Diamond, G., Ruff, H., et al. (1987). Developmental abnormalities in children with acquired immunodeficiency syndrome (AIDS): A follow-up study. *International Journal of Neuroscience, 32,* 661–667.

Watkins, J., Brouwers, P., & Huntzinger, R. (1992). Neuropsychological assessment. In M. Stuber (Ed.), *Children and AIDS.* Washington, DC: American Psychiatric Press.

Wechsler, D. (1991). *Manual for the Wechsler Intelligence Scale for Children—Third Edition.* New York: Psychological Corporation.

Woodruff, G., Driscoll, P., & Sterzin, E. (1992). Providing comprehensive and coordinated services to children with HIV infection in their families: A transagency model. In A. Crocker, H. Cohen, & T. Kastner (Eds.), *HIV infection and developmental disabilities* (pp. 241–245). Baltimore: Paul H. Brookes.

Working Group on Antiretroviral Therapy: National Pediatric HIV Resource Center. (1993). Antiretroviral therapy and medical management of the human immunodeficiency virus-infected child. *Pediatric Infectious Disease Journal, 12,* 513–522.

SECTION III

THE PSYCHOSOCIAL CONTEXT: PSYCHOSOCIAL ISSUES FOR DIFFERENT GROUPS

4

Cultural Sensitivity and Competence

African-American, Latino, and Haitian Families with HIV/AIDS

Nancy Boyd-Franklin, PhD
Julia del C. Alemán, MSW
Michèle M. Jean-Gilles, MA
Sandra Y. Lewis, PsyD

THE NEED FOR CULTURAL SENSITIVITY AND COMPETENCE

Culture represents a way of life embodied in a set of integrated customs, values, and beliefs. McGoldrick, Pearce, and Giordano (1982) have shown that in order to be effective service providers, health care professionals must develop cultural sensitivity toward the different sets of norms and beliefs held by their patients and families, and the ways in which these culturally determined attitudes aid or adversely affect the delivery of health and mental health services. A cultural competence model (Lewis, 1992) that enables clinicians to incorporate cultural awareness and sensitivity into their methods of intervention and service delivery includes the following elements:

- Making use of natural resources
- Understanding family values with regard to roles, strengths, child rearing, and extended family involvement

- Understanding the role of spirituality or religion in the life of the family
- Assessing the level of acculturation—that is, the degree to which the behaviors and practices of a family match the behaviors of the majority group
- Cultivating respect for difference and diversity
- Empowering families to use their own strengths and resources to produce change and to advocate for services
- Encouraging other health and mental health care providers and facilities to provide concrete assistance and services
- Understanding the impact of one's own culture/values upon the care partnership/relationship with families

In this chapter, we apply this model in exploring the impact of pediatric HIV/AIDS on three cultural groups greatly affected by the disease: inner-city African-American, Latino, and Haitian families. Since each of these groups has different historical and geographical origins, and their response to and experience with HIV/AIDS have been culturally determined to a large extent, they are discussed separately.

There is always a risk that cultural material will be applied in a stereotypical fashion. Practitioners therefore should view this material not as a rigid template, but as a lens that can be adjusted with each new family, or discarded altogether if exceptions are encountered. In fact, there is considerable intragroup variability within each culture: No entity can monolithically be referred to as *"the* African-American," *"the* Latino," or *"the* Haitian" family. African-American families may differ in terms of their geographical origin (i.e., region of the country), class, education, skin color, religious and spiritual beliefs, and attitudes toward medical and mental health services. In addition, many groups are classified as "Black" in this country and may be mistakenly considered African-American. These include West Indians or Afro-Caribbeans, Haitians, and Africans (who may be from various African countries and thus have various cultural expressions). Latino or Hispanic families may also come from a number of different places, including Puerto Rico, Cuba, the Dominican Republic, Mexico, Panama, Nicaragua, San Salvador, and numerous other countries in Central and South America.

A central aspect of the Multisystems HIV/AIDS Model discussed throughout this book is its cross-cultural perspective. With regard to inner-city, poor African-American, Latino, and Haitian families, the model addresses these three basic issues: (1) the many levels of systems (agencies, clinics, etc.) that have an impact upon and often complicate families' lives; (2) the multigenerational family aspect of this disease, particularly in cultures characterized by complex extended families; and (3) the range of different beliefs, values, and coping styles in families living with HIV/AIDS, and the ways in which these have challenged service providers to become more culturally competent.

AFRICAN-AMERICAN FAMILIES

African-American inner-city families have one of the highest incidence rates for AIDS in women and children (Brown, Mitchell, & Williams, 1992; Stuber, 1992; Macklin, 1989). Health and mental health practitioners often become involved with such a family at the point at which a child is diagnosed as HIV-infected. These practitioners are rapidly learning that the impact of the disease is not limited to the diagnosed child, but has consequences for the entire family network (Boyd-Franklin & Aleman, 1990; Walker, 1991). (See Chapter 7.)

Extended Family and Multigenerational Issues

For generations of African-Americans, the extended family has been a source of cultural pride and strength. In times of trouble, extended family members—grandparents, siblings, aunts, and uncles—informally adopt or "take in" children (Billingsley, 1968; Hill, 1977; Boyd-Franklin, 1989). These include children with pediatric HIV/AIDS whose parents may have died of AIDS or have been diagnosed as HIV-infected. Because nonrelatives are also often included in African-American extended families, caretakers may be friends of the family, former baby-sitters, neighbors, godparents, or members of the "church family." Often this caretaker role is filled by foster parents who have assumed responsibility for children with no family members available to care for them.

Caretaker Issues

Traditionally, the burden of HIV/AIDS in the African-American community has fallen on women—mothers, aunts, grandmothers, or even great-grandmothers of children with pediatric HIV/AIDS.

Sometimes a mother becomes HIV-infected through sexual contact with a drug-using partner. Most often, it is after giving birth that a mother learns that both she and her infant are HIV-infected. The maternal caretaking function becomes complicated by feelings of blame, guilt, anger, and shame. Conflicted feelings about transmitting the disease or her own deteriorating health may cause the mother to relinquish the role of caring for a sick child to a relative—in many cases, her mother or another older relative.

Older caretakers in the extended family often serve a central role in their families as "switchboards" for all family communications. Frequently, however, they are already raising young members of their families (grandchildren, great-grandchildren, nieces, nephews, younger siblings). The additional care of an HIV-infected child can overload them.

The family myth that grandmothers and other extended family caretakers are "towers of strength" is absolutely true, but it does not allow the caretakers to protest when their burdens become too great. As a result, help from extended family members, as well as from medical and social service systems, is usually not forthcoming. Too often, no one discovers the degree of burden until a caretaker has become completely overwhelmed and can no longer care for an HIV-infected child. To make sensitive family interventions, we must be aware of this abiding desire among African-Americans to hold together the extended family.

One African-American grandmother in her 70s shares the story of her family's experience with AIDS as follows:

> My first son had the [HIV/AIDS] virus. My granddaughter, who was one and a half, had it too. My daughter, who also had the virus, gave the children away. She left them at the Salvation Army. DYFS [New Jersey Division of Youth and Family Services] picked them up. The older boys asked for Grandma and Grandpa. There was no question. We came and picked them up that night. They are my flesh and blood. I have all six children.
>
> When my daughter got the virus she said to me, "I'm sorry I did this to you." I said, "No, you didn't do anything to me." I was there when she died. Me and my husband were both there. I held her head as she died. Now I am raising her six children—me and my husband.
>
> Later, when my son was dying, sometimes he would crawl up in my bed during the day when I was with the kids and just lay there. He would say, "I feel like you're here holding me." My neighbor used to say, "How could you let him sleep on your bed? Aren't you afraid you'll get it?" But I said to her, "If God meant for me to have it [AIDS], I would. He's my child. He's 42, but he's still my child. It's hard to cry in front of him; he thinks I'm punishing him. . . . I go off to cry."

Grandmothers are certainly among the heroines of the AIDS crisis, but they pay a high price. Mental health and health care providers must play a part in helping prevention of role overload and burnout among these "towers of strength." Their tasks are twofold: to help grandmothers open up and ask for assistance, and, more importantly, to help locate family members who can provide support or take over *before* the grandmothers become overwhelmed and burn out. Some families have lost so many members to AIDS and other illnesses that there truly *are* no longer supports available. African-American women have always depended on one another for support (Boyd-Franklin, 1989), but the AIDS crisis has created a serious problem in this area. For many families, this "sisterhood network" has been debilitated by drug abuse and disease and can no longer provide support. To help caretakers cope, Theresa Kreibick started a caretakers' support group (see Chapter 11). She learned, as we all have learned, that in the inner-city AIDS struggle we therapists must be pragmatic and offer what is needed without rigid preconceptions regarding our role.

Secrets Regarding HIV/AIDS

In many African-American families, the cause of death of a family member who has died of AIDS is treated as a toxic family secret (Boyd-Franklin, 1989) that is not appropriate to discuss with children (Boyd-Franklin & Alemán, 1990).

Concern about secrecy is common to families of all cultures who are living with HIV/AIDS. However, for many African-American families it has additional significance. For generations, being subjected to racism in this country has caused many African-American families to adhere to strict rules about the privacy of family-related matters. Common attitudes are conveyed in statements such as "It's nobody's business but our own" and "Don't air our dirty laundry in public." Also, because of negative experiences with the welfare system, many inner-city African-American families view outside agencies as "prying" into family business. Unlike Latino clients, who may be very responsive to "the doctor" and will seek therapy on a doctor's orders, African-American clients often respond with a great deal of suspicion toward therapy and other forms of "help." A part of this suspicion has to do with a mistrust of "White institutions" that have historically been associated with racism and discrimination. Grier and Cobbs (1968) have referred to this as "healthy cultural paranoia." In addition, therapy is viewed negatively by many members of the Black community. It is seen as "for crazy people," "for weak people," or "for White people." For many African-American clients who fear disclosure, therapy is also seen as very "public." This issue is even more complicated for people living with HIV/AIDS and their families.

Resistance to therapy is an important reality for both health and mental health professionals to be aware of. Unless these issues are recognized, service providers may become angry and frustrated in their treatment of African-American families in general, and particularly those living with HIV/AIDS.

Perceptions of HIV/AIDS
in African-American Communities

Researchers have documented in many African-Americans the misperception that HIV/AIDS is a "White gay man's disease" (Brown et al., 1992; Bouknight & Bouknight, 1988; Dalton, 1989; Flaskerud & Rush, 1989; Honey, 1988; Mays & Cochran, 1988; Mitchell, 1990; Peterson & Marin, 1988). Brown et al. (1992), Di Clemente, Boyer, and Morales (1988), Mays and Cochran (1987), Selik, Castro, and Papparoanou (1988), and Fullilove, Fullilove, Bowser, and Gross (1990) have all shown how this misperception leads African-American men and women to deny that injection drug use, needle sharing, prostitution, and heterosexual sex are also risk factors. Fordyce, Sambula, and Stonebruner (1989) have shown that mandatory reporting of HIV testing would therefore deter African-Americans and Latinos from being tested.

A key barrier to risk perception in minority communities is homophobia (Brown et al., 1992; Peterson & Marin, 1988), which leads to denial of homosexual or bisexual activities in both African-American and Latino communities. This is particularly true of men who have engaged in homosexual activity during incarceration or in their adolescence and believe that insertive anal and oral sex are not risky, whereas receptive behavior is (Brown et al., 1992, p. 25).

In the light of the many problems facing inner-city families in African-American communities, including poverty, homelessness, drug usage, and crime, the impact of HIV/AIDS has not been fully recognized. Magic Johnson's announcement of his HIV infection has had a profound emotional impact on African-Americans and has focused attention on heterosexual transmission. The question of whether this has resulted in safe-sex behavior in African-American communities, however, remains to be seen. There is a crucial need for culturally sensitive HIV/AIDS education in African-American communities (Williams, 1986; Mitchell & Heagarty, 1991; Rogers & Walter, 1987).

Spirituality as a Means of Coping with HIV/AIDS

Spirituality has been well documented as a strength in many African-American families (Hill, 1977; Billingsley, 1968; Boyd-Franklin, 1989; Levin, 1984). Unfortunately, many well-meaning clinicians who have limited experience with African-American families fail to view spirituality as an effective psychological coping mechanism to be utilized therapeutically. This is a serious oversight, particularly when a family's spirituality is its chief source of strength in times of crisis. Health and mental health professionals who ask an African-American caretaker of a pediatric AIDS patient, "How do you cope?" frequently hear the response, "I pray to the Lord."

Often the diagnosis of HIV or AIDS in an adult or a child exposes the family secret of drug abuse or homosexuality to the church community. It is important for those treating families in the African-American community to recognize ministers as a support for such families. For those African-American families who, because of the shame associated with HIV/AIDS, have withdrawn from their "church families," this crisis may be an important time to help them reconnect.

For African-American families, the spiritual view of death may be a release from the pain of this earth. This concept is often raised by caretakers to help HIV/AIDS children cope with their anticipated loss. Funerals and wakes are central rituals in the lives of African-American people; they serve as means of emotional release or catharsis, allowing survivors to express their tears and grief openly. It is highly significant when the clinician and other members of the hospital staff, with a family's permission, attend the funeral or other rituals (such as the viewing at the funeral home) when a child or an adult dies while the family is in treatment.

After the funeral, however, many African-American family members will seal over their grief in order to "go on with life." Frequently psychological symptoms or distress develop in family members who still need to experience and share their mourning after the funeral. Helping family members discuss the burdens of the disease and the pain of loss in therapy is often a very powerful intervention. But it is important for clinicians not to offer this type of family mourning session until they have established a solid bond with the family members. Personal tragedy is rarely shared with people outside the family until they are accepted and trusted.

LATINO FAMILIES

Latino and African-American families with HIV/AIDS share similar issues. For example, Latinos, like African-Americans, place emphasis on and take great pride in the extended family. Godparents (*compadres* and *comadres*) are very important and are seen as coparents to a child (García-Preto, 1982). In times of crisis, it is a common pattern to place a child with a grandmother, a sister, a *comadre* or *compadre*, or a neighbor (García-Preto, 1982; Ramos-McKay, Comas-Díaz, & Rivera, 1988). Many Latino families with HIV/AIDS are in fact complex extended families, in which several nuclear families share one home or live in one apartment building. One often hears *"Fulano es como la familia"*—that is, "So-and-so is like a family member." Among the issues particular to Latino families are heterogeneity among groups labeled Latino; respect for authority; language; socialization and sexual practices of men and women (the concepts of *machismo* and *marianismo*); and immigration-related issues.

According to statistics from the Centers for Disease Control (1989), although only 7% of the total U.S. population is Latino, Latinos account for 15% of all adult AIDS cases and 23% of pediatric AIDS cases. HIV/AIDS is a severe problem among Latinos, mainly because of injection drug use.

Diversity among Latino Families

The rapid spread of HIV/AIDS among members of the Latino community represents, in part, the failure of the larger system to provide strategies for education and prevention that are sensitive to cultural differences. There is an urgent need for better understanding of Latinos as a *heterogeneous* group, so that service providers can become culturally competent.

The terms "Hispanic" and "Latino" are often used to refer to an entire cultural group; this practice, however, discounts the actual heterogeneity among the various cultures. "Hispanic" is not a race. As noted earlier, Latino families may come from Puerto Rico, the Dominican Republic, Cuba, Spain, Colombia, Guatemala, Mexico, Belize, Argentina, Chile, Ecuador, Peru, Nicaragua, El Salvador, and many other Central and South American countries. Moreover, the diversity of Latino families is based on other factors as well—the era in which they emigrated, the area of the United States in which they settled, and the number of generations they have lived here.

Language

Most Latino families speak Spanish as their primary language. But other official and indigenous languages are represented among Latin Americans. For example, Portuguese is the official language of Brazil; Quechua, an indigenous language, is mainly spoken in Guatemala. Often the language is seen as a connection to the culture of the country of origin.

In the United States, there are many Latino communities, or *bar-*

rios where older family members may not speak any English. They may live, work, and have all of their needs met within their own families or communities. Often, children learn English before their parents and grandparents do. Contact with other children in the school system exposes them not only to the English language but also to "Anglo" (or mainstream American) values and mores. This can often be very problematic for families who wish to preserve their Latino culture.

The onset of HIV/AIDS abruptly forces a Latino family into contact with the medical, social service, and possibly the mental health systems. All of these systems expect patients to speak English and may not be equipped with translators. As a result, family members in these situations often become overwhelmed and frustrated. Typically, Latino family members want to accompany a patient to an emergency room or clinic visit. But medical, nursing, and social service staffs often ignore these relatives and take "the patient" away from them into an examining room or for a consultation. This is insensitive and frustrating to the family.

In addition, medical and social service staffs often use children as translators for parents or other older relatives. One can only begin to imagine the burden and stress placed, for instance, on a young boy who has to translate for his mother that his newborn baby sister is HIV-infected. HIV/AIDS programs should recruit professional staff members who are from the Latino culture and/or at least fluent in Spanish.

Respect for Authority

Latinos show respect for authority and place great trust in a physician, nurse, social worker, or psychologist as a professional. This stands in marked contrast to African-American families, who are very suspicious of authority figures and who often bring "healthy cultural paranoia" (Grier & Cobbs, 1968) to the treatment process. This trust in doctors and in the health care system among Latinos can and should be utilized to engage the family and extended family system.

Socialization and Sexual Practices of Men and Women

The socialization process of men in many Latino families centers on the concept of *machismo* (García-Preto, 1982; Ramos-McKay et al., 1988; Sluzki, 1982). Medina (1987) has described this concept as "the exaggerated importance of being a man." Boys are taught to be strong, and one often hears "*Los hombres nunca lloran*," or "Men never cry." Ramos-McKay et al. (1988) offer a description of *machismo* as the traditional male sex role: "[It] literally means maleness and virility." Culturally, "the male is associated with the provider or the one responsible for the welfare of the family. . . . In the family, machismo is usually associated with sexual prowess and power over women" (pp. 207–208). Later in this section and throughout this book (see especially Chapter 7), we illustrate how this sense of manhood and responsibility can be reframed for Latino men, particularly as it relates to sexual practices and safer sex.

The female counterpart to *machismo,* called *marianismo* (García-Preto, 1982; Ramos-McKay et al., 1988), reflects the religious influence on a culture where women are expected to emulate the Virgin Mary, *La Virgen Maria.* A woman is expected to remain "pure," a virgin, until she is married. Traditional Latino families place a high priority on virginity in the female, as well as submissiveness and obedience, especially in the role of wife (Medina, 1987; Espin, 1984).

Machismo and *marianismo* complicate conventional HIV/AIDS education and contribute greatly to unsafe sexual practices and HIV risk. It would be considered very forward and inappropriate for a Latina to discuss safe-sex issues, such as using a condom, with a man. A woman is not supposed to have any sexual knowledge, much less discuss these issues with her lover. Counseling a Latina to go back and discuss condom use with her husband or boyfriend without an awareness of the male's investment in *machismo* may result in her being beaten or abused in other ways.

Homosexuality and Bisexuality

Homosexuality is often a secret within Latino families. Homophobia is prevalent in Latino communities, where the homosexuality of a son is often considered a "shame" to the family. Bisexuality, however, is frequently practiced among Latino men (Carrier, 1976, 1985, 1988; Magaña & Magaña, 1992). Magaña and Magaña (1992, pp. 36–37), in their discussion of the sexual behaviors of Mexican men, make the following observations:

> It is estimated that approximately 30% of the Mexican males have engaged in sex with other men (Carrier, 1985). The men who engage in this activity are not necessarily primarily sexually oriented toward other men and usually engage in heterosexual activities also. Researchers in this area have speculated that the high rate of bisexual behavior among Mexican males may be influenced by cultural beliefs that allow men to participate in certain sexual acts with other males without conceiving of themselves as homosexual. As long as the male engages in anal intercourse and assumes the active role of penetrator, he is not seen as a homosexual and

does not risk any negative impact on his male image. Only the man who assumes the passive role and allows himself to be penetrated is considered homosexual (Carrier, 1985; Magaña & Carrier, in press).

Anecdotal reports from other groups of Latino men confirm these beliefs. Further research needs to be conducted to confirm the prevalence of these beliefs and practices among other groups of Latinos. This information has enormous implications for the spread of HIV/AIDS in the Latino community. As Magaña and Magaña (1992) have indicated, this has serious implications for HIV risk factors, because many of these men are also involved with women of childbearing age. These cultural factors should be taken into account when questioning Latino men about their sexual practices.

Other Issues Regarding HIV/AIDS in Latino Communities

Although HIV/AIDS has spread with alarming speed through Latino communities, public health, education, and prevention services have been slow to address the needs of this population (Magaña & Magaña, 1992; Amaro, 1988; Bakeman, Lumb, & Smith, 1986; Marin, 1989; Coates, Temoshok, & Mandel, 1984). In addition to the sex roles and sexual attitudes discussed above, there are many other important issues that make the treatment of HIV/AIDS as well as prevention very difficult. One such issue is the high fertility rate among Latinos (McCarthy & Valdez, 1986), which has contributed to the disproportionately high rates of pediatric HIV and AIDS (Magaña & Magaña, 1992; Amaro, 1988).

Poverty, homelessness, and drug use have also had an impact on the incidence of AIDS in the Latino community (Nyamathi & Vasquez, 1989; Magaña, 1991). Poverty is associated with high rates of injection drug use, which is implicated in 80% of Latino pediatric HIV/AIDS cases (Magaña & Magaña, 1992).

In addition, because of lack of cultural sensitivity, physicians and public health personnel have often not taken into account religious issues, such as attitudes about abortion (Rosenhouse-Pearson & Sabagh, 1983), birth control practices (Amaro, 1988), and sex education (Medina, 1987; Worth, 1987) among Roman Catholic Latina women.

Health, mental health, and social service providers who insist that Latina women use birth control (condoms) and/or have an abortion must realize that many of them experience conflict in regard to these practices, both of which are against the teachings of the Roman Catholic Church. In such cases, providers must intervene with greater sensitivity.

Latino Families in Therapy

In addition to *machismo* and *marianismo,* traditional Latino culture promotes the belief that a woman must sacrifice herself for the sake of her family. Often a Latina will make the ultimate sacrifice—her health and her life—by not asking the man to use a condom. For some Latina women, it seems they must place themselves at risk for contracting HIV to make the sexual situation comfortable for their male partners. AIDS also, as we can see from the following case example of Sandra, serves to loosen the cultural strictures of *marianismo.*

Case Example: Cultural Issues and Safe Sex

Sandra is a 35-year-old Latina who presented a chronic history of injection drug use starting at age 13. Sandra was diagnosed with HIV in 1986. She is asymptomatic at this time and her health is good.

Sandra grew up in a household in which her mother inculcated the traditional role of a woman as "mother and spouse," whose responsibility was to "make it right" for men. When Sandra was initially diagnosed, it would have been inconceivable for her to have challenged any of the men with whom she had sex about the issue of condom use. Although she was made aware that professional help was available to her, she did not believe anyone would understand, in her words, "where I was coming from." She was confused and in denial.

Sandra had learned from her mother that a woman's job was to bear children and that abortions were "against God's will." Some time after she was diagnosed she gave birth to two children. The children live with her sister, and Sandra has not been involved in their parenting.

Sandra expresses regret that she "left them" and "didn't do what I was supposed to," although she recognizes that, because of her drug use, this is the best thing for them. They have both been tested for AIDS, but Sandra has not divulged their status.

Through her church, Sandra joined a support group of Latina women whose lives had been affected by AIDS—either through their own HIV infection (two members) or that of loved ones.

Sandra's reluctance to discuss condom use and her decision to bring her pregnancies to term were validated by other group members, who had also been raised in traditional Latino households.

Sandra is now living with a Latino man who is himself HIV-infected. Her group experience has enabled her to be comfortable enough to discuss safe sex practices with him.

The concept of sacrifice inherent in *marianismo* often extends to a woman who, after separating from her lover or husband because of his drug abuse, takes him back once he becomes symptomatic with AIDS. Often she is forced by cultural prohibitions against expressions of anger. Frequently, it is children who express emotions for the rest of the family. In treatment a therapist will help a mother to express her own sadness, pain, and anger more directly.

A key source of conflict between Latino couples and health practitioners has to do with the issue of pregnancy. A man's ability to impregnate a woman is an important part of *machismo;* the ability to have children, particularly male children, is considered a testimony to his sexual prowess and virility (García-Preto, 1982). This is equally true for women: *Marianismo* is closely connected to the role of motherhood and with a woman's ability to have children with and for her husband. This can become very complicated when a couple is HIV-infected and the man insists that his wife not use birth control and have another child by him. Health and mental health practitioners who are unaware of these complex issues often become furious with a Latina who has one HIV-infected child and then becomes pregnant with her second or third.

Religious and Other Spiritual Support Systems

Although many Latino families are at least nominally Roman Catholic, a growing number belong to Pentecostal or other Protestant churches. Churches are often important community support systems, and priests or ministers are often consulted for important medical, particularly life-and-death, decisions. García-Preto (1982) has shown that many Latino families tend to personalize their religious beliefs. This *personalismo* is reflected in dialogue with the Virgin Mary and the saints. Sick family members and children will often be surrounded by candles and members of the family praying with crucifixes and rosary beads. Hospital staff members often have to be helped to understand the purposes of these rituals.

In many Latin cultures, there are also alternative spiritual belief systems: *espiritismo* (primarily a Puerto Rican folk system); *santeria* (folk healing beliefs in Cuba); and *curanderismo* (folk healing beliefs in Mexico and nearby countries).

Espiritismo as practiced by Puerto Ricans is described as "a belief system consisting of an invisible world, populated by spirits, which surrounds the visible world" (Ramos-McKay et al., 1988, p. 210). García-Preto (1982) has also described this system of spiritual beliefs, which utilizes a person known as an *espiritista,* who communicates between the dead and the living by interpreting dreams and other experiences. Ramos-McKay et al. (1988) and García-Preto (1982) have likened this practice to an indigenous form of psychotherapy. Hospital personnel need to be aware of this practice, because although many Puerto Rican families will state that they are Catholic if asked about religious or spiritual beliefs, they will also consult an *espiritista* if faced with a life-threatening illness such as AIDS. Comas-Díaz and Griffith (1981) discuss an intervention model that utilizes medical and mental health interventions and *espiritismo*, and allows the practitioner to accept and bridge both systems.

Cuban families often practice a folk belief system known as *santeria*, an Afro-Cuban religious and spiritual system that integrates Catholic saints with Yoruba deities. *Santeros* are mediums who initiate others into this faith healing system (Bernal & Gutierrez, 1988). These beliefs as well as *espiritismo* have spread through other Latino communities in the United States, largely through *botanicas*, which are very popular stores in these neighborhoods. In addition to food, individuals can also purchase special herbs, potions, candles, and statues or pictures of the saints at these stores (Bernal & Gutierrez, 1988). *Santeria* teaches that diseases have both natural and supernatural origins. Hospital personnel are often surprised to find statues of saints or beads around the necks or wrists of children and adults with HIV/AIDS. These are intended to protect the individuals from supernatural causes of illness.

Folk medicine is very common in many Latin countries, particularly in rural areas. In Mexico and other surrounding Central American countries, *curanderismo*/folk healing is practiced (Maduro, 1983). A *malruesto* (or hex) is commonly seen as one of the causes of a patient's illness. A *curandera* (folk healer) is often consulted, who may prescribe herbs or folk medicine.

Once again, it is crucial for medical practitioners to recognize that Latinos frequently use their folk beliefs while participating in the hospital medical system. Doctors and nurses need to inquire carefully about any other treatment that may be used. Often, upon investigation a physician will discover that these practices do no harm; they may even provide some of the nutrients and vitamins that are necessary to sustain very compromised immune systems.

Factors Related to Immigration Patterns and Status

Latinos differ greatly as to their country of origin, their citizenship, their immigration status, and their degree of acculturation. It is therefore important for the clinician to inquire carefully about these issues with the family.

Many first-generation Latino immigrants adhere very closely to their traditional values; their cultural, spiritual, and medical beliefs; and their language. Often one family member, usually the man, is sent to this country to establish residence. However, because women often find entry-level employment more quickly in this country, problems surface within the traditional male–female relationship. A family may, for example, arrive in this country illegally, and the woman may be sponsored by her employer so that she can obtain her "green card." This allows her to work in this country legally and to sponsor her husband and her children. Often families are separated for long periods of time, and children are left with extended family members in the country of origin while parents establish residence in the United States.

Puerto Ricans, as U.S. citizens, do not have the onus of immigration restrictions that affect other Latino families. They can travel back and forth freely between the island of Puerto Rico and the mainland United States. This has facilitated the spread of AIDS between the United States and Puerto Rico, however (Lambert, 1990). Families in Puerto Rico with a member with AIDS often come to the United States seeking better health care. For example, until fairly recently, there were very few hospitals or clinics on the island of Puerto Rico that specialized in the care of HIV-infected children.

Many Latino families from Central and South America, who have likely fled war-torn countries or oppressive regimes to come to the United States, are here illegally. When HIV or AIDS is diagnosed, it often creates great fear among family and friends that contact with a variety of systems—hospitals, clinics, and (if children are involved) the child welfare authorities—will expose others in the family and friend support network, who are also in the United States illegally. Moreover, undocumented families typically have no health insurance; for this reason, many Latino patients will not seek much-needed medical treatment. These issues require particular sensitivity among health and mental health service providers who are working with already stressed families.

HAITIAN FAMILIES

Immigration patterns and status are also critical issues for practitioners working with Haitian children and families with HIV/AIDS. Other important areas are language issues; psychosocial stressors upon the family; beliefs about the supernatural causes of illness, voodoo, and alternative health care; illness prevention and care measures; trust and confidentiality; and medical compliance.

Factors Related to Immigration Patterns and Status

It is important for practitioners to fully understand changes in the immigration patterns of Haitian families and their impact on how Haitian families interact with the medical care system, mental health facilities, and the broader social service system.

Giles (1990) describes three waves of Haitian immigrants to the United States in the last 30 years:

> The first wave—well-educated members of the Haitian upper class—began coming to the United States in the late 1950's to flee the harsh regime of President Francois Duvalier, "Papa Doc." The second wave of middle-class Haitians began arriving in the mid-1960's, and the third wave, composed largely of Haitian peasants and unskilled urban workers with little or no education, including the "boat people," began making its way to American shores in the mid-1970's. (pp. 317–318)

Schiller et al. (1987), Stepick (1987), and Bayardelle (1984) have also documented these immigration patterns. The majority of children who are HIV-infected themselves or who are being raised in families dealing with HIV/AIDS are part of this third immigration group. These Haitians are often very poor and include both immigrants and political refugees.

Giles (1990) identifies this third wave of immigration as "chain migration," whereby "extended family members pool their limited financial resources to send to the United States the family member considered most likely to find a job. That person then sends money to relatives in Haiti to support them and to enable certain others to migrate to the United States" (p. 318). This process has been well documented by Buchanan (1979), Laguerre (1984), and Seligman (1977). According to Fjellman and Gladwin (1985), many Haitian families help support the new arrivals until they can work on their own. This process of immigration creates a financial burden for the family members who come first to the United States. The immigration laws also lead to the disruption of families; often children are left behind and parents are unable to effectively monitor their care back home in Haiti (Giles, 1990; Laguerre, 1979, 1980).

For some Haitian families, their illegal immigration status is a major stressor (Giles, 1990; Laguerre, 1984; Seligman, 1977). These families, particularly the "boat people" who came during the 1980–1982 period, live with constant anxiety about being returned to Haiti. De Santis and Thomas (1990) and Massanz (1984) point out that the "boat people" were given a special classification of "entrant," which permitted them to reside in the United States. Yet their status put them in a "political limbo": "They were not permitted to return to Haiti, did not qualify for most federal assistance programs and could not bring family members to the United States and were constantly in fear of deportation." (Massanz, 1984, quoted in De Santis & Thomas, 1990, p. 4).

Haitians in the United States, many of them Black and poor, have been affected by many forms of stigma and discrimination. The illegal immigration status of some Haitian families has also contributed to biases. But perhaps the most stigmatizing issue for immigrants has been the identification of HIV/AIDS with the Haitian community. De Santis and Thomas (1990), Marchette (1984), Miller (1984), and Slevin and Colon (1984) have indicated that fear of deportation, particularly if HIV or AIDS is diagnosed (Montalvo, 1987; Nachman & Dreyfuss, 1986), greatly contributes to the avoidance of health care and all other social systems by some Haitian families. De Santis and Thomas (1990) point out that the Immigration Reform Act of 1986 requires that all applicants be tested for HIV before being processed for residency.

The public phobia about HIV/AIDS in the United States has had a negative impact on the acceptance of many Haitian families. Haitian women have told us that they have been turned down for employment as babysitters, housekeepers, day care workers, and private duty nurses because of fears about HIV contamination. Physicians, nurses, and social workers who treat these families often report angry responses when HIV/AIDS is diagnosed. Health, social work, and mental health practitioners must work with a family through these initial responses.

Language Issues

Because many Haitian families do not speak English, they are often at a true disadvantage when advocating for themselves, their children, and other family members.

Laguerre (1981) emphasizes the importance of the language problems for Haitians. Medical and mental health settings often assume that Haitians speak French. This is an unfortunate misconception, because, as Laguerre (1981) points out, French is used by only a small proportion of the elite in Haiti. The majority of Haitians in fact speak Haitian Creole. In this case, finding a physician, nurse, or a clinician who speaks French is not sufficient.

Hospitals and clinics in locations such as New York City, Miami, and Chicago, where large numbers of Haitian families reside, have struggled with this issue. Some have successfully recruited Creole-speaking nurses, physicians, and social workers, but the numbers of these professionals are still very small.

Since AIDS also carries a stigma within the Haitian community, many families feel guarded even with other members of their own community for fear that their confidentiality will not be maintained. Trust building is therefore very important in care partnerships/relationships with Haitian families.

Like Latino families, many Haitian families may feel that using children as translators shows disrespect for the parents and the culturally accepted generational hierarchy. It also places a tremendous psychological burden on the youngsters. It is important to ask Haitian parents whether they know a trustworthy English-speaking adult who can accompany them to meet with the physician. Clearly, this is a very important intervention with all immigrant families for whom language is an issue.

Beliefs about Supernatural Causes of Illness and Voodoo

Just as there is a tremendous diversity in African-American and Latino communities, so too there are differences in Haitian communities in terms of responses to health care, use of traditional folk healers, and voodoo doctors. These differences are based on a variety of factors, including urban versus rural origin, social class, education, and even skin color (Black vs. mulatto) (Laguerre, 1981).

Haitians believe that many types of illness are of "supernatural" origin and are caused by voodoo spirits (Laguerre, 1981). Illness is often viewed as a punishment by a spirit. De Santis and Thomas (1990) define voodoo as a "syncretism of African and Catholic religious beliefs and practices that shape[s] almost every aspect of Haitian culture and health culture" (p. 6). This has been documented by other researchers as well (Charles, 1986; Coriel, 1983a, 1983b; Gustafson, 1989; Kilpatrick & Cobb, 1990; Laguerre, 1980, 1981, 1984, 1987; Mathewson, 1975; Murray & Alvarez, 1973).

Many Haitian families have learned to deny any belief in these systems when dealing with traditional health care providers. The important factor here is that in the indigenous Haitian island culture, Catholic or other Christian individuals practice voodoo while simultaneously receiving "scientific" medical treatment (Laguerre, 1984; De Santis & Thomas, 1990).

As one explores the broader beliefs regarding voodoo, it becomes more clear how many Haitians families view a devastating illness such as HIV/AIDS. De Santis and Thomas (1990) point out that according to Haitian folk religion, each Haitian family subscribing to voodoo has the responsibility to protect individual members against the evil powers of other persons. . . . Children are generally considered innocent of evil doing, but they can be afflicted by illness as a means of punishing parents. Therefore, parents will often consult voodoo priests (houngans) or priestesses (mambos) to seek ways of protecting children from malevolent human beings or to restore harmony between themselves and the spirit world. (pp. 6–7)

For Haitian parents who discover the presence of HIV/AIDS in the family when a newborn child is diagnosed as having HIV antibodies, this knowledge is devastating on many levels. The family may assume that someone has used evil powers or spirits against their family by afflicting their child. Parents, on hearing this news from medical practitioners who do not speak their language or understand their beliefs, will often seek the aid of a voodoo priest.

Medical and social work practitioners may become alarmed when they see evidence of voodoo practices, such as placing special cloths or multicolored bead necklaces or bracelets on a child to protect him or her. One mother who was told that her child tested positive for the HIV antibodies became convinced that her child had become infected because "evil people" were harming her child. She also felt that she had not protected her child because she had not buried the umbilical cord and placenta in the ground after birth (De Santis & Thomas, 1990). Medical personnel unaware of this strongly held folk belief could not fully comprehend her grief and sense of guilt.

De Santis and Thomas (1990) and Laguerre (1981) caution medical and mental health practitioners against unilaterally counseling families against the use of voodoo. They prescribe a more prudent course of action—that is, "to accept such practices as adjuncts to biomedical efforts. . . . Acceptance of . . . Haitian ethnomedicine conveys respect for [Haitians] as knowledgeable parents and will make them exceptionally receptive to health teaching from biomedical health care professionals" (p. 11).

Once medical and mental health practitioners begin to recognize and accept the tendency among Haitians to choose a traditional medical doctor and a healer simultaneously, community outreach can promote a closer working relationship between the two healing systems.

Medical Beliefs and Illness Prevention Strategies

In addition to their beliefs about the supernatural causes of illness and voodoo, many Haitian families, particularly recent immigrants, hold other medical beliefs and practice other illness prevention strategies. A knowledge of these is essential for physicians, nurses, and nutritionists who are working with Haitian families, because the families will use these home remedies, often without consulting a physician. Whenever possible, cultural beliefs should be respected. When they conflict with medical care for HIV-infected children, however, a person who is fluent in Haitian Creole will be needed to help explain why another treatment or nutritional regimen is recommended. Often, members of the extended family must also be included to increase the likelihood of compliance.

De Santis and Thomas (1990) have documented the preventive strategies used to ensure the health of a newborn at birth. These researchers state that many of the Haitian mothers they interviewed believed in wrapping newborn babies in blankets as a way of preventing cold and air (*gaz*) from entering the infant's body. *Gaz* is believed to cause a variety of illnesses, such as tetanus, vomiting, and stomach pain (Murray and Alvarez, 1973). De Santis and Thomas (1990), in their sample of Haitian mothers, also found that 47% used home remedies (poultices, home-brewed teas, etc.) to treat common childhood illnesses. Some of the mothers also used purgatives (laxatives) to rid the stomach of parasites. De Santis and Thomas (1990), Alvarez and Murray (1981), De Santis (1988), Laguerre (1981), and Nachman, Widmayer, Archer, Moon, and Aleroth (1984) have documented that this periodic purging is quite common in Haitian families, particularly recent immigrants. There are also food restrictions based on the "hot–cold" theory of illness, which is prevalent in Haitian culture (Alvarez & Murray, 1981; Coriel & Genece, 1988; Dempsey & Gesse, 1983; Kilpatrick & Cobb, 1990; Laguerre, 1981; Nachman et al., 1981; Weiss, 1976). Some mothers, for example, may avoid cold food and drink in an attempt to prevent children from catching cold and bronchitis (De Santis & Thomas, 1990).

SUMMARY

In the 1980s and 1990s, the emerging "faces of the AIDS epidemic" brought practitioners into contact with many different cultural groups, of which they often had limited knowledge. Because HIV/AIDS is a multigenerational family disease, this has meant that physicians, nurses, social workers, and psychologists have had to obtain this cultural understanding rapidly in order to apply it effectively to their clinical interventions. This chapter has explored three cultural groups that have been greatly affected by the AIDS epidemic—African-Americans, Latinos, and Haitians—and has provided clinical examples to illustrate the ways in which this cultural material can be translated into effective interventions.

REFERENCES

African-American Families

Billingsley, A. (1968). *Black families in White America,* Englewood Cliffs, NJ: Prentice-Hall.

Bouknight, R. R., & Bouknight, L. G. (1988). Acquired immunodeficiency syndrome in the Black community: Focusing on education and the Black male. *New York State Journal of Medicine, 88,* 232–235.

Boyd-Franklin, N. (1989). *Black families in therapy: A multisystems approach.* New York: Guilford Press.

Boyd-Franklin, N., & Alemán, J. del C. (1990). Black inner city families and multigenerational issues: The impact of AIDS. *New Jersey Psychologist, 40,* 14–17.

Brown, G., Mitchell, J., & Williams, S. (1992). The African-American community. In M. Stuber (Ed.), *Children and AIDS* (pp. 21–31). Washington, DC: American Psychiatric Press.

Dalton, H. (1989). AIDS in blackface. *Daedalus, 118,* 205–227.

DiClemente, R. J., Boyer, C. B., & Morales, E. S. (1988). Minorities and AIDS: Knowledge attitudes and misconceptions among Black and Latino adolescents. *American Journal of Public Health, 78,* 55–57.

Flaskerud, J. H., & Rush, C. E. (1989). AIDS and traditional health beliefs and practices of Black women. *Nursing Research, 38,* 211–215.

Fordyce, E. J., Sambula, S., & Stonebruner, R. (1989). Mandatory reporting of human immunodeficiency virus testing would deter Blacks and Hispanics from being tested [Letter, comment]. *Journal of the American Medical Association, 262,* 349.

Fullilove, R. E., Fullilove, M. T., Bowser, B. P., & Gross, S. A. (1990). Risk of sexually transmitted disease among Black adolescent crack users in Oakland and San Francisco, California. *Journal of the American Medical Association, 263,* 851–855.

Grier, W., & Cobbs, P. (1968). *Black rage.* New York: Basic Books.

Hill, R. (1977). *Informal adoption among Black families,* Washington, DC: National Urban League Research Department.

Honey, E. (1988, June). AIDS and the inner city: Critical issues. *Social Casework,* 365–370.

Levin, J. S. (1984). The role of the Black church in community medicine. *Journal of the National Medical Association, 6,* 477–483.

Macklin, E. (Ed.). (1989). *AIDS and families.* Binghamton, NY: Harrington Park Press.

Mays, V. M., & Cochran, S. D. (1987). Acquired immune deficiency syndrome and Black Americans: Special psychosocial issues. *Public Health Report, 102*, 224–231.

Mays, V. M., & Cochran, S. D. (1988). Issues in the perception of AIDS risk and risk reduction activities by Black and Hispanic/Latino women. *American Psychologist, 43*, 949–957.

Mitchell, A. (1990, November). AIDS: We are not immune. *Emerge*, 30–44.

Mitchell, J., & Heagarty, M. (1991). Special considerations for minorities. In P. Pizzo & C. Wilfert (Eds.), *Pediatric AIDS* (pp. 704–714). Baltimore: Williams & Wilkins.

Peterson, J. L., & Marin, G. (1988). Issues on prevention of AIDS among Black and Hispanic men. *American Psychologist, 43*, 871–877.

Rogers, M., & Walter, W. (1987). AIDS in Blacks and Hispanics: Implications for prevention. *Issues in Science and Technology, 3*(3), 89–94.

Selik, R. M., Castro, K. G., & Papparoanou, M. (1988). Racial/ethnic differences in the risk of AIDS in the United States. *American Journal of Public Health, 78*, 1539–1545.

Stuber, M. (Ed.). (1992). *Children and AIDS*. Washington, DC: American Psychiatric Press.

Walker, G. (1991). *In the midst of winter*. New York: Norton.

Williams, L. S. (1986). AIDS risk reduction: A community health education for minority high risk group members. *Health Education Quarterly, 13*, 407–421.

Latino Families

Amaro, H. (1988). Considerations for preventions of HIV infection among Hispanic women. *Psychology of Women Quarterly, 12*, 429–443.

Bakeman, R., Lumb, J. R., & Smith, D. W. (1986). AIDS statistics and the risk for minorities. *AIDS Research, 2*, 249–252.

Bernal, G., & Gutierrez, M. (1988). Cubans. In L. Comas-Díaz & E. Griffith (Eds.), *Clinical guidelines in cross-cultural mental health* (pp. 233–261). New York: Wiley.

Carrier, J. M. (1976). Cultural factors affecting urban Mexican male homosexual behavior. *Archives of Sexual Behavior, 5*, 103–124.

Carrier, J. M. (1985). Mexican male bisexuality. In F. Klein & T. Wolf (Eds.), *Bisexualities: Theory and research* (pp. 359–375). New York: Haworth Press.

Carrier, J. M. (1988). Sexual behavior and the spread of AIDS in Mexico. *Medical Anthropology, 10*(2–3), 1–14.

Centers for Disease Control. (1989, February). *HIV/AIDS surveillance report*. Atlanta: Author.

Coates, T. J., Temoshok, L., & Mandel, J. (1984). Psychosocial research is essential to understanding and treating AIDS. *American Psychologist, 39*(11), 1309–1314.

Comas-Díaz, L., & Griffith, E. (Eds.). (1981). *Clinical guidelines in cross-cultural mental health*. New York: Wiley.

Espin, O. M. (1984). Cultural and historical influences on sexuality in Hispanic/Latin women: Implications for psychotherapy. In C. S. Vance (Ed.), *Pleasure and danger*. Boston: Routledge & Kegan Paul.

Garcia-Preto, N. (1982). Puerto Rican families. In M. McGoldrick, J. K. Pearce, & J. Giordano (Eds.), *Ethnicity and family therapy*. New York: Guilford Press.

Lambert, B. (1990, June 15). AIDS travels New York to Puerto Rico "air bridge."

Maduro, R. (1983). Curanderismo and Latino views of disease and curing. *Western Journal of Medicine, 139*(6), 64–70.

Magaña, J. R. (1991). Sex, drugs and HIV: An ethnographic approach. *Social Science and Medicine, 32*(9), 1–5.

Magaña, J. R., & Carrier, J. M. (in press). Mexican and Mexican-American male sexual behavior and spread of AIDS in California. *Journal of Sex Research*.

Magaña, J. R., & Magaña, H. (1992). Mexican-Latino children. In M. Stuber (Ed.), *Children and AIDS* (pp. 33–43). Washington, DC: American Psychiatric Press.

Marin, G. (1989). AIDS prevention among Hispanics: Needs, risk behaviors and cultural values. *Public Health Report, 104,* 411–415.

McCarthy, K., & Valdez, R. (1986). *Current and future effects of Mexican immigration in California*. Santa Monica, CA: Rand.

McGoldrick, M., Pearce, J. K., & Giordano, J. (Eds.). (1982). *Ethnicity and family therapy*. New York: Guilford Press.

Medina, C. (1987). Latino culture and sex education. *SIECUS Report, 15,* 1–4.

Nyamathi, A., & Vasquez, R. (1989). Impact of poverty, homelessness and drugs on Hispanic women at risk for HIV infection. *Hispanic Journal of Behavioral Sciences, 11,* 299–314.

Ramos-McKay, J., Comas-Díaz, L., & Rivera, L. (1988). Puerto Ricans. In L. Comas-Díaz & E. Griffith (Eds.), *Clinical guidelines in cross-cultural mental health*. New York: Wiley.

Rosenhouse-Pearson, S., & Sabagh, C. (1983). Attitudes toward abortion among Catholic Mexican American women: The effects of religiosity and education. *Demography, 20,* 87–98.

Sluzki, C. E. (1982). The Latin lover revisited. In M. McGoldrick, J. K. Pearce, & J. Giordano (Eds.), *Ethnicity and family therapy* (pp. 492–498). New York: Guilford Press.

Worth, D. (1987). Latina women and AIDS. *SIECUS Report, 15,* 5–7.

Haitian Families

Alvarez, M. D., & Murray, M. D. (1981). *Socialization for scarcity: Child feeding beliefs and practices in a Haitian village*. Port-au-Prince, Haiti: U.S. Agency for International Development.

Bayardelle, E. (1984, Winter). Haitian students in New York City public schools. *Bank Street College Bilingual Perspective*.

Buchanan, S. H. (1979, September). Haitian women in New York City. *Migration Today*, 19–25, 39.

Charles, C. (1986). Mental health services for Haitians. In H. P. Lefley & P.

B. Pederson (Eds.), *Cross cultural training for mental health professionals* (pp. 183–198). Springfield, IL: Charles C Thomas.

Coriel, J. (1983a). Parallel structures in professional and folk health care: A model applied to rural Haiti. *Culture, Medicine and Psychiatry, 7,* 131–151.

Coriel, J. (1983b). Allocation of family resources for health care in rural Haiti. *Social Science and Medicine, 17*(11), 709–719.

Coriel, J., & Genece, E. (1988). Adoption of oral rehydration therapy among Haitian mothers. *Social Science and Medicine, 27*(1), 87–96.

Dempsey, P. A., & Gesse, T. (1983). The childbearing Haitian refugee: Cultural applications to clinical nursing. *Public Health Reports, 98*(3), 261–267.

De Santis, L. (1988). Cultural factors affecting newborn and infant diarrhea. *Journal of Pediatric Nursing, 3*(6), 391–398.

De Santis, L., & Thomas, J. (1990). The immigrant Haitian mother: Transcultural nursing perspective on preventive health care for children. *Journal of Transcultural Nursing.*

Fjellman, S. M., & Gladwin, H. (1985). Haitian family patterns of migration to South Florida. *Human Organization, 44*(4), 301–302.

Giles, H. (1990, January–February). Counseling Haitian students and their families: Issues and interventions. *Journal of Counseling and Development, 68,* 317–320.

Gustafson, M. B. (1989). Western voodoo: Providing mental health care to Haitian refugees. *Journal of Psychosocial Nursing, 27*(12) 22–25.

Kilpatrick, S., & Cobb, A. (1990). Health beliefs related to diarrhea in Haitian children: Building transcultural knowledge. *Journal of Transcultural Nursing, 1*(2), 2–12.

Laguerre, M. S. (1979, September). The Haitian niche in New York City. *Migration Today,* 9–11.

Laguerre, M. S. (1980). *Voodoo heritage.* Beverly Hills, CA: Sage.

Laguerre, M. S. (1981). Haitian Americans. In A. Harwood (Ed.), *Ethnicity and medical care* (pp. 172–210). Cambridge, MA: Harvard University Press.

Laguerre, M. S. (1984). *American odyssey: Haitians in New York City.* Ithaca, NY: Cornell University Press.

Laguerre, M. S. (1987). *Afro-Caribbean folk medicine.* South Hadley, MA: Bergin & Garney Publishers, Inc.

Lewis, S. (1992). *Cultural competency model.* Presentation at the National Pediatric HIV Resource Center Core Curriculum.

Marchette, L. (1984). Barriers to health care for Haitian refugees. *The Florida Nurse, 32*(5), 4–12.

Mathewson, R. M. (1975). Is crazy Anglo crazy Haitian? *Psychiatric Annals, 5*(8), 79–83.

Miller, J. C. (1984). *The plight of Haitian refugees.* New York: Praeger.

Montalvo, T. (1987, February 2). Haitians still face bias, study shows. *The Miami Herald,* p. 4B.

Murray, G. F., & Alvarez, M. D. (1973). *Childrearing, sickness and healing in a Haitian village.* New York: Columbia University, Division of Social and Administrative Sciences. International Institute for the Study of Human Reproduction.

Nachman, S. R., & Dreyfuss, G. (1986). Haitians and AIDS in South Florida. *Medical Anthropology Quarterly, 17*(2), 32–33.

Nachman, S. R., Widmayer, S., Archer, J. D., Moon, K. H., & Aleroth, N. (1984, September). *Infant feeding practices among Haitian refugees in South Florida.* Paper presented at the Meeting of the American Anthropology Association.

Schiller, N. G., De Wind, J., Brutus, M. L., Charles, C., Fouron, G., & Thomas, A. (1987). All in the same boat? Unity and diversity in Haitian organizing in New York. In C. R. Sutton, & E. M. Chaney (Eds.), *Caribbean life in New York City: Sociocultural dimensions* (pp. 182–201). Staten Island, NY: Center for Migration Studies of New York.

Seligman, L. (1977). Haitians: A neglected minority. *The Personnel and Guidance Journal, 55*(7), 409–411.

Slevin, P., & Colon, Y. (1984, July 1). Cloud of despair still hangs over Haitians. *The Miami Herald,* pp. 1A, 16A.

Stepick, J. (1987). The Haitian exodus: Flight from terror and poverty. In B. Levine (Ed.), *The Caribbean exodus* (pp. 131–151). New York: Praeger.

Weiss, H. J. (1976). Maternal nutrition and traditional food behavior in Haiti. *Human Organization, 35,* 193–199.

5

HIV-Relevant Issues
in Adolescents

Jacqueline A. Bartlett, MD
Steven E. Keller, PhD
Haftan Eckholdt, PhD
Steven J. Schleifer, MD

HIV/AIDS continues to pose a catastrophic public health threat that is reaching crisis proportions among young people. Indeed, AIDS is the leading cause of death for 25-year-old males in the United States (*AIDS Weekly*, 1993).

Although adolescents constitute roughly less than 1% of all reported cases of AIDS, young adults between the ages of 20 and 29 account for almost 20% of AIDS cases. Given the long (5- to 10-year) incubation period for HIV, researchers assume that many of these individuals were infected as adolescents; on the basis of this statistic, they speculate that HIV transmission has occurred in adolescence for over 40,000 youngsters (Centers for Disease Control [CDC], 1992).

Analyses of the trends in diagnoses of HIV show that HIV transmission is growing among certain groups. AIDS diagnoses increase most between the adolescent (13 to 19 years old) and young adult (20 to 24 years old) groups, indicating that the highest rate of HIV transmission occurs among adolescents. Blacks and Hispanics are overrepresented among people diagnosed with AIDS, and the interactions between age and race show that more than half of all diagnoses among the younger age groups are African-American and Latino. The proportion of AIDS diagnoses are growing among women and among those who are infected heterosexually; while at the same time the proportion of AIDS diagnoses among the male homosexual transmission group is decreasing. These trends in the epidemiology of AIDS also interact with race and age, such that women and men have similar or equal rates of diagnosis among African-American and Latino cases, and the proportion of heterosexual transmissions is highest among younger African-Americans. These data suggest that adolescent African-American and Latino diagnoses may be a demographic epicenter of HIV.

Regional data on the epidemiology of AIDS show that an unexpectedly high proportion of adolescent (18%) and young adult (30%) AIDS diagnoses are reported in New Jersey and New York (AIDSPIDS, 1993), although only about 10% of the U.S. population in these age groups resides in this area (U.S. Bureau of the Census, 1992). This places adolescents and young adults residing in the AIDS epicenters of Newark and New York City at an alarmingly high risk for HIV exposure (Des Jarlais et al., 1990).

In this chapter, we focus on four HIV-relevant areas: (1) HIV/AIDS risk behaviors, (2) HIV/AIDS knowledge and its relationship to risk behaviors, (3) potential predictors of HIV/AIDS risk behaviors, and (4) suggested intervention/prevention strategies with adolescent patients. A major concern of the health care system is prevention of the spread of HIV. Identifying common and useful predictors of risk is critical to understanding how adolescents become exposed to and transmit HIV infection. It is also an essential factor in developing effective interventions and prevention strategies.

HIV/AIDS RISK BEHAVIORS

Exposure to HIV occurs through personal behaviors, including intimate sexual contact and shared-needle injection drug use. These behaviors, which play a critical role in the transmission of HIV, commonly begin during adolescence (Kandel et al., 1982; O'Reilly & Aral, 1985). Adolescents who experiment with drug use and/or sexual behaviors are potentially at risk for exposure to HIV, the etiological agent of AIDS. The frequency both of experimentation with sexual activity and of substance use in adolescents has been on the rise (Bailey, 1988; Orr et al., 1989; Zelnik & Shah, 1983). Therefore we can anticipate increased exposure and illness.

The occurrence of these behaviors in areas endemic for AIDS—particularly inner-city areas in the Northeast, California, and Florida—will carry more inherent risk. Although AIDS cases have been reported in all 50 states, the focus of this section is on the behaviors of inner-city minority adolescents, who are at the greatest risk for HIV exposure.

Sexual Behaviors

Although AIDS is more likely to be transmitted by heterosexual means in adolescents (16%) than in adults (6%) (CDC, 1994), about 22% of adolescent AIDS cases have been attributed to homosexual or bisexual routes of transmission, with an additional 13% of cases having histories of both (CDC, 1994). Minority youth groups residing in the mid-Atlantic states and on the West Coast are disproportionately represented in adolescent AIDS cases. These youngsters reside in areas endemic for AIDS, where risk behaviors carry more inherent risk for exposure.

Homosexual experimentation and homophobia have both been reported as common adolescent responses to emerging issues of sexuality and adult identification. Although it is believed that homosexual experiences are common in adolescence, the actual percentage of teenagers self-identified as homosexual is not known. The average age of homosexual self-identification in one study of Midwestern adolescents was 14 years (Remafedi, 1988), although attraction to people of the same gender may occur at puberty or earlier. However, in a large sample of inner-city minority adolescents (Keller et al., 1991) recruited from an adolescent medical clinic and from a large inner-city high school, reported rates of homosexual behaviors in the males were low to nonexistent: 0.5% in the adolescent clinic sample and absent in the 0% recruited from a high school. There were two females reporting homosexual behavior from the clinic and none from the school sample (Keller et al., 1991). This suggests either that homosexual risk of HIV transmission is low in the adolescent minority population attending school and therefore likely to be exposed to educational programs concerning HIV/AIDS risk, or that these adolescents were hesitant to disclose their homosexual encounters.

Although adolescent homosexuality may not constitute a widespread risk of HIV exposure, homosexual adolescents *are* likely to be at risk. Adolescent homosexuality in a societal climate of adult homophobia has many psychosocial and medical ramifications, including a reluctance to seek medical attention (Remafedi, 1988). Therefore, the frequency of such problems as sexually transmitted diseases in homosexual adolescents is not well documented. Furthermore, adverse responses to an adolescent's homosexual orientation from family members, friends, and/or peers are also common. The adolescent frequently responds to such disapproval and rejection by abusing alcohol or chemical substances and by running away from home. Prostitution among homeless, runaway, homosexual adolescents is common and often necessary for survival (Deisher, Robinson, & Boyer, 1982).

For these reasons, exposure to HIV is greatly increased in runaway and homeless adolescents.

Heterosexual behaviors in adolescents have been the focus of many recent investigations (Keller et al., 1989; Orr et al., 1989; Weber, Elfenbein, Richards, Davis, & Thomas, 1989; Zelnik & Shah, 1983). Inner-city adolescents have been reported (Keller et al., 1989) to become sexually active at an average age of 13 years.[1] This was found from a detailed sexual history of over 400 inner-city adolescents recruited from a high school and an adolescent medical clinic. Sexual risk for HIV transmission was defined by a youngster's score on the Composite Sex Risk Scale (CSRS), which utilizes interview data on behaviors that have been shown to be relevant to HIV transmission (condom usage; vaginal, anal, and oral sexual activity; fidelity; and knowledge of partners). Similar numbers of these primarily minority adolescents in both samples were sexually active (65.2% of the clinic sample, 54.5% of the school sample). The average number of sexual partners both in the past month and over an adolescent's lifetime was also quite similar for both samples (1 past month, 10 lifetime), as was the average number of definite high-risk sexual partners (i.e., injection drug users, bisexual persons).

Zabin and Clark (1981) report that onset of sexual intercourse usually precedes contraceptive use by at least 1 year. During that time sexual activity tends to be sporadic and "protection" inadequate or nonexistent (Zabin & Clark, 1981). Adolescents who become sexually active remain so for an average of 1 year before seeking "protection" (Zabin & Clark, 1981). Only about 25% of sexually active inner-city adolescents use condoms correctly and regularly, despite knowing how AIDS is transmitted (Keller et al., 1990).

These data reveal a high rate of unsafe heterosexual behaviors among adolescents, and particularly among inner-city minority youths. They suggest that abstinence and/or safe sexual practices must be fostered through programs aimed at these populations. In AIDS epicenters such as New York City and Newark, heterosexual cases of AIDS have outnumbered homosexual cases of AIDS for several years now. It is important, especially among adolescents in these epicenters, to focus on heterosexual risk. The early epidemiology of AIDS among gay men has given many heterosexuals a false sense of security—a feel-

---

[1] In 1979 the average age for first intercourse among U.S. adolescents in general was 15.7 years for males and 16.2 years for females (Zelnik, 1983). In a more recent study, the majority of boys were sexually active by age 13 and the girls by age 15 (Orr et al., 1989).

ing that they are not *really* at risk. Convincing adolescents to lower their HIV risk is very difficult. Even when they know a great deal about HIV transmission and the risks of growing up in an AIDS epicenter, they practice unsafe sex with multiple partners. During the course of a 2-year study we conducted, we found many examples of adolescents who had accurate overall knowledge about HIV/AIDS disease and risk reduction. It was often the case that they initially increased their condom use or practiced abstinence in an effort to reduce risk. However, by the end of the 2-year study many of the adolescents had progressively reduced their condom use to perhaps only half of the times they had sexual intercourse. Others reported at the beginning of the study that their sexual activity was infrequent (e.g., once every 2 months), with a condom being used every time. However, by the end of the study, some of the males reported that, although they thought about reducing the number of sex partners in an effort to reduce the risk of contracting HIV/AIDS, they did not use condoms at all.

Thus, despite adolescents having accurate knowledge about HIV/AIDS risk, both male and female adolescents revealed that they either continued to take risks in their sexual behavior or that they began to practice more risky behaviors as they got older.

Drug and Alcohol Use

Injection drug use with needle sharing has not been well studied in adolescents. Researchers found that 2–5% of high school students reported having injected cocaine, heroin, or other illicit drugs, and that 0.2–3% reported sharing needles used to inject drugs (CDC, 1990). These behaviors were reported more often by male students.

Noninjection drug use usually precedes the injection of drugs, and more detailed investigations of general substance use in adolescents have been undertaken (Macdonald, 1987; Keller, 1989; Welte & Barnes, 1987; Robinson et al., 1987; Smith, Ehrlich, & Seymour, 1991). Nationwide, about 25% of adolescents (ages 12–17 years) have had some experience with one or another drug (not including alcohol). The average age of beginning drug use has declined to 8.8 from 10.7 in some areas, and experimentation has been reported in children as young as 6 years (Smith et al., 1991).

In our study of inner-city adolescents, over half of the sample reported the use of alcohol (Keller et al., 1991). These adolescents were more likely to be among the sexually active subjects. Almost half (46%) of these same adolescents reported having used illicit substances (most commonly marijuana and/or cocaine). Drug usage was also reported more frequently by the sexually active subjects.

Robinson et al. (1987) reported that 22% of 10th-graders and 41% of 12th-graders had used marijuana. Macdonald (1987) reported that almost 66% of high school seniors admitted trying illicit drugs; 41–51% reported marijuana use, 9–17% reported cocaine use, and 26% reported the use of other drugs (smokable methamphetamine, psilocybin, and heroin). Moreover, 92% of seniors reported trying alcohol, with 5–7% reporting daily use. In a survey of over 27,000 subjects, Welte and Barnes (1987) found that 59% of Black and 63% of Hispanic adolescents reported the use of alcohol.

Drug use and alcohol use have also been associated with risk-taking behaviors, including sexual behaviors. Males are more likely to report substance use (Macdonald, 1987), and sexually active adolescents are more likely to report alcohol and/or drug use than sexually inactive ones. This may contribute to their failure to take proper precautions, such as using condoms (Keller et al., 1989). Adolescent use of alcohol has also been found to be associated with less use of contraceptives (Kraft et al., 1990). Although injection drug use is a well-known HIV risk, any substance use in adolescents may contribute to risk of HIV exposure.

HIV/AIDS KNOWLEDGE AND ITS RELATIONSHIP TO RISK BEHAVIORS

Until recently, education about AIDS was thought to be one of the best preventative measures. Public health officials conducted widespread public education campaigns, and schools included HIV/AIDS related facts in their health education classes.

Knowledge about HIV/AIDS has been investigated in both preadolescent and adolescent populations. Vermont school children had some knowledge about HIV/AIDS at a young age, and by fourth or fifth grade they were fairly knowledgeable, although misconceptions about AIDS persisted (Fassler, McQueen, Duncan, & Copeland, 1990). The majority of 7th- and 10th-grade students in Rhode Island knew that HIV/AIDS was transmitted through sexual intercourse rather than by casual contact (Brown & Fritz, 1988).

Thirty-one inner-city minority preadolescent children participated in a pilot study of HIV/AIDS knowledge that we conducted. Of the 31 children, 29 (94%) had heard of AIDS, and 13% had a family member with AIDS. Scores on an AIDS knowledge questionnaire ranged from 33% to 100% correct (mean 67% ± 14%). With respect to disease transmission, all except one child knew that sexual intercourse and sharing needles with an injection drug user would put them at risk for exposure. However, 73% thought that AIDS could be contracted by kissing someone with the disease, 35% thought that stress causes

AIDS, 35% thought that they could catch AIDS just by being around someone with AIDS, and 17% thought you could catch AIDS from the food they ate. Moreover, 52% thought that AIDS can be completely cured, and 24% thought that having AIDS was like having a bad cold. Misconceptions such as these were present in almost every child, with only one child obtaining a perfect score.

In adolescents, HIV/AIDS-related knowledge has been found to be variable (Keller, 1989; DiClemente, Zorn, & Temoshok, 1986; Kooman, Hunter, Henderson, & Rotheram-Borus, 1989). Keller et al. (1991) found that knowledge concerning HIV transmission, methods of prevention of HIV transmission, and general knowledge concerned with AIDS was high for all inner-city minority adolescents in one sample (both sexually active and inactive). The importance of HIV/AIDS-related knowledge, however, is its potential impact on behavior. In a further study of inner-city adolescents ($n = 400$), knowledge about HIV and AIDS was high, but risk behaviors were also common (Keller et al., 1990). Regression analyses controlling for age and sex revealed that none of the knowledge variables were associated with the level of sexual risk. Knowledge had no apparent relationship to behavior. This apparent denial of the impact of risk behaviors on adolescents' own personal lives has been found in more than one population (DiClemente, Forrest, & Mickler, 1989; Hudson, Petty, Freeman, Haley, & Krepcho, 1989; Sherr, 1990).

To conclude that knowledge has no impact whatever on behavior, however, would be premature. HIV/AIDS-related knowledge available to a person *prior* to the onset of risk behaviors may have greater impact on the development of these behaviors than knowledge gained after the fact. Norwegian adolescents surveyed after massive public education about HIV/AIDS demonstrated safe-sex practices to a greater extent than those surveyed before (Kraft et al., 1990). The sexually active postinformation group was more likely to use condoms (Kraft et al., 1990). This suggests that the influence of HIV/AIDS-related knowledge on behavior is greater when it is available before the development of the risk behavior, thus, offering such knowledge in the early years of school should be considered an essential component of any HIV/AIDS prevention strategy.

POTENTIAL PREDICTORS OF HIV/AIDS RISK BEHAVIORS

Krener and Miller (1989) suggested that behavioral aspects of developmental issues may be greatly influenced by the AIDS epidemic. To date, there is little information concerning what relationships exist among attitudes and beliefs, level of knowledge about AIDS, psychosocial factors, and behavior in adolescents. HIV/AIDS risk behaviors (both sexual behaviors and drug use) in adolescents have been reported to be associated with various psychosocial factors, including those dating from childhood (such as a past history of sexual abuse), current depressive disorders, and psychological stress or depressed mood (Keller, 1989; Newcomb, Maddahian, Skager, & Bentler, 1987; Gibbs, 1986).

Several studies have investigated risk factors for childhood-onset psychiatric disorders. Low socioeconomic status, overcrowding, paternal criminality, and maternal psychiatric disorder have all been identified as strongly associated with psychiatric disorders (Rutter & Quinton, 1977; Williams, Anderson, McGee, & Silva, 1990). Stress and parental psychopathology have been found to be important in children's symptoms and in utilization of mental health services (Jensen et al., 1990). Although it is not known whether risk factors for psychiatric or substance use disorders will predict the development of HIV/AIDS risk behavior, substance use itself (not necessarily injection drug use) is, as mentioned previously, associated with increased sexual risk behaviors (Keller, 1989; Gibbs, 1986; Kraft et al., 1990; Pope, Ionescu-Pioggia, Aizley, & Varma, 1990). In addition, mood disturbance and a history of sexual victimization are associated with sexual risk behaviors in adolescents (Brye, Nelson, Miller, & Krol, 1987; Burgess, Hartman, & McCormack, 1987; Rohsenow, Corbett, & Devine, 1988; Keller, Schleifer, Bartlett, & Johnson, 1988a, 1988b). Other correlates of increased sexual activity include behavioral problems, socioeconomic status, and race. Black adolescent females have been reported to be particularly vulnerable to early sexual activity, because of increased support in the social context for this behavior (Chilman, 1983). Those psychosocial factors associated with psychiatric and substance abuse disorders may also influence HIV/AIDS risk behaviors (Greenblatt, Kegeles, Schachter, & Miller, 1989).

Since alcohol and drug use are reported more frequently in sexually active adolescents, we must consider the potential contribution of these disinhibiting substances in promoting risk behaviors. Both alcohol use and drug use strongly predict high-risk sexual behaviors. The moderate amounts of alcohol and/or marijuana used by most adolescents, however, would suggest that the contribution of these factors to risk-taking behaviors is not limited to direct disinhibiting effects. It also may identify *behavioral* traits (e.g., risk-taking behaviors), as well as adverse life conditions (e.g., sexual victimization; Brye et al., 1987; Burgess et al., 1987), that are more likely to be associated with high-risk sexual behaviors.

INTERVENTION/PREVENTION STRATEGIES

The ability to curb HIV transmission is dependent on an effective approach to preventing spread of the disease among the young and minorities. Multiple factors, including behavior, knowledge, and psychosocial factors, can influence exposure, AIDS onset, and disease course.

The most commonly suggested method of risk reduction is the use of condoms. As stated previously, there is a considerable literature indicating that adolescents rarely use condoms and that their attitudes about condom usage are not positive.[2] Correct condom usage is now reported in about 25% of sexually active adolescents (Keller et al., 1990), almost twice the percentage reported earlier in the AIDS epidemic. However, the earlier reports included special high-risk groups, including runaways, adolescents in detention centers, and those in family planning clinics. These data therefore suggest that methods used to date to encourage condom use in adolescents have not been successful.

Another commonly suggested strategy in halting the spread of HIV is public education. Again, however, the literature indicates that passive education has little influence on risk behaviors in adolescent populations. AIDS-specific knowledge does not appear to predict sexual behavior in adolescents (Keller et al., 1991). Although passive education, including the use of pamphlets, didactic instruction, and the news media, may have increased the level of AIDS-specific knowledge, *the desired change in risk behaviors as a result of this increased knowledge has not occurred.* Unfortunately, adolescents often do not modify their behavior on the basis of their knowledge because they fail to personalize that knowledge.

In an attempt to alter risk behaviors, several approaches have been utilized. In a program of one-on-one counseling (Keller), based upon the individual subjects' reported behaviors, trained interviewers have adolescents verbalize their understanding of the actual risks of HIV infection associated with their specific reported behaviors. On the basis of their knowledge of AIDS, the subjects are asked to comment on their actions, and specifically to predict the potential consequences to themselves of such behavior. Data from 20 subjects who returned for a 6-month follow-up interview revealed a change in behavior, as reflected in lower sexual risk scores on the CSRS. Although the effectiveness of the program can only be definitively determined as larger samples

---

[2]However, there is some evidence indicating that condom usage is on the increase.

are studied, and ultimately by a decline in HIV rates, the decline in sexual risk behavior is encouraging. Furthermore, since behavioral change in adolescents is likely to be time-limited, and since long-term behavioral change is at present the most important strategy in halting the epidemic, ongoing counseling offered at 6-month intervals is highly recommended.

REFERENCES

AIDS Weekly. (1993, December 6).

AIDSPIDS. (1993). *AIDS public information data set through December 1992.* Atlanta, GA: Centers for Disease Control and Prevention, Division of HIV/AIDS.

Bailey, G. W. (1988). Current perspectives on substance abuse in youth. *Journal of the American Academy of Child and Adolescent Psychiatry, 28*(2), 151–162.

Brown, L. K., & Fritz, G. K. (1988). Children's knowledge and attitudes about AIDS. *Journal American Academy Child Adolescent Psychiatry, 27*(4), 504–508.

Brye, J. B., Nelson, B. A., Miller, J. B., & Krol, P. (1987). Childhood sexual and physical abuse as factors in adult psychiatric illness. *American Journal of Psychiatry, 144,* 1426–1431.

Burgess, A. W., Hartman, C. R., & McCormack, A. (1987). Abused to abuser: Antecedents of socially deviant behaviors. *American Journal of Psychiatry, 144,* 1431–1436.

Centers for Disease Control (CDC). (1990). HIV-related knowledge and behaviors among high school students, selected U.S. sites, 1989. *Morbidity and Mortality Weekly Report, 39,* 51–52.

Centers for Disease Control (CDC). (1992, January). *HIV/AIDS surveillance report.* Atlanta: Author:

Centers for Disease Control and Prevention (CDC). (1994). *HIV/AIDS Surveillance Report, 5,* 1–12.

Chilman, C. (1983). *Adolescent sexuality in a changing American society.* New York: Wiley.

Deisher, R., Robinson, G., & Boyer, D. (1982, October). The adolescent female and male prostitute. *Pediatric Annals, 11*(10), 819–825.

Des Jarlais, D. C., Ehrhardt, A. A., Fullilove, M. T., Hein, K., et al. (1990). AIDS and adolescents. In H. G. Miller, C. F. Turner, & L. E. Moses (Eds.), *AIDS: The second decade.* Washington, DC: National Academy Press.

DiClemente, R. J., Zorn, J., & Temoshok, L. (1986). Adolescents and AIDS: A survey of knowledge, attitudes and beliefs about AIDS in San Francisco. *American Journal of Public Health, 76,* 1443–1445.

DiClemente, R. J., Forrest, K., & Mickler, S. (1989). *Differential effects of AIDS knowledge and perceived susceptibility on the reduction of high risk behaviors among college adolescents.* Paper presented at the Fifth International Conference on AIDS, Montreal.

Fassler, D., McQueen, K., Duncan, P., & Copeland, L. (1990). Children's perceptions of AIDS. *Journal of the American Academy of Child and Adolescent Psychiatry, 29*(3), 459–462.

Gibbs, J. T. (1986). Psychosocial correlates of sexual attitudes and behaviors in urban early adolescent females. *Journal of Social Work and Human Sexuality, 5,* 81–97.

Greenblatt, R. M., Kegeles, S. M., Schachter, J., & Miller, J. (1989). *Predictors of condom use and STDs in a group of sexually active adolescent women.* Paper presented at the Fifth International Conference on AIDS, Montreal.

Hein, K. (1989, May). AIDS in adolescence: Exploring the challenge. *Journal of Adolescent Health Care, 10*(Suppl. 3), 10S–35S.

Hudson, R. A., Petty, B. A., Freeman, A. C., Haley, C. E., & Krepcho, M. A. (1989). *Adolescent runaways' behavioral risk factors, knowledge about AIDS and attitudes about condom use.* Paper presented at the Fifth International Conference on AIDS, Montreal.

Jensen, P. S., Bloedau, L., et al. (1990). Children at risk: Risk factors and clinic utilization. *Journal of the American Academy of Child and Adolescent Psychiatry, 29*(5), 804–812.

Kandel, D. B. (1982, July). Epidemiological and psychosocial perspectives on adolescent drug use. *Journal of the American Academy of Child Psychiatry, 21*(4), 328–347.

Keller, S. E., Bartlett, J. A., Schleifer, S. J., Johnson, R. L., Pinner, E., & Delaney, B. (1991). HIV-relevant sexual behavior among a health inner-city heterosexual adolescent population in an endemic area of HIV. *Journal of Adolescent Health, 12,* 44–48.

Keller, S. E., Glaser, R., Schwartz, S., Schutzer, S., & Schleifer, S. J. (1990, January). *Immunology for the neuroscientist.* Paper presented at the Winter Conference on Brain Research, Aspen, Colorado.

Keller, S. E., Schleifer, S. J., & Bartlett, J. A. (1989, May). *A psychoimmunological model of AIDS risk.* Paper presented at the annual meeting of the American Psychiatric Association, San Francisco.

Keller, S. E., Schleifer, S. J., Bartlett, J. A., Johnson, R. L., & Thompson, C. (1988a, May) *AIDS risk behavior in adolescents.* Paper presented at the 141st Annual Meeting of the American Psychiatric Association, Montreal.

Keller, S. E., Schleifer, S. J., Bartlett, J. A., & Johnson, R. L. (1988b, December 23). AIDS risk behavior in adolescents [Letter]. *Journal of the American Medical Association.*

Kooman, C., Hunter, J., Henderson, R., & Rotheram-Borus, M. (1989). *General and personalized knowledge of AIDS among adolescents.* Paper presented at the Fifth International Conference on AIDS, Montreal.

Kraft, P., Rise, J., & Bente, T. (1990). *The HIV epidemic and changes in the use of contraception among Norwegian adolescents. AIDS, 4,* 673–678.

Krener, P., & Miller, F. B. (1989). Psychiatric response to HIV spectrum disease in children and adolescents. *Journal of the American Academy of Child and Adolescent Psychiatry, 28*(4), 596–605.

Macdonald, D. I. (1987). Patterns of alcohol and drug use among adolescents. *Chemical Dependency, 34,* 275–288.

Newcomb, M. D., Maddahian, E., Skager, R., & Bentler, P. M. (1987). Substance abuse and psychosocial risk factors among teenagers. *American Journal of Drug and Alcohol Abuse, 13*(4), 413–433.

O'Reilly, K. R., & Aral, S. O. (1985, July). Adolescence and sexual behavior: Trends and implications for STD. *Journal of Adolescent Health Care, 6*(4), 262–270.

Orr, D. P., Wilbrandt, M. L., Brack, C. J., Rausch, S. P., & Ingersoll, G. M. (1989). Reported sexual behaviors and self-esteem among young adolescents. *American Journal of Diseases in Children, 143,* 86–90.

Pope, H. G., Ionescu-Pioggia, M., Aizley, H. G., & Varma, D. K. (1990). Drug use and life style among college undergraduates in 1989: A comparison with 1969 and 1978. *American Journal of Psychiatry, 147,* 988–1001.

Remafedi, G. J. (1988, March). Preventing the sexual transmission of AIDS during adolescence. *Journal of Adolescent Health Care, 9,* 139–143.

Robinson, T. N., Killen, J. D., Taylor, B., Telch, M. J., Bryson, S. W., Saylor, K. E., Maron, D. J., Maccoby, N., & Farquhar, J. W. (1987). Perspectives on adolescent substance use: A defined population study. *Journal of the American Medical Association, 258,* 2072–2076.

Rohsenow, D. J., Corbett, R., & Devine, D. (1988). Molested as children: A hidden contribution to substance abuse? *Journal of Substance Abuse Treatment, 5,* 13–18.

Sherr, L. (1990, April). Fear arousal and AIDS: Do shock tactics work? *AIDS, 4*(4), 361–364.

Smith, D. E., Ehrlich, P., & Seymour, R. B. (1991). Current trends in adolescent drug use. *Psychiatric Annals, 211*(1), 74–79.

U.S. Bureau of the Census. (1992). Statistical abstract of the United States. In *The national data book* (112th ed.). Washington, DC: U.S. Department of Commerce, Economics and Statistics Administration.

Weber, F. T., Elfenbein, D. S., Richards, N. L., Davis, A. B., & Thomas, J. (1989). Early sexual activity of delinquent adolescents. *Journal of Adolescent Health Care 10,* 398–403.

Welte, J. W., & Barnes, G. M. (1987). Alcohol use among adolescent minority groups. *Journal of Studies on Alcohol, 48,* 329–336.

Williams, S., Anderson, J., McGee, R., & Silva, P. (1990). Risk factors for behavioral and emotional disorder in preadolescent children. *Journal of the American Academy of Child and Adolescent Psychiatry, 29*(3), 413–419.

Zabin, L. S., & Clark, S. D. (1981). Why they delay: A study of teenage family planning clinic patients. *Family Planning Perspectives, 5,* 205–217.

Zelnik, M., & Shah, F. K. (1983). First intercourse among young Americans. *Family Planning Perspectives, 2*(15), 64–70.

6

· · · · · · · · · · · ·

Women and HIV/AIDS

· · · · · · · · · · · ·

Julia del C. Alemán, MSW
Patricia Kloser, MD, FACP
Theresa Kreibick, PsyD
Gloria L. Steiner, EdD
Nancy Boyd-Franklin, PhD

Women of childbearing age represent approximately 12% of the nation's more than 355,936 reported AIDS cases as of December 1993 (44,357 adult and adolescent women; Centers for Disease Control and Prevention [CDC], 1994). They are among the fastest-growing groups of newly infected adults (Barth, Pietrzak, & Ramler, 1993). Although researchers have gathered an impressive body of information on HIV/AIDS in men and children, they have published far less on the subject in regard to women. Researchers who focus on HIV/AIDS in the pediatric population in particular have ignored the medical and mental health implications for women, despite the fact that the overwhelming number (89%) of HIV cases in children result from mother–infant transmission. Given the growing prevalence of HIV and AIDS in women, researchers must begin to investigate the unique effects of HIV/AIDS on this population (Minkoff & DeHovitz, 1991). Many communities do not offer competent health services to women. This combined lack of knowledge and resources has raised fundamental questions about the progression of HIV/AIDS in women (Anastos & Palleja, 1991), and its direct impact on HIV-infected women's mortality (Chu, Buehler, & Berkelman, 1990). Selik, Chu, and Buehler (1993, p. 2991) have identified the following mortality figures: "Among young women, HIV infection was the leading cause of death in nine cities, with the proportion of deaths due to HIV ranging from 15% in Baltimore to 43% in Newark, New Jersey." Vermund (1993) has further shown that these statistics do not represent a peak in HIV-infection mortality rates, which continue to rise.

One component of the Multisystems HIV/AIDS Model stressed throughout this book—namely, that HIV/AIDS is a multigenerational family disease—necessitates that health care professionals place greater emphasis on the needs of infected women. These include both their individual needs and their needs as caretakers in families living with HIV/AIDS. One cannot separate the impact of HIV/AIDS on children and families from its impact on women. Although the main focus of this chapter is on women who both are infected with HIV/AIDS and are mothers, here and in other chapters we also examine the role of noninfected women relatives and "nonblood" family members who often take over the caretaking responsibilities when mothers become more symptomatic and develop full-blown AIDS. (See especially Chapter 4 and Chapter 7.)

Too often, women with HIV infection are not seen as health casualties in their own right. As Amaro and Gornemann (1991) and Anderson, Landry, and Kerby (1991) report, they tend to be seen as "vessels of infection" (i.e., as transmitters of the disease to their children) or as "vectors of transmission" (i.e., as prostitutes and sex workers who infect men who buy sex for money or drugs) (Anderson et al., 1991, p. 24). This narrow view among medical and health service providers negates the devastating impact of HIV/AIDS on the women themselves.

EPIDEMIOLOGY

AIDS was first recognized as a threat to women in Third World countries—particularly in Africa and the Caribbean basin—where heterosexual transmission was identified. In many countries in central Africa, AIDS is the leading health hazard; it is responsible for hundreds of thousands of deaths and vast numbers of infected people (Merson, 1993). In these countries, where the mode of transmission is primarily heterosexual, the rate of infection in these areas is equal for men and women.

As the disease spreads geographically, a high incidence of infected women is being found in Southeast Asia and Central America (Merson, 1993). In these regions, injection drug use is a factor in HIV transmission, although the primary means is still heterosexual transmission. In the developed nations of the West, the incidence of HIV-infected women is also increasing. Now, over 37% (3 million) of the

8 million adults in the world who are HIV-infected are women (Merson, 1993).

In the United States, the current ratio of infected heterosexual men to women is about 2.4 to 1, with women comprising about 12% of AIDS cases (Merson, 1993). (See Chapter 2 of this volume for more information on prevalence rates.) The epidemic falls largely on women in their reproductive years (15 to 44 years of age), who are members of minority groups (75% are African-American or Latina), and who live in large cities in the Northeast (Barth et al., 1993). Barth et al. have stated that "most HIV infected women become infected by sharing needles during injection drug use or by having sex with men who are drug users" (p. 3). The percentage of children with HIV-infected mothers who are infected at birth is also increasing. Of those who are HIV-infected, the following percentages inject drugs: 68% of the African-American women, 59% of the White women, and 43% of the Latinas (Merson, 1993).

Recently, rapid growth has occurred in smaller cities and rural areas, where women comprise 28% of cases (Merson, 1993). Given an 18% increase in the rate of sexual activity in girls aged 15–17 years since 1982, adolescent females now constitute an increasingly significant risk group. Because of the latency period, HIV infection is not likely to be discovered until symptoms are manifested—usually 7–10 years later, when a woman infected as an adolescent is in her 20s (Merson, 1993).

Although no one can predict the course of the epidemic, several trends have become evident. First, the absolute number of infected women is increasing; second, in certain geographic areas the percentage of infected women is increasing; and third, these increases are appearing among women who do not inject drugs and who contract the disease heterosexually. Indeed, the seropositivity prevalence in the heterosexual male population of a community largely determines the probability that a female sexual partner will be exposed to and/or contract the disease. Women who are not injection drug users are experiencing the highest rate of growth in infection, and it is believed that worldwide by the year 2000, women will surpass men in the number of cases.

Many AIDS and women's health activists, together with some health care professionals, believe that prevalence figures understate the extent of cases of HIV/AIDS in women in the United States. Until January 1, 1993, the CDC definition of AIDS excluded infections associated with HIV that are specific to women, such as cervical cancer, vaginal candidiasis, and pelvic inflammatory disease.

However, in January 1993, the CDC revised the criteria for the diagnosis of AIDS to include all HIV-infected women who have invasive cervical cancer, pulmonary tuberculosis, and recurrent pneumonia. It has also expanded the AIDS definition to include all HIV-infected persons who have < 200 CD4 T-lymphocytes or a CD4 T-lymphocyte percentage of total lymphocytes of < 14% (CDC, 1993a). These changes are very important: Prior to this reclassification, the lack of early recognition and treatment of HIV infection, rather than biological differences, resulted in shorter survival time for women. This explanation is supported by Turner, Markson, McKee, and Fanning (1991), who reported at the 1991 International AIDS Conference in Italy that no differences were found in survival rates between women and men of equal socioeconomic status. Their finding suggests that the greater severity and shorter disease course reported in women may have been a function of unequal access to treatment prior to January 1993.

MEDICAL ASPECTS

More attention has been paid recently to the medical issues that relate specifically to HIV infection in women. The time of infection is unknown for most women, and the person who caused the infection may likewise be unknown. The symptoms associated with seroconversion and the initiation of HIV infection—fever and malaise, which usually occur 6–12 weeks after infection—are often overlooked, as they resemble common flu-like symptoms. Seroconversion may go unnoticed for many years, and the infected woman during this asymptomatic period usually feels entirely well.

A woman in the early stage of HIV infection can transmit the virus to her sexual partners, drug-sharing partners, and any unborn children. An undiagnosed woman may only learn of her own infection when she gives birth to a sick baby who is identified as HIV-infected, or through the illness of a sexual partner who dies of AIDS (Kloser, 1991). Sometimes the discovery may arise from a routine physical exam.

The symptoms of HIV can be quite mild and may be confused with other conditions not associated with HIV disease. Mild fever, weight loss, swollen glands, fatigue, vaginal discharge, diarrhea, thrush, skin rashes, cough, headache, weakness, and vague aches or pains are some of the symptoms frequently ignored by women (Kloser, 1991). Health care providers likewise can easily misdiagnose anemia, hepatitis, oral or vaginal candidiasis, and weight loss as being stress-related in young menstruating women. When these conditions do not go away, and recur singly or together, most women do seek medical attention and discover their seropositivity. However, some women are still not examined thoroughly or diagnosed properly, because some health care workers are unaware that *any* woman who has been sexually active is at risk for HIV infection (Kloser, 1991).

During the symptomatic stage of the disease, a woman's immune system falters, with CD4 counts dropping to the 500 mm^3 range or below. The woman may have recurrent and persistent gynecological symptoms, including but not limited to vaginal candidiasis, an abnormal Pap smear, or severe herpes genitalis. This stage of the disease may last several years, during which the patient is usually able to function as a parent and sexual partner or in a job, and is able to infect others via high-risk activities.

The immune system deteriorates as the illness progresses. Usually by the time a woman has CD4 counts less than 200 mm^3, she manifests some symptomatology, which may include anemia, thrush, hairy leukoplakia, diarrhea, weight loss, fever, sweats, lymphadenopathy, vaginitis, shingles, herpes genitalis, venereal warts, dermatitis, hair loss, nail changes, neuropathy, or myopathy. An AIDS diagnosis is made when an opportunistic infection, such as pneumocystic pneumonia, some form of *Candida,* esophagitis, lymphoma, cryptococcal meningitis, toxoplasmosis, extrapulmonary tuberculosis, or cervical cancer occurs. At this stage of disease, many women may show extensive gynecological disturbances—namely, abnormal Pap smears with evidence of dysplasia, including squamorous intrepithelial lesion, cervical epithelial neoplasia, or human papillomavirus infection; abnormal menses; or persistent vaginitis (Allen & Marte, 1992). Herpes may recede with treatment, although condyloma and genital warts can be quite aggressive and difficult to treat. At this disease stage, although some are able to work, most women experience disability ranging from partial to complete.

The addition of the diagnosis of invasive cervical cancer to the expanded AIDS definition is particularly significant for the treatment of HIV-infected women. Laga et al. (1992) and Schafer, Friedmann, Mielke, Schwartlander, and Koch (1991) have found an increased prevalence of cervical dysplasia (a precursor lesion for cervical cancer) among HIV-infected women. CDC (1993a) reports that in a number of studies cervical dysplasia was found in approximately 22% of the women. A number of studies have also shown that "HIV infection may adversely affect the clinical course and treatment of cervical dysplasia and cancer" (CDC, 1993a, p. 381; see Maimen et al., 1990; Klein,

Adachi, Fleming, Hogyf, & Burk, 1992; Rellihan, Dooley, Burkey, Berkland, & Longfield, 1990; Schwartz, Carcanglu, Bradham, & Schwartz, 1991).

The end stage of AIDS is usually characterized by a CD4 count below 50 mm³ and a history of opportunistic infections. Many women at this stage have multiple infections and exhibit severe gynecological conditions. They are also usually completely disabled and are unable to care for themselves or others. Although unlikely to engage in sexual activity and injection drug use, a woman, if she chooses to do so, is still capable of transmitting the infection. However, her life expectancy at this point is usually measured in months.

The cause of death is not always an opportunistic infection; more commonly death, results from bacterial infection or from a chronic illness such as wasting. In many cases, the cause of death is unknown.

HIV TESTING FOR WOMEN

There is considerable anxiety and fear related to HIV testing, particularly in high-risk groups (Anderson et al., 1991; Stevens, Victor, Sherr, & Beard, 1989). Since many women discover their HIV-infected status at the birth of their children, Amaro (1990) has recommended that HIV testing become a part of routine prenatal care for women at risk of HIV infection. This has major personal and public policy implications. Stevens et al. (1989), in a study conducted in England, reported that only half of the 80% of women who thought HIV testing should be available at prenatal clinics would agree to be tested.

There are political issues involved as well. Amaro (1990), Bayer (1990), and Mitchell (1989) have discussed the implications for women's reproductive rights in routine HIV testing of pregnant women. Medical practitioners frequently encourage and even coerce HIV-infected women to seek abortions. However, fears of contagion on the part of abortion service personnel limit the availability of this procedure for HIV-infected women. Since poor African-American women and Latinas are particularly likely to experience violations of basic reproductive rights (Anderson et al., 1991), further investigation is needed to explore the relationship between those rights and HIV infection (Amaro, 1990).

The confidentiality of substance abuse and HIV antibody test results is also an important concern for women. Barth et al. (1993) discuss the complexities of this issue, particularly since test results can be used in child abuse reports and can lead to permanent loss of custody of children.

TRANSMISSION AND RISK FACTORS

Most (49%) women in the United States with HIV/AIDS have contracted HIV through their own injection drug use. Most of the rest have done so through heterosexual contact with an infected partner (36%); a small proportion have been infected by contaminated blood products; and there are rare cases of infection through artificial insemination, organ transplantation, and work-related methods (e.g., contact with blood products in a laboratory). In a few cases the mode of transmission is unknown (CDC, 1993b).

Heterosexual Transmission

In heterosexual transmission, HIV-infected males are nearly twice as likely to transmit HIV to females as HIV-infected females are to transmit it to males. A British study of heterosexual couples with one HIV-infected partner found a 12% female-to-male rate of transmission and a 20% male-to-female rate (*AIDS Line,* 1992). Anatomical and physiological features give the female the disadvantage of having a larger surface of mucous membrane in the vagina and the likelihood of receiving a larger volume of the virus in the male ejaculate. The presence of tears or inflammation in the woman's genital area, including the vulva, vagina, cervix, perineum, and anus, further increase the risk of transmission from male to female. The risk of female-to-male transmission increases with men who have genital sores. This is the usual mode of transmission among heterosexuals in Third World countries (e.g., countries in central and east Africa), where injection drug use is not common, although it is less frequent in the United States and Western Europe.

Pregnancy and Reproductive Choices

Pregnancy rates in HIV-infected women remain high. Many women decide against becoming pregnant when they find out they are seropositive. But in cases where women do not know their status or are in denial, the rates have not diminished (Minkoff, 1989). At University Hospital, New Jersey Medical School, Oleske et al. (1991) report the highest cord blood seropositivity rates in the country at 4.65% (cited in Kapila & St. Lous, 1991).

An HIV-infected woman may decide to become pregnant or to continue her pregnancy out of a need to experience a life-affirming act or in hopes that her baby will live on as a legacy. Pregnant women who are HIV-infected but asymptomatic do relatively well. However, pregnant women with advanced disease may not do well, and pregnancy may be discouraged for them as dangerous to both mothers and fetuses. In postpartum care, women who are HIV-infected are discouraged from breast feeding, since the virus can be passed to infants through breast milk (Minkoff & Feinkind, 1989).

As discussed above, reproductive choice can be a critical issue for many HIV-infected women. The perception of these women as vectors of disease who produce "innocent victims"—HIV-infected children—pervades all levels of society, even those programs that provide services to these women.

There are also subjective, internal factors that influence an HIV-infected woman's decision to terminate or continue a pregnancy. For some women, identity and self-worth are linked to reproductive capacity; that is, in certain instances, motherhood is the primary source of self-expression and self-esteem. Health care workers need to become culturally sensitive to African-American and Latina women who place high value on their roles as mothers and caretakers—a value system that can influence their decision-making process during or prior to pregnancy.

The fact that there is approximately a 75% chance that a child will not be HIV-infected lends some statistical support to this view. However, many point out negative aspects of the decision to become pregnant. For one, since many of these women are substance abusers, there is the possibility that their children's nervous systems will be impaired, as well as a 25% chance of HIV infection. Another argument is that since the mothers' life expectancy is predictably short, society is left to deal with the social and psychological consequences of large numbers of orphans.

Bermon (1993) stresses the importance of counseling and its impact on the reproductive decision-making process. She emphasizes the importance of a pregnant patient's right to access to all information about the impact of HIV infection on pregnancy that remains unknown to her. If the woman decides to continue her pregnancy, a genogram or family tree is then constructed to define the woman's support system, and the many difficult and painful issues are explored with her: the possibility that she may become ill during her pregnancy and the need to decide who will care for her child if she becomes ill, is hospitalized, or dies while her child remains healthy. However, it should also be noted that clinics and other abortion providers, when made aware of her diagnosis, may refuse to terminate the pregnancy of an HIV-infected woman because of unrealistic fears of contagion.

Other Risk Factors

Prostitution

Prostitution is a key risk factor for women. Studies have shown that prostitutes are often aware of the risks regarding HIV/AIDS but do not take precautions (Anderson et al., 1991; Amaro & Gornemann, 1991; Bellis, 1990; Shedlin, 1989). Many are also drug users. Bellis (1990), in a study of prostitutes who injected drugs, IV drug users found that 88% were sharing needles; 57% had sexual partners who used injection drugs; and 80% shared needles with their partners. Bellis (1990) also found that condom use was extremely low among these subjects (26%). Other studies show that the frequency of condom use among prostitutes varies (39–74%) (Freund, Leonard, & Lee, 1989). However, most sexual contacts go unprotected (Anderson et al., 1991).

The association between poverty and prostitution is well established. A more recent trend is that women who work in the "sex industry" place themselves at risk for contracting HIV as a way to obtain drugs. Mays and Cochran (1988) stated that "we have not offered the sex industry worker an economic substitute should she choose abstinence. For her, safe sex may already be an economic compromise" (p. 952).

Substance Abuse

Drug abuse is a significant risk factor even for women who are not prostitutes, and particularly for women of color (Anderson et al., 1991; Feucht, Stephens, & Roman, 1989). Early studies by Chaffee (1989) and Fullilove, Fullilove, Bowser, and Gross (1990) found injection drug use to be a risk factor in 71% of AIDS cases among women. Even a noninjection drug, such as crack, facilitates transmission because crack use is often accompanied by high-risk sexual behavior, and thus may put more women at risk for HIV infection. In addition, crack is often linked in an exchange for unprotected sex (Fullilove et al., 1990).

Alemán (1990) has reported the need of many substance-abusing women to be connected to a male, even if only symbolically. The woman's relationship with the addicting substance and/or drug paraphernalia can function as a symbolic substitute for a male, as a "transitional object."

Risk Factors among Lesbians

Lesbians have not generally been recognized as women at risk for HIV/AIDS. In fact, as of May 1993, the CDC surveillance report does

not list female-to-female transmission as a risk behavior for contracting HIV (CDC, 1993b). There are great misunderstandings and misconceptions about lesbian relationships, and education and prevention
have been almost nonexistent for this segment of the female population. Some lesbians engage in oral, vaginal, and anal intercourse with
men by choice, force, or necessity, and can become infected in this
manner. Other risk factors for infection can include drugs and shared
needles, blood transfusions, artificial insemination, and the exchange
of blood and vaginal secretions during sexual contact with women.

One of us (Alemán) has found in her psychotherapy of HIV-
infected lesbians that many have contracted HIV through needle sharing, and many have children. In many instances their parental rights
are ignored. They may experience discrimination and be mislabeled
as "unfit parents" for two reasons—because of their HIV status and
their sexual orientation. These discriminatory beliefs must be
challenged by health and mental health service providers.

PSYCHOSOCIAL STRESSORS

The psychosocial problems presented by HIV-infected women need
to be examined within the historical context of socially imposed barriers, including racism and sexism. HIV has helped highlight how this
growing segment of the population has been systematically neglected
and denied access to the many systems and services that could positively affect their lives. Because HIV-infected women have been viewed
mainly as sources of transmission to children and others (Mitchell,
1989), their own right to treatment access is only just being recognized,
as suggested by the recent change in the CDC criteria for AIDS to include recognition of a gynecological condition (cervical cancer) in HIV-
infected women (see above).

Throughout this book, we have explored the stresses inherent in
a disease that can simultaneously strike multiple family members. For
the HIV-infected mother and child, the anguish is especially acute. She
must contend with her own feelings of failure as a mother, not only
because she has infected her offspring (albeit unknowingly), but also
because she will not live to provide protection for her children as they
grow up. She also has to deal with the practical problems of housing,
child care, health insurance, health care, and employment or obtaining other sources of income. The nutritional needs of HIV-infected children require impoverished women to stretch an already limited food
stamp budget.

Like any patient with HIV/AIDS, an infected mother may become "emotionally cut off" (Bowen, 1976) from her extended family support system because of her own shame and her family's anger about behaviors (drug use, sexual activity) that may have resulted in her diagnosis. Health care providers may also blame mothers for infecting their children, and often prefer to interact with grandmothers, aunts, or foster mothers, who are seen as "heroines" for caring for HIV-infected children.

A woman may not seek medical treatment for fear that someone might recognize her in the clinic and find out that she is "sick." She may distrust health care systems. If the woman has HIV-infected children of school age, she may also be fearful that the children will become targets for discrimination if her and their diagnosis is discovered.

An additional factor compromising an HIV-infected woman's health and ability to seek and receive treatment may be the stress associated with the role of caretaker for an HIV-infected child, spouse, or significant other. As the primary family caretaker, she may postpone medical treatment to the point where she is too debilitated to benefit from medical interventions.

Women in heterosexual relationships with abusive males are also unlikely to seek proper care. As discussed in Chapter 4, the female may be fearful that a discussion of safe-sex practices with her partner may lead to physical assault if the man perceives such a discussion as a threat to his masculinity.

An HIV-infected woman may experience an inability to express anger at the partner who infected her through sexual transmission. Although this often becomes a precipitant for depression, an HIV-infected woman may also be hesitant to seek treatment for depression, because of her fear of stigmatization.

The delivery of health care services to HIV-infected women must reflect the formulation of sound public policies that show a better understanding and sensitivity to the issues and concerns of women in general, and are not limited to treating them as "vectors" of disease. It is also extremely important in the final stages of the disease, even when a woman appears totally isolated and cut off, to explore her former extended family network and (if at all possible) to help her complete "unfinished business" with her own family of origin. Since the end stages are often marked by neurological decompensation and AIDS-related dementia, it is important that the painful but necessary issues of child care and legal custody be raised by health and mental health practitioners while a mother can still make her wishes known and know that her children will be cared for.

The increase in the numbers of women with children who are dying of AIDS has created a crisis in social service agencies in regard to finding homes for these children, especially if a mother does not have close relationships with her own extended family members. Another excruciatingly painful issue has been the process whereby a mother with AIDS must discuss the realities of her own death and dying with her children, who may or may not be infected. This requires special sensitivity on the part of health and mental health care providers. Often it is not a one-step disclosure, but a process that can produce strong emotional reactions on the part of the mother and children. Nurses, physicians, social workers, and psychologists who are working to help families through this painful time will have to be available to all family members and help them to convey the multitude of emotions—love and caring, loss, sadness, and anger—that may arise.

Finally, it sometimes happens that a mother is dying in one hospital and her child is dying in another with no opportunity to say goodbye. A major change in health care policy that would prevent such a tragedy by allowing a mother and her child or children to share a hospital room or a hospice facility must be explored.

BARRIERS TO TREATMENT INTERVENTIONS

Many factors contribute to the problems that women, particularly poor African-American women and Latinas, face in entering drug treatment programs. One of the major barriers is the lack of integration of HIV services and drug-related services (Barth et al., 1993). These divisions in the medical care system are exacerbated for mothers with HIV/AIDS. For example, it is not unusual for pediatric care to be provided in one facility while care for women is provided on infectious disease or OB/GYN units in another facility. Faced with limited time and energy, overburdened single mothers will often choose care for their children over care for themselves.

Although substance abuse has been identified as a risk behavior in the transmission of HIV among women, women have difficulty obtaining drug treatment, including less access to drug treatment programs (Chaffee, 1989; Cohen, Hauer, & Wotsy, 1989; Karan, 1989; Amaro & Gornemann, 1991). Some treatment programs will not accept pregnant addicts at all, and only a very small number of methadone treatment programs nationwide are designed specifically for pregnant women. Drug programs that are not designed to provide child care force a mother seeking treatment to place her children either in kinship (extended family) care or foster care. Mabon House in New York, and Mandela House near Oakland, California, were among the first residential treatment programs for drug-using mothers.

Indeed, some states, by criminalizing substance abuse during pregnancy, are making it even more difficult for women seeking treatment for drug abuse. Consequently, many substance-abusing pregnant women, who may also be HIV-infected, do not seek medical treatment for fear that they will be convicted as criminals (Siegel, 1990), or that their children might be removed from their homes. Often women in recovery following drug treatment programs can spend years trying to regain custody of their children and reunite their families.

Some HIV-infected women, often young, who stop their injection drug use are among the most cooperative clinic patients, and become very involved in good nutrition and a healthy lifestyle. Many such women become involved in Narcotics Anonymous, Double Trouble, or other support groups, and eventually become advocates for their sisters. Relapse is less frequent for those who opt for detoxification with the help of support groups, although the struggle to remain drug-free is a daily one, especially in the inner city. Unfortunately, many women are unable to maintain their resolve, despite their best intentions.

Since many prescription drugs have street value, and some women support their habit in part by selling and trading pills, a clinician may play an unwitting part in this pattern of abuse. Some preventive AIDS education messages have been effective in reducing the amount of sharing of needles, but trading drugs for sex still occurs.

It is important for the mental health clinician working with a woman who injects drugs not to be judgmental, or to insist on her entering a recovery program until a relationship has been established. A woman may stay away from medical care because previous attempts have been met with poor treatment as a result of her injection drug use, or because of embarrassment after a relapse. The clinician must try to avoid condemning a client for a relapse, while also not colluding in the woman's drug use or efforts to avoid treatment. The timing of the intervention is often critical.

CASE EXAMPLES: INCORPORATING MULTIGENERATIONAL FAMILY SYSTEMS CONCEPTS

In dealing with emotional and psychological difficulties related to HIV/AIDS, a psychotherapist typically focuses on the individual or her immediate family. But, generally, the losses and deaths related to HIV/AIDS and the subsequent need for grief work can only be fully appreciated when the therapist has a picture of the total family system. A multigenerational family genogram is a useful tool for tracking patterns of multiple losses in families. Below, in Figure 6.1, a genogram depicts an intergenerational pattern of substance abuse and its relation to HIV/AIDS; in Figure 6.2, a genogram illustrates injection drug use and AIDS as having devastating effects on an entire generation in one family.

Injection drug use, as discussed throughout this book, is a major risk behavior for HIV for both men and women. In our work with women and their families, we are struck by the evidence that many in the generation of parents or grandparents had a familial pattern of alcohol abuse. This original familial pattern of alcohol abuse expanded as both injection and noninjection drug use became more common in the mid-1960s. Because dealing drugs provides for the survival needs of some poverty-stricken families, recovery from substance abuse is a complex and difficult process.

Case 1: The Relation of Multigenerational Substance Abuse to HIV/AIDS

A 56-year-old African American woman, Mrs. S., mother of seven adult children requested psychotherapy so that she could talk about why her children were dying of AIDS. She said that two of her seven children had died of AIDS, and that she wanted "to get strength" so that she could continue to take care of her 43-year-old daughter, who had been recently diagnosed with HIV and was symptomatic at the time.

Over several sessions, the therapist developed a genogram of the family (Figure 6.1), which helped Mrs. S. understand some of the intergenerational behavioral patterns—specifically, abuse of alcohol and street drugs—that had placed many of her family members at risk for contracting HIV.

Mrs. S. and her husband (now deceased) were alcoholics, as were her father and one sister, and one brother abused drugs. She and her husband had five children together—four daughters and a son. The oldest daughter was married to a man who was an injection drug user and developed AIDS, the daughter contracted AIDS through heterosexual transmission, and both of them died of the disease. The son, a substance abuser, fathered four children, with two of his mates being drug abusers. The second daughter married an alcoholic, and they had a son who abused drugs. Her third daughter abused drugs and had three children by three different men who used drugs, one of whom was in prison for pushing drugs. It was the oldest daughter's diagnosis of HIV that led Mrs. S. to seek psychological treatment. The youngest daughter and her husband were both drug abusers. Mrs. S.

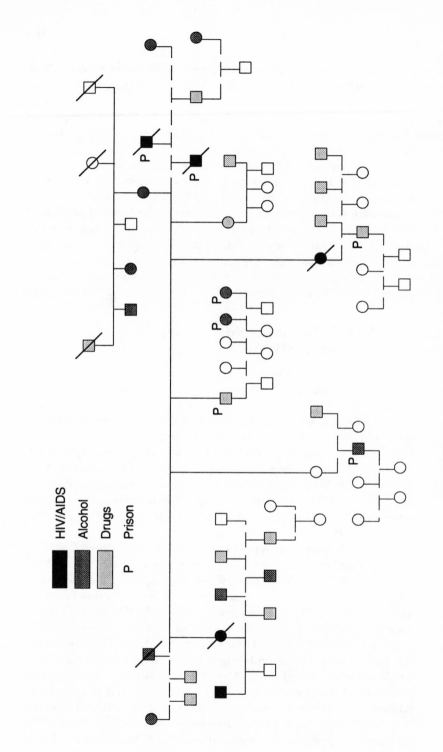

FIGURE 6.1. Genogram of Mrs. S.'s family.

also had two other sons by two other men. One was an injection drug user, went to prison, and died of AIDS; the younger son used drugs and was married to an alcoholic.

During the next few months of weekly sessions, Mrs. S. disclosed that her alcoholic husband had violent rages. Once he had thrown an electric fan at her, which precipitated her leaving the family out of fear for her life. The children were sent by their father to live with relatives in the South, where they were reportedly abused. After a few years Mrs. S. returned to her children, but she held deep feelings of guilt for "abandoning" them. As they began to be diagnosed as having HIV/AIDS, Mrs. S. believed that it was God's punishment for her having left her children.

Working with the genogram helped Mrs. S. deal with feelings of parental guilt. Gathering information for the genogram was an empowerment technique. In the process, Mrs. S. realized she knew a substantial amount of information about her children and her family of origin, which she had not acknowledged until that point. The genogram helped her to feel more comfortable and less threatened in disclosing some of the secrets concerning the family's substance abuse patterns.

After a number of sessions, Mrs. S. expressed to the therapist a sense of relief. She developed an understanding of familial substance abuse as a risk factor for HIV/AIDS. She began to stop being the family enabler who provided bail money for grandsons incarcerated for selling drugs. She also began to urge family members with drug involvement to move toward detoxification and substance abuse treatment. However, she was still unable to do any grieving for the death of her children, and continued to have difficulties in accepting her third daughter's illness. At this time a new therapist, who was familiar with Mrs. S.'s 43-year-old daughter from a support group she had conducted at a medical treatment unit at the hospital, began working with her.

During this time the daughter was diagnosed with full-blown AIDS, and Mrs. S. began to use the therapy as a way to cope with her daughter's rapid physical and emotional changes. Many times Mrs. S. would telephone the therapist to ask whether she could just talk for a few minutes, because she was "too tired and overwhelmed" to come to the sessions. One afternoon, Mrs. S. telephoned the therapist requesting help with her daughter, because the daughter, although extremely sick, was refusing to go to the hospital. The therapist persuaded Mrs. S. to obtain permission from her daughter so that the therapist could intervene. Mrs. S's daughter called the therapist, and the therapist finally convinced the daughter to come to the hospital. The therapist contacted the attending physician, who agreed to meet the daughter in the emergency room. After a few weeks of hospitalization, the daughter died.

This case underscores the importance of maintaining a family systems perspective in doing psychotherapy with one woman affected by AIDS. The systems perspective and the genogram helped Mrs. S. assume ownership of her family. She became the "family expert" on substance abuse intervention and on the relation between substance abuse and HIV/AIDS.

The second genogram (Figure 6.2) illustrates how injection drug use and HIV/AIDS can affect an entire generation of one family. This genogram also makes it clear why change, which is linked to issues of substance abuse and independent living, has been so difficult for this family.

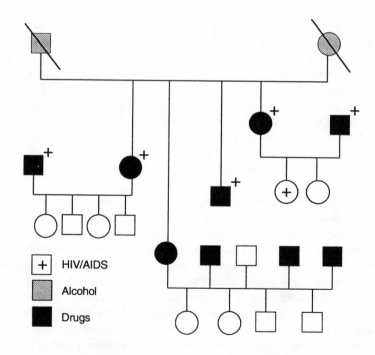

FIGURE 6.2. Genogram of Mary's family.

Case 2: Effects of Drug Use and HIV/AIDS on One Generation

Mary, a 39-year-old woman, is raising four children of her own and two nieces, a 4-year-old (infected with HIV) and a 2-year-old—the daughters of her younger sister, who died of AIDS. Both of Mary's parents were severe alcoholics, such that the family was frequently homeless and in dire financial straits during Mary's childhood. Mary's younger brother, like her younger sister, was an injection drug user who died of AIDS. An older sister is still living but is HIV-infected. The family members have a history of violent interactions with each other, especially when under the influence of alcohol or other substances, frequently resulting in stabbings and beatings so severe as to require hospitalizations.

Mary refuses to be tested for HIV, because she believes that as long as she does not know she will not be affected by HIV. "When people find out that they has the virus," she says, "then they gets thin and die."

Mary used to shoot drugs with the younger sister who died of AIDS, and for a time continued to do so with her older sister and brother-in-law, both of whom are HIV-infected. The father of Mary's first child was an injection drug user with whom she shot up and with whom she had unprotected sex. Mary continues to be sexually active with several partners and refuses to utilize safe-sex practices.

Interventions with this family have required a multisystems model of care. Managing chronic homelessness and obtaining adequate food for the children need to be addressed on an almost daily basis. Budgeting and money management skills are also being taught. Interventions with the children have involved substance abuse education and prevention. Mary had one detoxification while living with her older sister and brother-in-law. She was able to stay drug-free for about a month, continuing in outpatient treatment and strongly resisting the family's pressures to resume drug use. However, because of extreme family pressure not to change or recover, Mary relapsed. Fortunately, the therapist helped Mary understand that relapse did not mean total failure, so that she could continue her recovery.

Until recently, Mary had never left home or lived independently. Much work had to be done to assist Mary to move to a new, independent, drug-free situation with her children and nieces. Since the move, Mary has been using alcohol but avoiding other substances, despite a boyfriend who uses heavily. The therapist continues to work with Mary on issues related to alcohol use and economic survival for her and the children.

This genogram graphically illustrates the interface between HIV/AIDS and familial substance abuse patterns. Such a genogram also provides a diagnostic tool for identification of persons at highest risk for future diagnosis of HIV, and it furnishes information related to family structure and functioning that needs to be addressed if recovery from substance abuse is to occur.

THE NEED FOR FAMILY-FOCUSED SERVICES

Clearly, there is a need for family-focused medical care to allow HIV-infected women and their children to obtain their medical care in the same facility and from the same team of doctors. Barth et al. (1993) have also argued for family-focused drug treatment, particularly for HIV-infected women and their families. They state that "substance-abusing and HIV infected parents have as much right as other parents to care for their children" (p. 13)—a right that should be abridged not as a result of a positive drug or HIV antibody test, but only when it is clear that a parent is unfit and unable to care for a child.

Although this tenet seems self-evident, it is frequently violated by child protective services, drug treatment programs, hospitals, clinics, judges, and the courts, rendering it extremely difficult for recovering women and men to retrieve their children from placement. Sudia (1990) and Barth et al. (1993) have shown that when supportive services are provided, a woman will often use her parenting as a motivation for maintaining a drug-free lifestyle. Family-centered intervention can make a crucial difference in recovery. This is particularly true of HIV-infected women faced with the life-threatening illness of their children.

Since the correlation between drug addiction and child abuse is very high, child protective services are often at odds with presently or formerly drug-addicted HIV-infected women and their children. We need a monitoring approach that promotes family preservation. We also need models of "shared care" that provide "child protection without parent—child separation" (Barth et al., 1993, p. 41). Within the United States, the Texas Baptist Children's Home houses mothers and children in "family cottages." Supportive services are provided for women in the areas of parenting education, housing, job and educational training, and child support. This model could be tailored to develop drug treatment homes to meet the needs of HIV-infected recovering addicts and their children, particularly isolated, single-parent mothers (Barth et al., 1993).

CONCLUSION

A woman's increased risk for HIV infection, and the quality and availability of medical treatment she receives if infected, is influenced by
her low status in the family and society. It is necessary that women's
human and health rights be protected. They need to be empowered
to protect themselves from infection. But they also need greater access to competent medical care. This chapter has emphasized the need
for the inclusion of women within a multisystems model of care and
the necessity of a shift to a family-focused treatment model.

REFERENCES

AIDS Line. (1992). (Academy of Medicine of New Jersey), pp. 4, 7.

Alemán, J. del C. (1990). *AIDS and women.* Unpublished manuscript.

Allen, M., & Marte, C. (1992, March 15). HIV infection in women: Presentations and protocols. *Hospital Practice,* pp. 113–120.

Amaro, H. (1990, August 12). *HIV prevention with pregnant women: Preliminary findings from the MOM's project.* Paper presented at the 98th Annual Convention of the American Psychological Association, Boston.

Amaro, H. A., & Gornemann, I. (1991). Health care utilization for sexually
transmitted diseases: Influence of patient and provider characteristics. In
J. Waserheit, S. O. Aral, & K. K. Holmes (Eds.), *Research issues in human
behavior and sexually transmitted diseases in the AIDS era.* Washington, DC: American Society of Microbiology.

Anastos, K., & Palleja, S. (1991). Caring for women at risk for HIV infection.
Journal of General Internal Medicine, 6(Suppl.).

Anderson, J., Landry, C., & Kerby, J. (1991). *AIDS: Abstracts of the psychological behavioral literature.* Washington, DC: American Psychological
Association.

Barth, R. P., Pietrzak, J., & Ramler, M. (Eds.). (1993). *Families living with drugs
and HIV: Intervention and treatment strategies.* New York: Guilford
Press.

Bayer, R. (1990). AIDS and the future of reproductive freedom. *Milbank Quarterly, 68,* 179–204.

Bellis, J. D. (1990). Fear of AIDS and risk reduction among heroin-addicted
female street prostitutes: Personal interviews with 72 California subjects.
Journal of Alcohol and Drug Education, 35, 26–37.

Bermon, N. (1993). Family and reproductive issues: Reproductive counseling.
AIDS Clinical Care, 5(6), 45–47.

Bowen, M. (1976). Theory in the practice of psychotherapy. In P. J. Guerin
(Ed.), *Family therapy: Theory and practice.* New York: Gardner Press.

Centers for Disease Control (CDC). (1993a, January). 1993 revised classification system for HIV infection and expanded surveillance case definition

for AIDS among adolescents and adults. *Morbidity and Mortality Weekly Report, 41*(RR–17), 1–19.

Centers for Disease Control (CDC). (1993b, July). *HIV/AIDS surveillance report.* Atlanta: Author.

Centers for Disease Control and Prevention (CDC). (1994). *HIV/AIDS Surveillance Report, 5,* 1–10.

Chaffee, B. H. (1989). Prevention and chemical dependence treatment needs of special target populations. *Journal of Psychoactive Drugs, 21,* 371–379.

Chu, S., Buehler, J., & Berkelman, L. (1990). Impact of the HIV epidemic on mortality in women of reproductive age. *Journal of the American Medical Association, 264,* 225–229.

Cohen, J. B., Hauer, L. B., & Wotsy, C. B. (1989). Women and IV drugs: Parenteral and heterosexual transmission of human immunodeficiency virus. *Journal of Drug Issues, 19,* 39–56.

Feucht, T. E., Stephens, R. C., & Roman, S. W. (1989). The sexual behavior of intravenous drug users: Assessing the risk of sexual transmission of HIV. *Journal of Drug Issues, 20*(2), 195–213.

Freund, M., Leonard, T. L., & Lee, N. (1989). Sexual behavior of resident street prostitutes with their clients in Camden, New Jersey. *Journal of Sex Research, 27,* 25–46.

Fullilove, R., Fullilove, M., Bowser, B., & Gross, S. (1990). Crack users: The new AIDS risk group? *Cancer Report and Prevention, 14*(3), 363–368.

Kapila, R., & St. Lous, M. E. (1991). Anonymous human immunodeficiency virus surveillance and clinically directed testing in a Newark, N.J. hospital. *Archives of Internal Medicine, 151,* 965–968.

Karan, L. D. (1989). AIDS prevention and chemical dependence treatment needs of women and their children. *Journal of Psychoactive Drugs, 21,* 395–399.

Klein, R. S., Adachi, A., Fleming, I., Hogyf, J., & Burk, R. (1992, July). *A prospective study of genital neoplasia and human papillomavirus (HPV) in HIV infected women.* Paper presented at the VII International Conference on AIDS/III STD World Congress, Amsterdam, Netherlands.

Kloser, P. (1991, April). HRSA Women and AIDS Conference, Washington, DC.

Laga, M., Icenogle, J. P., Marsella, R., Manoka, A., Nzila, N., Rdey, R., Vermund, S., Hemaud, W., Nelson, A., & Reeves, W. (1992). Genital papillomavirus infection and cervical dysplasia: Opportunistic complications of HIV infection. *International Journal of Cancer, 50,* 45–48.

Maimen, M., Fruchter, R. G., Serur, E., Remy, J. C., Feuer, G., & Boyce, J. (1990). Human immunodeficiency virus infection and cervical neoplasia. *Gynecology and Oncology, 318,* 377–382.

Mays, V., & Cochran, S. (1988). Issues in the perception of AIDS risk and risk reduction activities by Black and Hispanic/Latina women. *American Psychologist, 43*(11), 949–957.

Merson, M. (1993, September 7). Presentation at the World Health Organization's Second International Conference on Children and Mothers with AIDS, Edinburgh, Scotland.

Minkoff, H. (1989). AIDS in pregnancy: Current problems. *Obstetrics and Gynecology and Fertility, 12,* 211–225.

Minkoff, H., & DeHovitz, J. (1991). Care of women infected with the human immunodeficiency virus. *Journal of the American Medical Association*, *266*(16), 2253–2258.

Minkoff, H., & Feinkind, L. (1989). Management of pregnancies of HIV-infected women. *Clinical Obstetrics and Gynecology*, *32*(3), 467–475.

Mitchell, J. L. (1989). Drug abuse and AIDS in women and the affected offspring. *Journal of the National Medical Association*, *81*, 841–842.

Rellihan, M. A., Dooley, D. P., Burkey, T. W., Berkland, M. E., & Longfield, R. N. (1990). Rapidly progressing cervical cancer in a patient with human immunodeficiency virus infection. *Gynecology and Oncology*, *36*, 435–438.

Schafer, A., Friedmann, W., Mielke, M., Schwartlander, B., & Koch, M. A. (1991). The increased frequency of cervical dysplasia-neoplasia in women infected with the human immunodeficiency virus is related to the degree of immunosuppression. *American Journal of Obstetrics and Gynecology*, *164*, 593–599.

Schwartz, L. B., Carcanglu, M. L., Bradham, L., & Schwartz, P. E. (1991). Rapidly progressive aquamous carcinoma of the cervix coexisting with human immunodeficiency virus infection: Clinical opinion. *Gynecology and Oncology*, *41*, 255–258.

Selik, R., Chu, S., & Buehler, J. (1993). HIV infection as leading cause of death among young adults in U.S. cities and states. *Journal of the American Medical Association*, *269*(23), 2991–2994.

Shedlin, M. G. (1989). An ethnographic approach to understanding HIV high-risk behaviors: Prostitutional and drug use. In R. J. Battjes & Z. Amsel (Eds.), *AIDS and intravenous drug use: Future directions for community-based prevention research* (National Institute on Drug Abuse Research Monograph Series No. 93). Rockville, MD: National Institute on Drug Abuse.

Siegel, L. (1990). The criminalization of pregnant and child-rearing drug issues. *Newsletter of Division 35 American Psychological Association*, *17*(4), 6–10.

Stevens, A., Victor, C., Sherr, L., & Beard, R. (1989). HIV testing in antenatal clinics: The impact on women. *AIDS Clinical Care*, *1*, 165–171.

Sudia, C. (1990). *In-home services for crack-using mothers in Detroit*. Washington, DC: U.S. Department of Health and Human Services.

Turner, B. J., Markson, L. E., McKee, L., & Fanning, T. (1991). *Survival patterns of women and men with AIDS: Impact on health care prior to AIDS*. Paper presented at the International AIDS Conference, Florence, Italy.

Vermund, S. (1993). Rising HIV-related mortality in young Americans. *Journal of the American Medical Association*, *269*(23), 3034–3035.

SECTION IV

THERAPEUTIC APPROACHES WITH HIV-INFECTED CHILDREN AND THEIR FAMILIES

7

· · · · · · · · · · · ·

Family Systems Interventions and Family Therapy

· · · · · · · · · · · ·

Nancy Boyd-Franklin, PhD
Julia del C. Alemán, MSW
Gloria L. Steiner, EdD
Elizabeth W. Drelich, MSW
Bradley C. Norford, PhD

The diagnosis of HIV/AIDS puts a family in crisis. Therapeutic interventions must be designed to develop a partnership between the family members and health and mental health service providers, in order to mobilize family support networks and provide a flexible system of care. In this chapter we explore two therapeutic approaches to working with families that have been stricken with HIV/AIDS: (1) family systems interventions and (2) family therapy.

"Family systems interventions" are direct, often short-term, problem-focused interventions that mobilize family support systems at various key points in the process of medical care. Such critical junctures may include the time of diagnosis; emergency room care; "do not resuscitate" (DNR) decisions; and death of a family member. It is our experience that a family systems perspective helps to facilitate the delivery of family-focused care by medical, nursing, social service, and mental health staff.

"Family therapy" refers to ongoing family treatment sessions conducted by a health or mental health professional—that is, a family therapist, a social worker, a psychologist or psychiatrist, or a nurse with specialized mental health training. Such treatments often require a referral to a family therapy unit, a community mental health center or clinic, or a professional with specialized family therapy training.

The dual-approach family systems model that we utilize can be taught to practitioners of all disciplines. Its flexibility and its goal-directed focus allow service providers to make key interventions (problem-solving or longer-term therapy) strategically, and to "seize the moment" when a family is ready to address a certain issue. (See Chapter 4 for culture-specific family therapy case examples.)

FAMILY SYSTEMS INTERVENTIONS

Walker (1991) describes the introduction of a family systems model to a pediatric AIDS unit. She and the other members of her team, who worked closely with the staff of the pediatrics unit, developed a family interview with the following goals:

> (1) to give staff members a more positive view of the family's struggle with the disease by helping them "walk in each family member's shoes"; (2) to identify family resources (via genogram) and useful family coping systems and (3) to demonstrate strategies for creating a more cooperative loop between families and staff. (p. 289)

In addition, this family systems team worked with the pediatric staff to structure a family case conference to promote a supportive and collaborative relationship between families and staff; to offer "alternative narratives" and "positive redescriptions" for family members; and finally to encourage the staff to think of the family as a "living system," in which death is only one aspect of the total family experience. For families that are living with HIV/AIDS and are already stigmatized by poverty, racism, and drug use, creating positive alternative narratives and thinking in terms of the "living system" are extremely important.

Walker (1991) has found that it is necessary to help these women and their families try to reclaim their lives by establishing positive hope and goals both for themselves and their children. Drawing upon the work of Gilligan, Ward, and McClean (1988), she has stated that

> a woman repairs her life best in a positive context of care, where she can create a positive narrative about herself. In this narrative, she begins

to see herself as a woman competent to tend her children and able to create a rich tapestry of meaningful relationships. (p. 291)

Since many of these families come to hospitals and clinics expecting to be judged or labeled, positive reframing must be a major family systems goal.

The Concept of Empowerment

All therapeutic interventions with families coping with AIDS must begin with the concept of empowerment. Inner-city African-American, Latino, Haitian, and Caribbean families that are stricken with HIV/AIDS are overwhelmed by the losses and the demands of this multigenerational family disease. They have a particular need to feel a greater sense of mastery over their lives. It is extremely important to make the distinction here between "empowerment" and "helping." Helping involves doing something *for* a person or a family; empowerment involves giving the family members the tools to do the interventions themselves. Boyd-Franklin (1989) and Imber-Black (1988) have shown that it is incumbent upon medical, social work, and mental health practitioners who may have limited contact with a family to give its members the skills and information they need to produce change. Often these interventions can serve as a model to the family for future interventions (see Chapter 13).

Family Responses to the Process of the Disease

Rolland (1984, 1987a, 1987b) has described the following time phases of all chronic and life-threatening illnesses: (1) crisis, (2) chronic, and (3) terminal. As Tiblier, Walker, and Rolland (1989) and Macklin (1989) have shown, each of these phases for HIV/AIDS families requires different coping skills and adaptations. This, of course, is complicated for many families, for whom HIV/AIDS is a multigenerational family disease (Boyd-Franklin & Alemán, 1991). Often family members will be in different phases simultaneously; this puts further stresses on the family and extended family. Also, as Tiblier (1987) has shown, when a family member becomes symptomatic (the chronic and terminal phases), increased care and treatment are necessary, and it is increasingly difficult for members to conceal the presence of AIDS in their families. As demonstrated throughout this book, many family members also experience guilt and shame in response to children who have HIV/AIDS (Kaplan, 1988; Helmquist, 1984).

Crisis Intervention

A crisis that erupts during the course of the medical or clinical treatment of a family is often the best time to make a family systems intervention. Once it is clear that families offer important resources, staff members can mobilize them during crisis interventions. One critical opportunity for a family intervention is the point when a new or frightening medical treatment is introduced. It is also important that there be staff members who speak a client's language and understand the culture in such a way that they can intervene during a crisis to pull together the client's extended family. As Chapter 4 has shown, this type of extended family organization, which is very common among Latino, African-American, Haitian, and Caribbean families, can be mobilized to effect beneficial change.

Intervention When Illness Becomes Chronic

As HIV infection progresses to full-blown AIDS and a patient becomes sicker, family systems interventions may be needed to deal with several different reactions on the part of family members. Among these may be burnout, anger, guilt (especially on the part of a parent who has transmitted HIV to a child), and frustration.

Interventions at the Terminal Stage

Painful and difficult decisions on intensive care units (ICUs) offer another opportunity for family systems intervention. Decisions about DNR orders can be very stressful for both families and medical and nursing staff. If the family members feel overwhelmed and unable to accept the burden of making such a decision, it is very helpful if a member of the child and family's case management team can be involved in this intervention. ICU staff members often have difficulty addressing this issue with a family that they do not know well. The family members, however, can derive some small degree of comfort if a staff member with whom they have had an ongoing relationship, and who they know cares about them as well as the patient, helps in the decision-making process.

FAMILY THERAPY

Family Beliefs and Attitudes about Illness

The assessment of family beliefs and attitudes about HIV/AIDS is a major component in determining approaches to mental health care delivery, and specifically in determining issues to be addressed in family therapy. The family therapist must assess the following:

- How does the family feel about HIV/AIDS? Is it considered a shameful secret or a medical disease?
- Who in the family and the extended family has been told the diagnosis?
- How supportive are family members? Is one family member (e.g., a mother or grandmother) overfunctioning and carrying the burden alone?
- How do the family members feel about the treatment plan? Do they feel it is invasive or helpful?
- How much is understood about what will happen in the course of the illness?
- Is the family denying the severity of the disease and the likelihood of death?
- Do the family members need medical information? Do they need greater psychological support? Do they need multisystems interventions?
- How well do the different family members communicate with one another? Is their own support system intact?

The answers to these questions help in identifying and mobilizing family strengths and resources.

Mobilizing Family Strengths and Resources

Families suffering from the stigma associated with HIV/AIDS often tell us they "have no one." As Walker (1991) has noted, "HIV diagnosis may mean that the family is separated from normal healing rituals, family gathering, friendship groups and Church groups. Such isolation inevitably increases stress (p. 47).

Once the family trusts the practitioner, a "genogram" (diagram of family members and significant others) (Boyd-Franklin, 1989; McGoldrick & Gerson, 1985) and an "eco map" (diagram of other systems and agencies that affect the family) (Hartman & Laird, 1983) can be constructed. The purpose of this process is to help the individual or family members define their current support system and to reconstruct the former supports that are no longer available. In today's world, when divorce, remarriage, and complex relationships are common, an illness such as HIV/AIDS adds to the complexity of family interactions. Often families must be helped to develop new rituals to draw together those who need support, particularly in the terminal phase of the illness (Imber-Black, Roberts, & Whiting, 1988).

Many of our HIV/AIDS families in Newark have taught us very important lessons about the importance of these rituals, many of which can be prescribed for other families.

Case Example: A New Family Ritual

Mrs. Joan Glover, a 65-year-old African-American grandmother, was the mother of Sandy Turner, a 35-year-old AIDS patient. Mrs. Glover was raising Sandy Turner's children, the youngest of whom, Imani (aged 6), was HIV-infected.

Mrs. Glover had been divorced from Ed Turner (aged 71), who was Sandy's father, for many years. She had since remarried Tom Glover (aged 70), who was a very involved stepfather to her children and stepgrandfather to her grandchildren.

When Sandy was dying of AIDS, Mrs. Glover went often to see her in the hospital. She reported to her therapist that the symptomatic phase of the illness had been very difficult for her family. Although Mrs. Glover had been raising Sandy's children for many years, Sandy had continued to live alone in a rented room. As Sandy entered the final phase of her illness, Mrs. Glover requested that she move into the Glover home. Mr. Glover strongly supported her in this process.

Mrs. Glover shared with our staff the rituals that she had evolved while Sandy lived in her home. One centered around having family (and extended family) meals. This ritual presented some complications within her family system. Her ex-husband, Sandy's father, had been very hesitant to visit his daughter. He stated that he "didn't know what to say to her." Mrs. Glover replied, "You don't have to say anything. Just be there and show her that you care." Mrs. Glover invited him to one of the family dinners. Mr. Turner asked whether he could bring his current girlfriend. Mrs. Glover replied, "Bring her and bring them all. Just come." In describing this family ritual, Mrs. Glover became animated. She talked about how her older son had videotaped these events. When asked why she had begun this ritual, Mrs. Glover replied, "Because it made her [Sandy] happy."

These ritual dinners for the extended family have taught us a great deal about the ways in which families can be helped to cope with grief and anticipatory loss. Many adult HIV/AIDS patients have been "cut off" from their families of origin during periods of drug use. Their return to their families, coupled with the tragedy of their illness, presents many difficult re-entry questions. We have learned a great deal from Mrs. Glover and have been able to help other families develop their own rituals for bringing together the "significant others" in the lives of persons with HIV/AIDS.

Secrecy and Disclosure Issues for Families

HIV/AIDS patients and their families are realistically concerned about the social stigma and ostracism that the diagnosis brings. Family therapists must be aware of these difficult realities and prepare to reach out to significant family and extended family members throughout the course of therapy. This may require some home-based sessions in order to reach key family members. Family therapists must also establish trust with African-American and other ethnic minority families.

The perceived need for secrecy affects how families disclose the disease (Boyd-Franklin, 1993; Black, 1993; Tasker, 1992). As stated throughout this book, disclosure is a *process,* not just for children but for their families also. Often when health or mental health service providers first raise the issue of disclosure with family members, they are very reluctant to discuss these issues with a child. This reluctance should be taken very seriously by professionals working with a family. The most common concern expressed by family members relates to the worry that a young child will quickly tell others, which will lead to further rejection and stigmatization of the child and family. This is a very realistic concern. Children, particularly when young, are very likely to talk openly with peers, other family members, schoolmates, teachers, friends, neighbors, and other members of the community, and admonishing a child not to share this information outside the family is often ineffective.

Professionals working with these children and families must anticipate the possibility of an initial refusal to disclose. Adult caretakers may still be reeling from the shock of an HIV diagnosis in the child and may still be engaged in various levels of denial. Talking to the child about the illness is often very threatening in these cases. Caretakers may also feel insecure about their own knowledge of HIV/AIDS, and may need the support of their health or mental health care provider in discussing these issues with a child. A trusting relationship with professionals is most likely to carry a family through the various stages of coping with this illness.

Another factor to be considered is the presence of other secrets in the family (e.g., the nature or mode of transmission; the degree to which the disclosure of HIV/AIDS has been shared with other close family and extended family members). Clinicians and health care providers must be aware that they often interact with only a very small part of the family system. The relative or caretaker (mother, father, grandmother, aunt, foster mother, etc.) who brings the child for treatment may be the only person in the extended family who knows the diagnosis. Often other family members are told that the child has another disease, such as leukemia. Therefore, the caretaker's reluctance to discuss the diagnosis with a child may be related to the degree to which the secret has been kept from other family members. This possibility should definitely be explored when family members resist disclosure.

The following family therapy case example, which illustrates the aftereffects of AIDS transmitted through drug usage, reveals the guilt, fears, and family myths that surround HIV/AIDS.

Case Example: Fears and Myths

Eric, an 11-year-old African-American male, was referred for therapy for frequent disruptive behavior in school and persistent sadness. The referral came 4 months after the death of his mother, Charlene, from AIDS. Eric and his family were seen in therapy for 2 years; Eric also attended a weekly group therapy for boys with behavior problems. During treatment Eric and his family moved from avoidance and silence regarding the illness and death of Eric's mother to sadness and anger, and eventually to open discussion of the matter. Although only about 10 sessions were spent dealing directly with these issues, the lifting of the veil surrounding Charlene's death eventually opened the door for intervention into other related issues plaguing family members.

Following his mother's death, Eric's maternal aunt, Donna, assumed caretaking of Eric, and his three siblings. (Eric's father had died 6 months after Eric was born.) Donna, who was 36 years old and single, had no children of her own and was several years younger than Eric's mother. Donna was a very responsible individual who had been close to the children throughout their childhood.

Eric's older sister, Delanya, was a 15-year-old "parentified child" who did well in school and assisted in the care of the younger children. She seemed to be in a great deal of private pain at the start of therapy, but refused to discuss her mother's death. Eric's younger half-brother, David, was a quiet, friendly 9-year-old who usually presented as sad and with symptoms of attention deficit disorder. Eric's younger half-sister, Michelle, was an outgoing, cheerful 3-year-old. She seroconverted and has tested negative for HIV since that time.

During the first 6 months of therapy, Eric was generally seen individually or with his aunt. Although neither AIDS nor the death of his mother was a central focus during this initial period, it became clear that these topics were not discussed in the family. It appeared that Eric was acting out the family's pain and silence. The whole family was invited to attend several sessions around the first anniversary of Charlene's death. All resisted discussing the topic. Eric, David, and

Delanya insisted that they rarely thought about their mother any more and that her death was not a relevant issue to therapy. At this point it was decided that family therapy would be best way to help Eric work through the loss of Charlene.

Secrecy was a central issue in the next few sessions. During this time, it was discovered that Donna was giving the children an implicit message that she did not want anyone to bring up Charlene's death. Before sessions or when the subject of Charlene's death came up at home, Donna would sometimes say to the children, "Now don't go talking all about your mother or you'll get me all upset." Indeed at the beginning of treatment, Donna had said to the therapist, "I hope that you do not plan to spend much time having Eric and me discuss AIDS and Charlene's death. We have been over that enough already." In actuality, they had discussed the subject very little.

In another session, Delanya and Eric expressed fear that people who learned that their mother had died of AIDS would view the family badly. Delanya was resentful at Donna and Eric for coming to therapy. Although Delanya soon became comfortable with the fact that the therapist would maintain confidentiality, she expressed fear that David and Eric would become comfortable discussing the topic in therapy and then be more likely to talk to one of their friends about their mother's having AIDS.

Eventually, as the topic became more readily available for discussion, issues of anger and guilt emerged. Eric in particular felt bad about discussing his mother in sessions. He felt that they were behaving disloyally by discussing family business with an outsider. Delanya eventually expressed anger about her mother's risky behavior, which had resulted in her leaving her children behind. Delanya also had a great deal of anger at her mother for not getting treatment early in her illness and for not continuing with regular treatment. Moreover, Eric and Delanya admitted guilt about their behavior when their mother had left for the hospital on the day of her death. Apparently she had awakened them early in the morning to do some favors for her and then to say goodbye. They related that they did not comply and got upset with her for waking them. They said that they did not realize the seriousness of her condition at that time and were shocked to learn of her death later that day. David then revealed for the first time his lack of response that morning, and cried about his insensitivity. In therapy, they worked on how they would have liked to have said goodbye to her.

Family myths surrounding AIDS and fears of abandonment also began to emerge during the 6 months following the first anniversary of Charlene's death. None of the children expressed a belief that they had caused their mother's death. However, Delanya expressed her conviction that if she had tried harder to convince her mother to get regular treatment, she would have survived much longer and perhaps even gotten rid of the virus. The children also believed that more compassionate behavior on their part on the day of their mother's death would have enabled her to live longer.

Eric indicated that many of his fights at school started because another student would make reference to his mother. In discussing the matter further, however, it became clear to Eric that none of his peers actually knew his mother or had any awareness of her illness. However, at the time of the insults he felt that everyone must be aware.

During one session, the family was very concerned because Michelle had a cold. They were fearful that her cold would make her vulnerable to recontracting HIV. Apparently, all family members were concerned about this possibility and had watched over Michelle carefully and fearfully during the past year.

Fifteen months after Charlene's death—shortly before Donna became engaged to her boyfriend, Alex—all three older children voiced their concern that Donna and Alex would one day marry, and that Donna would then move away and leave them behind. Alex began attending family sessions from that point on. Later, as they grew closer to Alex, Eric and Delanya became concerned that Donna and Alex might break up and they would lose him. On the second anniversary of Charlene's death, a few weeks before Donna and Alex were married, the children began to show apprehension about the upcoming wedding. David expressed concern that, during sex, Alex would give HIV to Donna, and she would die. (Alex and Donna both explained that they had tested negative for HIV.)

Once the wedding passed the family wound down treatment over the next 2 months although occasionally returned for follow-up sessions. They emerged from therapy with the ability to communicate more effectively with one another about their issues and were better able to handle adversity.

WHAT THE FAMILIES HAVE TAUGHT US

The families we have worked with have taught us a great deal. They have shown us the strength of their spirit, their survival skills, and the kinship bonds of their extended families.

Above all, we have been impressed by the strong spirituality of both the African-American and the Latino families we have treated.

We are reminded of the words of a Black grandmother who told us, "God never gives you more than you can bear, and I can do all things through God, who strengthens me." Too often, African-Americans' spiritual strength is dismissed by therapists as religiosity or grandiosity. When faced with grief and loss, these families have confirmed for us that their capacity to cope with the disease and the devastating impact of loss often comes from this spiritual bond. Latino families have shown us also that there are many routes to help. They will see a medical doctor, an *espiritista,* and a family therapist all in the same week if they feel that it will help a family member who is dying of AIDS. These are strengths that family therapists can utilize in their work (Boyd-Franklin, 1989). (See Chapter 4 for a more in-depth discussion of cultural issues and family treatment.)

Even "dysfunctional families" (i.e., those with multigenerational drug and alcohol abuse) have strengths if we are willing to look for and use them. Too often therapists adopt a blaming or labeling stance, particularly toward drug abusers and former addicts. By dismissing such families as "dysfunctional," mental health service providers fail to see the potential strengths such families have to offer.

REFERENCES

Black, L. (1993). Aids and secrets in families. In E. Imber-Black (Ed.), *Secrets in families and family therapy* (pp. 355–369). New York: Norton.

Boyd-Franklin, N. (1989). *Black families in therapy: A multisystems approach.* New York: Guilford Press.

Boyd-Franklin, N., & Alemán, J. del C. (1991). Black inner-city families and multigenerational issues: The impact of AIDS. *New Jersey Psychologist, 40*(3), 14–17.

Boyd-Franklin, N. (1993). Racism, secret-keeping and African-American families. In E. Imber-Black (Ed.), *Secrets in families and family therapy* (pp. 331–354). New York: Norton.

Hartman, A., & Laird, J. (1983). *Family centered social work practice.* New York: Free Press.

Helmquist, M. (1984). *The family guide to AIDS: Responding with your heart.* San Francisco: San Francisco AIDS Foundation.

Imber-Black, E. (1988). *Families and larger systems.* New York: Guilford Press.

Imber-Black, E., Roberts, J., & Whiting, A. (Eds.). (1988). *Rituals in family and family therapy.* New York: Norton.

Gilligan, C., Ward, J. V., & McClean, J. (Eds.). (1988). *Mapping the moral domain: A contribution of women's thinking to psychological theory and education.* Cambridge, MA: Harvard University Press.

Kaplan, L. (1988, January). AIDS and guilt. *Family Therapy Networker,* pp. 40–41, 80.

Macklin, E. (Ed.). (1989). *AIDS and families.* Binghamton, NY: Harrington Park Press.

McGoldrick, M., & Gerson, R. (1985). *Genograms in family assessment.* New York: Norton.

Rolland, J. S. (1984). Toward a psychosocial typology of chronic and life-threatening illness. *Family Systems Medicine, 2*(3), 245–263.

Rolland, J. S. (1987a). Family systems and chronic illness: A typological model. *Journal of Psychotherapy and the Family, 3,* 143–168.

Rolland, J. S. (1987b). Chronic illness and the life cycle: A conceptual framework. *Family Process, 26*(2), 203–221.

Tasker, M. (1992). *How can I tell you?* Bethesda, MD: Association for the Care of Children's Health.

Tiblier, K. (1987). Intervening with families with young adults with AIDS. In M. Wright & M. L. Leahey (Eds.), *Families and life-threatening illness.* St. Louis, MO: Springhouse.

Tiblier, K., Walker, G., & Rolland, J. (1989). Therapeutic issues when working with families of persons with AIDS. In E. Macklin (Ed.), *AIDS and families* (pp. 81–127). Binghamton, NY: Harrington Park Press.

Walker, G. (1991). *In the midst of winter.* New York: Norton.

8

· · · · · · · · · · · · ·

The HIV-Infected Child in Therapy

· · · · · · · · · · · · ·

Sylvia W. Pollock, PhD
Cheryl L. Thompson, PhD

With the incidence of pediatric HIV/AIDS increasing at such an alarming rate, psychotherapists in clinic settings and in private practice will inevitably encounter these children as clients. There is an abundance of literature describing psychotherapeutic issues with chronically ill children and their families, much of which has relevance for children with HIV/AIDS. However, there are also factors that make this illness different from any other. Psychotherapeutic process must be viewed from the perspective of the profound impact of this illness on the child, family members, and caregivers—and on therapists themselves.

Pediatric chronic illnesses have psychosocial sequelae, such as the impact of chronicity, an unpredictable disease course, and difficult and painful medical procedures (Stein & Jessop, 1982). There are often recurring hospitalizations resulting in absences from school, which disrupt the normal course of academic and social events. In general, the ability to engage in developmentally appropriate activities can be compromised by the illness and/or necessary medical interventions (Breslau, 1985; Perrin & Gerrity, 1984; Perrin, Ramsey, & Sandler, 1987). Psychological adjustment is often measured by the extent to which the child can adaptively cope with the reality of the illness and the resulting disability (Pless & Pinkerton, 1975; Zeltzer & LeBaron, 1986).

HIV/AIDS amplifies the impact of psychosocial stressors. In addition to those generally associated with chronic illnesses, HIV/AIDS is accompanied by an omnipresent stigma, which often elicits guilt, shame, anger, and fear of disclosure. The persistent desire to maintain the secret can erode the child's and family's resilience. These unique features differentiate the therapeutic treatment of pediatric HIV/AIDS patients from treatment of children with other chronic terminal illnesses.

This chapter first addresses four key tasks in providing psychotherapy for HIV-infected children: (1) developing a sense of safety in the therapeutic setting as a component of a working alliance; (2) understanding the child's perception of the illness; (3) sensitive handling of the disclosure of diagnosis; and (4) understanding of the impact of HIV/AIDS on the psychotherapeutic process. Case material is presented, detailing the course of individual psychotherapy with an HIV-infected child, which illustrates the powerful impact of this illness on every aspect of life. A discussion of issues raised by the case follows.

FOUR TASKS IN PSYCHOTHERAPY WITH HIV/AIDS CHILDREN

Developing a Sense of Safety

Two obvious but important points need to be stated. First, the treatment of HIV-infected children has a great deal in common with the principles of effective psychotherapy in general. Second, while not every child with HIV infection needs to be in therapy all of the time, nearly every infected child does require mental health services at some point in the course of the illness. When psychotherapy is appropriate, the first task is the establishment of a "safe environment."

Safety in this context refers to the sense of trust and cooperation between the child and therapist so that together they can examine painful issues and learn to tolerate frustrations and delays. It requires some capacity on the part of the child for self-observation and some awareness of the problems to be addressed (Ornstein, 1976). A relationship with a sense of safety cannot occur without the presence of a positive alliance between the therapist and the parents or caregivers. When the parents or caregivers do not trust or the therapist, there can be collusion with the child's resistance or unconscious sabotage of the psychotherapy.

For most HIV-infected children the process of establishing a sense of safety requires more time than usual, because it is complicated by a number of factors. There is often an unarticulated sense of shame, secrecy, or blame associated with HIV/AIDS. Children are watchful and guarded, a common occurrence when they are undergoing medical treatments. They may also have experienced disruptions in their lives because of the impaired health or death of parents or siblings. They may have been moved to new homes with extended family members and/or to foster care placements. Loss and grief are integral parts of their lives. Their fears of loss and abandonment can be so great that understandably they maintain distance from the therapist. As in the treatment of traumatized children, even when trust is finally established, the guardedness and wariness can re-emerge in the therapy when the child feels threatened again (Herman, 1992).

Sometimes secrecy and safety become confused. Families and caregivers resort to secrecy about the illness as a way of attempting to keep children safe from discrimination and hurt, which in turn can complicate the establishment of a therapeutic alliance. For example, the caregivers of some HIV-infected children are adamant against children knowing their own diagnosis. In the service of this stance, children are told not to discuss with anyone their visits to the immunology clinic, the frequent blood tests, or the sometimes painful procedures. Children then become caught between the therapist's well-intended wish to provide a safe place to encourage dialogue, and their desire to remain loyal to the caregiver's wish to see them protected. Joint sessions with children and caregivers may be necessary to allow some discussion of the child's beliefs about why he or she requires treatments, while still respecting the caregiver's position about the diagnosis.

The establishment of therapeutic safety can be complicated merely by the proximity of the therapy office to the site of medical treatment. When therapy is hospital-based, seeing the building and other familiar landmarks can remind children of unpleasant procedures. Therapists need to spend more time than usual differentiating between the functions of each location and assuring children that there are "no needles."

In younger children magical thinking abounds. They sometimes fear that expressing anger about painful medical tests can lead to retaliation. Children have reported that they believed that they were receiving subsequent shots because they were vocal when blood was being drawn at an earlier time.

Understanding the Child's Conception of the Illness

Whether or not an HIV-infected child knows the diagnosis, one of the most important issues that must be addressed in psychotherapy is the child's understanding of the causality of illness and the meaning of that illness in the child's life. Find out what children understand about what causes headaches, stomachaches, colds, and why they have them. Why do they feel less energetic than their peers? If they attend a clinic regularly, what do they understand about why they attend? Any exploration of the meaning of an illness for a child must be based on an understanding of illness causality from a cognitive-developmental perspective.

Cognitive development is viewed as a sequential progression, characterized by increasing differentiation, refinement of mental functions, and an increasing degree of organization (Piaget, 1960, 1963; Werner, 1948/1961). The child's linguistic comprehension and usage are linked with underlying cognitive structures and processes. Children's thinking about illness causality follows a similar developmental sequence, and they evolve schemas for explaining symptoms and treatments (Bibace & Walsh, 1981).

In a recent study conducted through the Children's Hospital AIDS Program, Newark, New Jersey, HIV-infected children aged 4 through 12 were interviewed regarding their understanding of both illness in general and HIV infection in particular (Pollock, 1990). Their reasoning about illness causality, including that of HIV/AIDS, followed a developmental sequence similar to sequences noted in studies with healthy subjects (Bibace & Walsh, 1980, 1981) and with other chronically ill subjects (Young, McMurray, Rothery, & Emery, 1987). Thus, an assessment of a child's thinking about illness causality in general is a helpful tool in planning how to frame new information about symptoms or treatments for the HIV-infected child.

Whether or not they know their diagnosis, HIV-infected children describe experiencing uncomfortable physical symptoms, making it essential for the therapist to know what they understand about illness causality in general. Most commonly children complain of headaches, stomachaches, and fatigue. These issues may surface in therapy. Infected children have talked about their brains crashing around inside of their heads, or banging from one side to the other. Some have talked about bad guys fighting in their stomachs or germs blowing up. And they describe wanting to sleep all day long, feeling tired in school, or feeling bad all of the time.

Misinformation and distortion are more likely to occur when a child's level of causal reasoning is ignored. For example, an explanation of airborne viruses is complicated, at best. When children incorporate that information, they do so at their own level of cognitive development. Airborne viruses could then be understood as a characteristic of the wind—it's in the wind and the wind flies up your nose and you have a cold.

It cannot be assumed that children's silence about HIV/AIDS indicates an absence of causal thinking and/or self-made explanations. Children may be accurately reading cues from parents and/or caregivers and not discussing their physical condition. The establishment of effective communication is critical in order to impart information, to extract information about symptoms and the efficacy of treatments, and to correct misinformation. Communication takes place in ways other than verbally. For example, human figure drawings elicited during therapy can provide revealing glimpses of children's thinking. Several large blobs flying in the air from a mother to a child can be used to portray the virus being transmitted perinatally. Pac-Man-like faces, some with smiles and some with frowns, illustrate "bad guys" and the cells that help fight them. Or a body with a number of large round objects inside of the stomach can illustrate a mistaken belief that pills are collecting in the stomach and causing the illness. It is easy to understand why a child with this misperception might resist medication.

Disclosure of the Diagnosis

Often the most difficult issue encountered in the treatment of children with HIV/AIDS has to do with disclosure of the diagnosis. Should a child be told? If so, when and by whom? How much information should be given? What if questions about death should arise? As a result of these painful questions, doctors and parents are often reluctant to tell a child anything about the diagnosis. Sometimes there are conflicts among family members or disagreements between medical staff members and other caregivers as to whether or not children should know that they have HIV/AIDS. Sometimes there are concerns about the child's capacity to manage the information and know that it is at times necessary to maintain secrecy.

The decision to disclose this diagnosis is an extremely complex one, and in fact belongs to a child's parent or caregiver. Mental health clinicians as well as medical staff can play critical roles in the decision-making process; however, it is often the child's therapist who is consulted by family members and health care providers as to the timing of the disclosure. The final decision should be made only after careful consideration of the child's level of functioning, the stage of the illness, and the family's wishes and needs.

Three principles emerge as guidelines about disclosure: (1) The truth is generally less threatening to a child than fear of the unknown; (2) information needs to be presented at a level that is developmentally appropriate for the child; and (3) disclosure is a process, not an event (Pollock & Boland, 1990). In addition, the stage of the illness is an important variable, particularly as it relates to issues of cognitive impairment such as memory loss. It is best to avoid making the disclosure during periods of acute medical crisis, when physical exhaustion, pain, and fear may complicate the child's and family's reactions. It may also be helpful to wait until a positive working alliance has been established between the child, the therapist, and the child's family.

"The truth" about this diagnosis can elicit such terror, rage, shame, and guilt that there is often reluctance to talk with children even about the necessity for medical treatments. In the absence of information, children devise their own complicated, often incorrect, and self-punitive explanations. Sometimes they believe they have the virus because they have been defiant or disobedient at home. Other times, they believe that they have been infected by the very procedures designed to help them, such as blood tests or infusion treatments. This is likely due to confusion between clean and contaminated needles. Children also believe that medical staff, in collusion with caregivers, are threatening them with the diagnosis to scare them into behaving. Although some families remain reluctant to disclose the diagnosis, the problems inherent in not doing so come up again and again, such as at entry into school, the onset of menses, or the beginning of sexual activity.

As was noted earlier, it is critical to determine a child's cognitive-developmental level prior to giving any information about the diagnosis. Developmental level cannot be determined by age alone and is complicated by unknown premorbid functioning, as well as the possibility of neurological and developmental delays secondary to HIV/AIDS. Exploring a child's understanding of his or her condition through questions such as "What do you think is wrong with you?", "What do you think is making you sick?", or "How do you get this sickness?" usually yields valuable baseline information about the child's understanding and beliefs about illness causality. Before the diagnosis is disclosed, it is also important to explore the child's knowledge of HIV/AIDS by asking questions such as "What have you heard about HIV?", "What have you heard about people with AIDS?", "What happens to people with HIV/AIDS?", "What do they say about AIDS in school?", or "What do your friends say?"

Once the child has been told, parents, caregivers, and medical and mental health personnel sometimes believe that the work is done. In fact, it is only beginning. Denial and distortion are frequent occurrences during periods of disclosure. Children may believe that an error has been made, that they have been "cured," or that they have a different illness. Often they recollect that they have been told they have cancer. Misunderstandings such as these are probably results of both cognitive and emotional factors. A major task of therapy is to help the child work through feelings and beliefs about the illness, feelings about grief and loss, and simultaneous concerns about death and dying and about life and living. The need for ongoing processing is critical. Renewed checking with the child is especially warranted as new symptoms emerge and/or new treatments are instituted.

As the diagnosis is disclosed, some families of infected children isolate themselves in an attempt to maintain control over the children, the information, and the presenting symptoms. Secrecy is equated with safety. If no one knows, the child and family members will be safe from discrimination. Their isolation can be intensified by blame or fear of contagion expressed by other family members as well as friends. Caregivers may feel that they and their children are contaminated; they can become angry about the many real and anticipated losses they face (Boland, Mahan-Rudolph, & Evans, 1989). Issues of fear of contamination and the need for isolation can be addressed through psychological support for caregivers (Steiner, 1990). In families challenged by racism, poverty, and the intrusive scrutiny of entitlement programs, there are often strict rules that must be overcome about the privacy of family-related matters (Boyd-Franklin & Alemán, 1990).

Understanding the Impact of HIV/AIDS on the Clinical Process

This illness is an inexorable force in the psychotherapeutic process for both the child and the therapist. It is a template that configures the overall nature and each individual element of treatment. It poses unique challenges for everyone.

The following case vignette highlights some of the psychodynamic, psychosocial, and medical issues presented in the individual treatment of an HIV-infected child. The vignette illustrates the complexity of the therapeutic process—namely addressing the powerful stigma, fear, and the need for denial—in the context of the shifting dominance of the illness. It also celebrates the incredible strength and courage with which children cope with their feelings and live their lives in the midst of this devastating disease.

Tanya (a pseudonym) is an 8½-year-old third grader who was diagnosed with full-blown AIDS at age 7. She had an extensive history of asthma and upper-respiratory infections, and the presence of *Pneumocystis carinii* pneumonia was discovered during a hospital stay following a severe asthma attack. Her mother was informed of the diagnosis and she subsequently told her daughter. The family was referred for therapy by the staff of the immunology department.

The source of Tanya's infection remains unclear, as all other natural family members test negative for the HIV virus. The possibility of sexual abuse has been investigated, with inconclusive results. Tanya was adamant that "no one ever did nothin' bad to me" and rejected all questions about sexual abuse. She was angry that "they don't believe me." Tanya's mother, who is intelligent and insightful, initially found the lack of a specific transmission factor to be source of pain and frustration. Over time she has tried to put those questions behind her and focus on maintaining Tanya's health.

Tanya, who is an attractive African-American child, had just been told of her diagnosis at the time of therapeutic intake. She presented with symptoms of severe anxiety and depression. Although she was cooperative and related well, her affect was blunted. She appeared tired with a chronic heavy cough. Her appetite was poor. In a discussion of the diagnosis during her first appointment, the therapist underscored the message that therapy was a safe place to talk, one which was condoned by her family.

She lives with her mother, stepfather, and 3-year-old sister Danielle (also a pseudonym). Her natural father lives in another city. He sees Tanya only infrequently though he does call, and there is a strong cultural belief in family closeness. However, one of Tanya's maternal aunts completely severed contact with the family when she learned of the diagnosis; in fact, she moved out of state. This was painful for Tanya's mother, as this was her closest sister. Other family members have distanced themselves in more subtle ways by calling and visiting with decreased frequency. Tanya's mother continues to invite them to her home because she cannot go out when Tanya is sick, but they complain about having to travel and insist that Tanya's family come there. These relatives appear not to understand the extent of Tanya's illness and comment that "she doesn't look sick."

For Tanya, the concern about the source of her infection fluctuates. When therapy began it was her primary focus for many sessions. She challenged medical facts, developing her own theory. "Maybe I got it because of my asthma—maybe they go together." She wondered if other children in school who had asthma also had HIV disease. She expressed concern about other children becoming infected as she had, "not knowin' how." In general her level of understanding of the causality of the illness is sophisticated for her age. She has accurately incorporated information about viruses and contagion. However, the lack of a specific means of contact seems to be a disorganizing element in her thinking.

School is primarily a source of gratification for Tanya. She is a competent student and has been placed in accelerated classes. There is no evidence of her having neuropsychological complications. Her teacher and the school nurse have been informed of her diagnosis, and antiviral medication is administered in school. Her attendance is irregular, however, as a result of frequent infections, all-day visits to the clinic, and frequent hospitalizations. As a precaution, she and her therapist role-play her answers to questions about her absences. She is confident in her ability to field questions about missed school from peers. "I got a cough and they know about my asthma. I just say that's why I wasn't in school."

One major theme in Tanya's play is her fear of being alone during medical tests and procedures. While this fear is not uncommon in children with chronic illnesses, it is amplified by the stigma attached to HIV disease. For Tanya this fear is further complicated by an incident that took place when she was being transported by ambulance to the hospital and there was not enough space for her mother to ride with her. In the playroom she repeatedly fills a toy ambulance to the top with plastic people "so the sick girl won't have to be alone." She assures the therapist that the ambulance driver does not know what is really wrong with the girl "in case he'd be scared and not drive her." When she is hospitalized her mother stays with her during most days. Tanya's physician, knowing of her fear, is careful to describe procedures to her. However, in her play children are often unceremoniously thrown out of hospital rooms when the "real sickness" is revealed.

She often muses about wishing other children could know about her disease, underscoring the burden of secrecy. However, when she was asked what she thought might happen if they did learn of her illness, her anticipated consequences were dire. "Nobody would want to sit near me or play with me." In one session she announced that she had been working on a group science project and told a boy "by accident." It was her perception that he was not surprised, and that he agreed to keep the secret. She appeared to be testing the waters of disclosure.

When Tanya is visited by her therapist during hospital stays, she often asks to borrow some small toy from the playroom at the mental health center. She tends to minimize the severity of her condition, attributing the need for hospitalization to "my asthma." The asthma has became a vehicle for talking about her compromised health.

Following inpatient stays, Tanya seems rested and energized, but it is then that she is most philosophical about her condition. It appears that those experiences have eroded her adaptive denial and caused her to confront the realities of her fragile condition. She has become keenly aware of the reason for other children's hospitalizations and is accurate in knowing who is HIV-infected. She has discussed occupational choice from the perspective of HIV/AIDS, wondering, for example, if she could be a nurse "even though I got the virus." She assured herself, "I know I can be a teacher 'cause in school you can't tell." She also talked about feeling tired and "sick all the time" during the hospitalization and contrasted those times with an awareness of well-being.

Several children she knew from the immunology clinic have died over the course of her treatment. Although she never discussed those losses directly, she has spoken with renewed determination about wanting to "live forever." Those moments, while serving as a painful reminder for the therapist of this child's shortened life, have also provided the opportunity to encourage Tanya to think about her life with realistic expectations. She has discussed with her therapist what would really make her happy, and what she would like to do with her life right now. Often her responses are simple wishes, able to be enacted, thus empowering her to effect happiness for herself.

Pain management is a concern now that the decision has been made for Tanya to receive monthly infusions of gamma globulin. Although she has not openly resisted the treatments, she complains adamantly about "getting stuck." Her complaints have been acknowledged as valid, and strategies are employed to give her some control and to reduce unpleasant experiences. Tanya has responded well to a combination of imagery and relaxation techniques, envisioning the infusion as "the good guys" destroying the virus, in Pac-Man fashion.

During the course of treatment the family has contemplated moving, a prospect complicated by the illness. Tanya is enrolled in a school in which disclosure to the nurse and teacher was a positive experience, and in which Tanya was well supported in the classroom. The idea of having to work this out in a new school raises anxiety for everyone. In addition, no one in their apartment building knows of Tanya's illness and the family feels it safest to maintain this secret. There has always been fear that somehow because of the move the diagnosis would be revealed and become a source of pain and discrimination for the family. It is well known among families of infected children that landlords sometimes refuse to rent housing if they learn of a child's infection. Now the family has decided not to move, though neither the neighborhood nor the hallways of their building are safe.

Tanya's life experiences have left her with some special sensitivities. Symptoms or illnesses in others arouses anxiety in her. She expressed great concern when her mother contracted the flu, and was worried about her therapist's having a routine cold. In addition, she is often concerned about her being the source of illness. For example, her sister's cough led to concerns that Danielle might have "caught" her asthma. She is also painfully aware of policies and political statements concerning AIDS. Although she confuses some details, she knows when AIDS funding is being threatened both nationally and locally. She expresses concern that "people might not get their right medicine."

Tanya remains in weekly therapy. There has been a marked reduction in signs of anxiety and depression, though they tend to reappear when her health is compromised. She is gaining autonomy and has made a remarkable adjustment to life with AIDS. In many ways she possesses a maturity beyond her years.

DISCUSSION

This case illustrates many elements that frequently arise in the treatment of children with HIV/AIDS, such as the challenge of establishing a safe working alliance amid stigma and fear of disclosure, the importance of helping HIV-infected children develop some understanding of their illness based on their own level of cognitive development, and the definition of goals and sources of happiness, despite the illness. The presenting problems were typical—depression, anxiety, disturbed appetite, and blunted affect. Therapy provided the opportunity for her to process her understanding of HIV/AIDS and its impact on her life.

In spite of what appeared to be some resolution and acceptance of the illness, there was an underlying sense of herself as "bad" and as potentially causing problems for others because of the infection. For infected children the sense of shame and personal defectiveness can be profound and is often exacerbated by the stigma and the need for secrecy associated with HIV/AIDS. These issues can appear in psychotherapy in play or drawings as themes about being "bad." Feelings of rejection or exclusion can be revealed metaphorically through play.

Tanya comes from an intact and supportive family. For many children whose parents, caregivers, or siblings are also infected, there is the omnipresent potential for multiple losses. As AIDS-related deaths do occur in the family, children are often left without caregivers and must move. The system becomes stressed and people barely recover from one loss before the next occurs.

Routine activities, such as the prospective move discussed in Tanya's case, reflect the complications of daily life. The move was particularly anxiety producing for Tanya's family because they lived in fear that her illness would be discovered, making housing unavailable to them. For Tanya, AIDS was the secret about her that might make her family somehow undesirable, again contributing to her sense of shame and defectiveness.

Any illness causes some anxiety and stress. This one is a major stressor in anyone's life. Psychotherapy can provide one of the few safe opportunities to deal with the fear and anxiety associated with HIV/AIDS and the multiple loss of family members. This opportunity becomes increasingly important and data suggest that stress can accelerate the course of the disease through suppression of the immune system. Specific behavioral and personality factors may contribute to the increased risk of disease in certain individuals (Schleifer, Keller, Bond, Cohen, & Stein, 1989; Schleifer, Keller, McKegney, & Stein, 1979; Vollhardt, 1991).

Routine childhood illnesses can precipitate excessive anxiety in HIV-infected children because of their compromised immune systems. For Tanya, even minor symptoms in herself or others caused her great anxiety. Often, infected children are fearful when they become ill; they resort to denial and dissociation. This reaction to illness highlights the need to maintain a critical balance among these variables—a commitment to the principles of reality, the need to support adaptive denial, the family's need for secrecy, and the therapist's responsibility to protect the family's right to confidentiality. In actuality, this need for therapeutic balance becomes an ethical dilemma (Gray, 1990).

The presence of HIV/AIDS raises special issues for the therapist. As they are with any child in psychotherapy, the most basic tasks include the development of a therapeutic alliance, providing an experience of constancy, and establishing a safe context in which the child can work through traumatic losses (Anthony, 1986; Yorke, 1986). These tasks become complicated by the stigma, the wish for secrecy and fear of disclosure, the continuing risk of additional deaths, and the threat of the child's own declining health and impending death. The risk of overidentification and the concomitant loss of an objective stance is omnipresent.

As in work with traumatized children, there are often intense dilemmas about whether to address issues directly with the child, or use a slower, indirect approach. This is experienced as a "conflicted protectiveness" (Thompson & Kennedy, 1987). There are risks with each stance. Opening the subject too much risks irritating already painful psychic wounds. And yet a slower, less directive approach may serve the needs of the therapist more than those of the child, and can be experienced by the child as collusion with the silence and secrecy. A straightforward acknowledgment of the hopelessness of trying to alter the course of the disease is a necessity—albeit a painful one.

Although denial can have healthy adaptive aspects for the child, it is not helpful for the therapist. An awareness of the illness must remain ever-present, even though it may not be introduced directly into sessions by the child. For example, academic problems may signal the onset of AIDS encephalopathy. Fatigue and changes in alertness can have medical significance. A child's decision to tell friends about the diagnosis may have implications beyond that child's awareness and may require intervention.

There is also the constant risk of anger on the part of the therapist because the patient, a victim in so many dimensions, can become symbolic of social injustice. What does it mean for the therapist to be treating a patient with a terrible and feared disease? Failure to monitor these feelings can result in a diminished sensitivity to the patient's unique dynamics. For example, when children are perinatally infected by mothers actively using injectable drugs, families often focus their anger about AIDS on the person who was actively using drugs. When the mother dies, it is often complicated for the infected children to express sadness and love for her, the presumed source of their infection, when others remain angry.

Another genuine concern for a therapist of HIV-infected children is fear of transmission. In spite of an intellectual understanding of the facts of HIV transmission, anxiety does occur. Such anxiety can be experienced when a child coughs, sneezes, has ruptures of the skin, or offers to share food or drink with the therapist. These issues need to be addressed from the perspective of reality and good hygiene, that is, for the therapist to feel comfortable, and for the child to be protected from the possibility of opportunistic infection as well as placing others at risk of infection.

SUMMARY

A major therapeutic goal in any child treatment is the return to as normal a course of development as is possible. HIV infection pervades each clinical issue and becomes a leitmotif in treatment. The presence of this illness places increased demands on both therapist and child. Developmental concerns and experiences cannot be viewed without consideration of the unique complexities of this illness. AIDS commands that kind of attention. Given the projected increase in the incidence of pediatric AIDS, these children will appear more frequently as patients in mental health centers and in private offices. The clinical issues unique to their treatment will become better understood as, unfortunately, the number of these children increases.

REFERENCES

Anthony, E. J. (1986). Children's reaction to severe stress. *Journal of the American Academy of Child Psychiatry, 25*(3), 299–305.

Bibace, R., & Walsh, M. (1980). Development of children's concepts of illness. *Pediatrics, 66*(6), 912–917.

Bibace, R., & Walsh, M. (1981). Children's conceptions of illness. In R. Bibace & M. Walsh (Eds.), *Children's conceptions of health, illness, and bodily functions* (pp. 31–48). San Francisco: Jossey-Bass.

Boland, M. G., Mahan-Rudolph, P., & Evans, P. (1989). Special issues in the care of the child with HIV infection/AIDS. In B. Martin (Ed.), *Pediatric hospice care: What helps* (pp. 116–144). Los Angeles: Los Angeles Children's Hospital.

Boyd-Franklin, N., & Aleman, J. del C. (1990). Black, inner-city families and multigenerational issues: The impact of AIDS. *New Jersey Psychologist, 40*(3), 14–17.

Breslau, N. (1985). Psychiatric disorders in children with physical disabilities. *Journal of the American Academy of Child Psychiatry, 24*, 87–94.

Gray, J. (1990). Pediatric AIDS research: Legal, ethical and policy influences. In J. Siebert & R. Olson (Eds.), *Children, adolescents, and AIDS* (pp. 179–227). Lincoln: University of Nebraska Press.

Herman, M. (1992). *Trauma and recovery.* New York: Basic Books.

Ornstein, A. (1976). Making contact with the inner world of the child. *Comprehensive Psychiatry, 17*(1), 3–36.

Perrin, E., & Gerrity, P. (1984). Development of children with a chronic illness. *Pediatric Clinics of North America, 31*, 19–31.

Perrin, E., Ramsey, B., & Sandler, H. (1987). Competent kids: Children and adolescents with a chronic illness. *Child: Care, Health and Development, 13*, 13–32.

Piaget, J. (1960). *The child's conception of physical causality.* Patterson, NJ: Littlefield, Adams.

Piaget, J. (1963). *The child's conception of the world.* Paterson, NJ: Littlefield, Adams.

Pless, I. B., & Pinkerton, P. (1975). *Chronic childhood disorders: Promoting patterns of adjustment.* Chicago: Year Book Medical.

Pollock, S. W. (1990). *Concepts of illness in HIV infected children.* Unpublished doctoral dissertation, Seton Hall University.

Pollock, S. W., & Boland, M. G. (1990). Children and HIV infection. *New Jersey Psychologist, 40*(3), 17–21.

Schleifer, S. J., Keller, S. E., McKegney, F. P., & Stein, M. (1979, March). *The influence of stress and other psychosocial factors on human immunity.* Paper presented at the meeting of the Psychosomatic Society, Dallas.

Schleifer, S. J., Keller, S. E., Bond, R. N., Cohen, J., & Stein, M. (1989). Major depressive disorder and immunity. *Archives of General Psychiatry, 46,* 81–87.

Stein, R. E., & Jessop, D. J. (1982). A noncategorical approach to chronic childhood illness. *Public Health Reports, 97,* 354–362.

Steiner, G. L. (1990). Children, families and AIDS: Psychosocial and psychotherapeutic aspects. *New Jersey Psychologist, 40*(3), 11–14.

Thompson, C. L., & Kennedy, P. (1987). Healing the betrayed: Issues in psychotherapy with child victims of trauma. *Journal of Contemporary Psychotherapy, 17*(3), 195–202.

Vollhardt, L. T. (1991). Psychoneuroimmunology: A literature review. *American Journal of Orthopsychiatry, 61*(1), 35–47.

Werner, H. (1961). *Comparative psychology of mental development.* New York: Science Editions. (Original work published 1948)

Yorke, C. (1986). Reflections on the problem of psychic trauma. *Psychoanalytic Study of the Child,*

Young, M., McMurray, M., Rothery, S., & Emery, L. (1987). Use of the Health and Illness Questionnaire with chronically ill and handicapped children. *Children's Health Care, 16*(2), 97–104.

Zeltzer, L., & LeBaron, S. (1986). Fantasy in children and adolescents with chronic illness. *Journal of Developmental and Behavioral Pediatrics, 7*(3), 195–198.

9

. . . .

Nonpharmacological Pain Management for Children with HIV/AIDS

Working with Hypotherapeutic Techniques

. . . .

Marge Iurato Torrance, PsyD
Olivia R. Lewis, MA
Mary Ellen La Brie, RNC
Lynn Czarniecki, RN, MSN

All sciences alike have descended from magic and
superstition, but none has been so slow as hypnosis
in shaking off the evil associations of its origins.
—*Hull (1933, quoted in Gibson & Heap, 1991, p. 134)*

Until recently, most health care professionals ignored the topic of children's pain. Like many adults, practitioners have often assumed that children do not feel pain as intensely as adults do. Some also believe that children are unable to understand medical procedures. As a result, these practitioners treat children as passive victims and do not include them in the process of decision and consent. When medical procedures are painful (e.g, venipuncture or injections), health care professionals may believe that just carrying out the procedures quickly or even forcefully, even when a child is frightened and screaming, is the best and kindest available option. In many of these cases, the child's pain is undertreated or not treated at all. This is frequently traumatic for the child, the family, and the staff.

Studies of infants and children undergoing painful procedures suggest that they not only feel pain, but can experience it as severely as adults do (Anand & Hickey, 1987b; Beaver, 1987). Babies display both physiological and psychological changes directly related to difficult and painful interventions. However, children tend not to talk about their pain. They may believe that their doctors and nurses know they have pain; they may also fear what will happen to them if they report their pain, or they have been taught by their families to be stoic (e.g., "Big boys don't cry"). Unfortunately, professionals tend to assume that children who do not complain or who deny they have pain do not experience it. For this reason, children experiencing acute or chronic discomfort frequently do not get the relief from their pain that they need.

Without proper treatment, pain can have deleterious effects on a child. Studies have shown that infant patients with untreated pain have more postoperative complications and a longer hospital stay (Anand & Hickey, 1987a; Anand, Sippell, & Ansley-Green, 1987). Children undergoing cancer treatment report the most difficult part of having cancer is the repeated painful procedures associated with the diagnosis and treatment of the disease (Zeltzer & Ellenberg, 1980). Professionals' attitudes and personal beliefs about pain—how bad it is, what it represents, how much one should endure, and whether it should be treated at all—can pose barriers to relieving pain in children. One reason why medical professionals often do not treat children's pain adequately is their concern about the effects of pharmacological interventions. For example, fears that opioids will cause respiratory depression or addiction in children is a frequently cited reason for not treating the children's severe pain. At the same time, health care professionals have a limited understanding of the utility and range of available alternatives (i.e., nonpharmacological interventions) to reduce or even obliterate the experience of pain.

Although more research needs to be conducted on pediatric pain, McGrath (quoted in Adler, 1990, p. 11) claims that children's pain, whether acute or chronic, is more "plastic" than that of adults, and thus easier to transform or to modify. This more hopeful difference has motivated those who work with children to develop more humane and effective pain management techniques. In this chapter, we describe some nonpharmacological interventions—particularly hypnotherapy and hypnotherapeutic techniques—that can be used safely, economically, and effectively with children who are ill, to alleviate their pain and distress. Olness and Gardner (1988) report the proven merits of hypnotherapy for managing the pain of children. Other researchers have found hypnotherapy successful with an array of childhood illnesses, from migraine headaches to sickle cell anemia (Olness & Mac-Donald, 1987; Usberti, 1984; Zeltzer, Dash, & Holland, 1979). These techniques can also be effectively applied to children with HIV/AIDS.

PAIN IN CHILDREN WITH HIV/AIDS

Children with HIV/AIDS experience pain related to their disease—its diagnosis, course, and treatment. Their pain can be acute (as in pancreatitis); it can be chronic or intermittent (as in headaches); or it can be related to medical procedures. Table 9.1 lists various causes of pain in pediatric HIV/AIDS that fall into each category.

Treatment of pain in children with HIV/AIDS can ameliorate their suffering, improve their quality of life, and even alter their clinical course. Proper alleviation of pain can restore appetite and activity to a sick child, preventing such other complications as anorexia and depression. Enhancing a child's skills in coping with painful procedures can not only relieve suffering but improve adherence to the medical treatment plan.

TABLE 9.1. Common Causes of Pain in Children with HIV/AIDS

Acute	Chronic/intermittent	Procedural
Headaches resulting from meningitis or sinusitis	Headaches (other)	Venipuncture
Diarrhea, pancreatitis	Abdominal infections, hepatosplenomegaly, tumor	Lumbar puncture
Dental caries/abscesses	Severe spasticity/neuropathy	Injections
Oral thrush/esophagitis	Persistent oral thrush	
Cellulitis/dermatitis	Persistent dermatitis	
Herpetic lesions		
Osteomyelitis		
Aftermath of surgery		

THE PAIN MANAGEMENT ASSESSMENT

Developing a plan to manage a child's pain must begin with a careful pain management assessment. The ideal assessment may take as long as 2½ hours, although in clinic settings an assessor typically has much less time. First the interviewer scans the environment for routines and practices that could be used or improved to reduce pain and anxiety. These may include using appropriate pharmacological treatment, preparing ("setting up") equipment before the child enters the treatment room, and reducing waiting time. It is important to inform the child and the family of exactly what will happen during the appointment. For chronically ill children, including those with HIV/AIDS, clear and appropriate education about the disease eliminates a considerable amount of confusion, and creates some predictability and feelings of control. The interviewer should also assess individual patient characteristics, such as the child's cognitive and social development; personality traits; characteristic coping strategies; previous experience with medical procedures, painful procedures, and pain; and favorite activities and interests.

Patients who suffer acute or chronic pain are likely to be very focused on the pain. In the assessment, the interviewer necessarily accepts the child's subjective evaluation of both the pain and its relief. The assessor helps the child to fully describe the parameters of the sensation of pain: its onset, intensity, and duration, as well as how it compares to other pain the child has previously experienced. A pain scale can be used to provide a concrete referent (Bager & Wells, 1989). Depending on the cognitive level of the child, the scale can be one of faces, numbers, or colors. This initial discussion gathers essential information and directs the child's attention to the specific boundaries of the pain, helping the child to focus attention on specific aspects of the pain rather than remaining overwhelmed with the diffuse pain experience. Paradoxically, helping the child focus on the pain can help the child to diminish it.

There are other important aspects of pain to be considered. The assessor needs to find out whether there are any secondary gains that may be lost when the pain is alleviated. For example, a child in pain may be receiving extra parental attention or special privileges. Such questions as "How will life be different when the pain is gone?" or "Is there anything good about it?" probe both motivation and the secondary-gain aspects of pain (Kohen, 1991). Professionals working with children with psychobiological pain must always be aware that pain can be a manifestation of such hidden psychological issues as sexual abuse or assault. It has been observed that both children and adults visiting the emergency room with unexplained stomach pain or headaches may be exhibiting pain symptoms related to sexual trauma. Of course, psychological interventions for a child with chronic pain presuppose a thorough medical evaluation.

Family dynamics also play an integral part in the child's presentation of pain. The assessor needs to explore (1) the family's perception and expectations of the pain, (2) who in the family assumes the caretaking role, (3) how calm the family is during medical procedures, (4) the reactions of family members to painful procedures, and (5) which family member can be enlisted to coach the child through a procedure or painful episode. In the midst of a discussion about the management of pain, the family and child need to be made aware that pain can help in signaling disease processes that require medical care. The experience of pain can be reframed to the family and to the child as a helpful signal or an unnecessary sensation (Kohen, 1991).

HYPNOTHERAPY AS A PAIN MANAGEMENT TECHNIQUE

Pain has three components: affective–motivational, sensory, and evaluative (Gibson & Heap, 1991). Hypnosis can affect all three components. Hypnotic suggestions may affect the closing of the spinal and thalamic "gates" of pain, making the sensorium less ready to receive the stimuli carried by the small efferent nerves reacting to a painful stimulus. "In essence, this results in a blocking of pain messages to the brain proper" (DePiano & Salzberg, 1986, p. 53). Hypnotically induced analgesia is a partial modification of the sensory component, not an all-or-nothing phenomenon (DePiano & Salzberg, 1986; Gibson & Heap, 1991). Therefore, a hypnotherapist never suggests that the pain will disappear, but rather that it will decrease or change.

Teaching pediatric patients effective techniques to deal with procedural pain can generalize, so that these children become more skilled in reducing other kinds of pain. The techniques that decrease pain give children an increased sense of control and mastery over the process. It is essential to teach more than one pain reduction technique, so that a child can develop a repertoire of coping strategies. This decreases the likelihood of discouragement and hopelessness when one technique fails.

The teaching of these techniques is supported by current studies in pain management with adults. Keefe, Dunsmore, and Burnette (1992) found that "self-efficacy," the belief in one's own ability to perform, correlated positively with higher tolerances for pain and increased endogenous opioid activation when faced with pain. Studies of adults reveal that those patients who believe that control over pain is internal rather than external report lower levels of pain (Keefe et al., 1992).

Families, patients, and members of the medical staff may have many misconceptions about hypnosis and need careful instruction about its use. Frequently families are more comfortable in conceptualizing hypnotic techniques as self-relaxation and visualization, or as methods that draw on one's ability to use imagination and to focus out of self. In the teaching of strategies such as self-hypnosis, it is essential that the instructor not only believe in its effectiveness but also have personal experience with using hypnosis to decrease pain. Orne has defined hypnosis as an altered state of consciousness occurring as a function of a person's ability "to focus attention, fantasize vividly, to suspend disbelief, and to 'think with' suggestions" (quoted in Soskis, 1986, p. v). The hypnotherapist works to create a "holding environment" in which the process of hypnosis can occur (Diamond, 1984). It has been posited that all hypnosis is self-hypnosis, and that the hypnotherapist simply acts as a guide, coach, or facilitator. In the teaching of self-hypnosis for pain control, it is particularly important that the child or adolescent understand that the process is under his or her control and can be used at times when the clinician is not present. Where parents are enlisted to coach, their function as assistants to the child should be emphasized. Whenever possible, a parent or caregiver can help the child practice the techniques. It is ideal for the child to practice two or three times per day. However, real life is frequently far from ideal; in our inner-city hospital experience, many children practice only when in the clinic.

One can teach and use simple distraction techniques with children, such as bubble blowing or singing. These simple techniques can be employed easily by medical personnel. However, using full hypnotic techniques requires appropriate training. Hypnosis is an altered state of consciousness and is used to "teach the patient an attitude of hope in the context of mastery. The patient learns to be an active participant in his or her own behalf, to focus on *creating a solution rather than on enduring a problem,* and to discover and use resources for inner control as much as possible" (Olness & Gardner, 1988, p. 89; emphasis added). In teaching children self-hypnosis, the hypnotherapist is simply enabling them to use a skill they already possess in a purposeful manner. Children are taught to decrease their pain by using their abilities to focus their attention away from their immediate environment or to change their perception of pain.

TRANCE INDUCTION

Children enter hypnotic states every day as they become absorbed in play, fantasy, and favorite activities; in so doing, they diminish their awareness of external surroundings. One need only observe a child absorbed in a Nintendo game to view a naturalistic example of a child in trance. To induce trance following the assessment, the hypnotherapist teaches the child how to facilitate entering this altered state of consciousness known as trance. This teaching or coaching process is called "trance induction." Children and young adolescents require an age-appropriate induction technique; methods appropriate for adults and older adolescents will probably not be stimulating enough. This explains in part why "cookbook" approaches to teaching children self-hypnosis are not useful (Erickson, 1991b).

Preliminary Induction Techniques for Children

1. *Eye fixation:* The child visually focuses on a fixed point.
2. *Eye roll:* The child is asked to roll his or her eyes up to the top of the head and to hold them up while slowly closing the eyelids. This is effective both in focusing attention and in facilitating closing the eyes. It should be noted that young children may not be comfortable closing their eyes; fortunately, closing the eyes is not a necessary component of trance (Spiegel & Spiegel, 1978).
3. *Focus:* Frequently children need no formal induction; hypnosis requires only that their attention be captured and focused.

Induction Techniques for Toddlers and Young Children

1. *Physical contact:* Touch, massage, rocking.
2. *Visual and auditory distractions:* Storytelling, particularly with pop-up books if the reader is dramatic and engaging with the child.
3. *Breath control:* Bubble blowing and singing to help a child breathe slowly and calmly (Kuttner, 1991).

Induction Techniques for School-Aged Children

1. *Imaginary trip:* The child closes her his or her eyes and describes an imaginary trip to a real or fantasized place. The exercise of describing to someone else the details of another place obliges the child to lose awareness of the immediate surroundings.

2. *"Magic glove":* An analgesic technique; through the use of touch and suggestion, the child begins to have reduced sensations in his or her hand and arm (see below for a fuller description). This analgesic effect may be transferred to any area of the body where the child wishes to reduce pain (Olness & Gardner, 1988).

3. *Superheroes/heroines:* The hypnotherapist suggests that the child can either be a superhero/heroine or take one along to help with the painful experience.

4. *Switch technique:* Use of imaginary controls, numbered dials, and switches to help the child "turn down" the pain (Erickson, 1991a).

A PAIN MANAGEMENT PROGRAM

This section describes the development of a nonpharmacological pain management program for children who have HIV/AIDS. We (two of us are psychologists and two are nurses) developed the program to help children deal with procedural pain in the outpatient HIV clinic. *Using hypnosis as an intervention or treatment requires training and appropriate supervision.*[1] At the time the program was proposed, medical staff members showed a burgeoning interest in helping children with pain.

The outpatient clinics were chosen because children regularly attended a monthly clinic for either blood work or infusions. After we held an in-service program on hypnosis and pain management techniques for the medical staff, staff members introduced certain supplies into all treatment rooms. These included materials for blowing bubbles and a "wand" or "moon stick" (a Plexiglas wand filled with floating, shiny moons, stars, and glitter dust). The introduction of these supplies had a dual function. One was to make manifest to the staff that pain needed to be, and could be, managed. The other was to offer the staff members simple tools they could use to help children in pain. Both the wand and the bubbles functioned as distraction techniques, particularly with children under 4 years of age. Some children learned to blow bubbles for the first time in these treatment rooms; they were so busy with the acquisition of this new, entrancing skill that they "for-

---

[1]Courses are offered by the Society for Behavioral Pediatrics of Philadelphia, the Society for Clinical and Experimental Hypnosis of Liverpool, NY, and the American Society of Clinical Hypnosis of Des Plaines, IL, in the use of hypnosis for pain management in children.

got to notice" the pain of the procedure. Blowing bubbles demands a physiologic response that is incompatible with tension and hyper-ventilation; the required exhalation forces even, calm breathing.

The psychologists taught self-hypnosis to those children who were older or required more intervention than simple distraction. The nurses identified appropriate patients according to several criteria: those who (1) became very agitated and upset during procedures, (2) were very quiet and noncomplaining, or (3) were new patients who had not yet experienced the regular procedures at the clinic. They introduced the hypnotherapists to the parents or caretakers as professionals who were teaching children ways to help them through the procedures. They emphasized the professionals' role as guides or coaches. Usually, the hypnotherapists spent 15–20 minutes explaining the use of techniques to each family and patient. Depending on the age and comfort level of the patient, some of the teaching time would be spent alone with the child. Some time was spent discussing some of the physiology of pain in simple terms, to help the child understand that the pain message must get to the brain in order for him or her to feel the pain. Comparing the brain with a computer and helping the child imagine a computer screen in his or her head, with pain dials to permit the child to turn the pain down to the preferred level, frequently proved an effective technique.

The use of language is critical for setting positive expectations. One can use such phrases as "Would you mind if it didn't bother you so much?", as well as consistently suggesting that change will occur ("You will be surprised to notice that it will be different") (Kohen, 1991). For children, unlike adults, there need be no formal induction or deepening of trance. A simple induction that may be used with many children is the eye roll, described above. As noted there, this is effective both in focusing attention and in facilitating closing the eyes.

The use of touch is very helpful in inducing trance when a child is comfortable with touch. One must always ask permission to use touch with a child. The "magic glove," also mentioned above, is a technique in which the hypnotherapist first suggests that there is a way that has helped other children to feel different during procedures. After being sure that the child's attention is fully engaged, the therapist carefully puts an invisible "magic glove" on the child, suggesting that, wherever the glove is placed, the child will feel lessened sensations. It is important to suggest that the glove can be transferred to another location with just a touch. In work with the "magic glove," the analgesic effect can be tested with something sharp, in case there is a need for more "magic."

CLINICAL EXAMPLES

Adam, 16 years old, appeared stoic and withdrawn during medical procedures. The staff was concerned about his lack of reaction to blood drawing and intravenous (IV) infusions. In a half-hour interview, Adam revealed that he experienced a great deal of pain but felt that he should not bother staff and relatives with complaints. He reported his pain level as 8 on a scale of 0–10. During the assessment he evidenced an ability to focus intensely, a voracious appetite for reading comic books, and an interest in collecting model cars. With little input from the hypnotherapist, Adam developed the idea of using the imagery of taking a trip in a sports car during the infusion procedure.

The hypnotherapist chose the eye roll as an induction technique, because Adam had kept his eyes fixed on her during the assessment interview. He used slow inhalation and exhalation as a breathing technique to relax. The hypnotherapist invited Adam to start his trip when ready. He was freely able to describe his trip, from getting into the car to stopping at various sites during the trip. His ability to focus on the trip and to exclude the painful procedure was demonstrated by his lack of awareness of the insertion of the IV needle, which was delayed until Adam began his imaginary trip. When the procedure was completed, the hypnotherapist gently helped Adam to refocus his attention on the present.

Rachel, 4 years old, was extremely fearful, agitated, and uncooperative during medical procedures. Before the introduction of this program, four or five staff members had to hold her down for procedures; this resulted in great distress for Rachel, her family, and the staff. A 20-minute assessment made it clear that Rachel was bright and could understand the concept of learning "magic tricks" to help with the pain. Although she learned the "magic glove" technique and used the wand to focus, her favorite strategy was bubble blowing. During the preparation for the procedure, her bubble blowing helped to keep her calm, focused, and physically engaged. When the procedure occurred she interrupted her bubble blowing, gave one loud scream, and instantly returned to blowing.

Lesa, 13 years old, became depressed and withdrawn the night preceding each clinic visit. Although cooperative, her regressive behavior concerned the staff. In the assessment interview, Lesa identified her internal emotions during procedures as corresponding to a crying face and her displayed emotion as corresponding to a happy face. Lesa came into the clinic carrying a hand-held video game; it seemed to be the one activity that held her interest. During the 20-minute assessment, the hypnotherapist introduced her to the techniques of self-hypnosis. Specifically, she was taught to imagine her brain as a computer screen on which she could "turn down" the pain. No formal induction was used, but she closed her eyes naturally and began the process on her own. During the procedure she remained relaxed, with eyes closed. While in trance she decided not to use the technique of turning down the pain; instead, she created an original video game in which she and the hypnotherapist were players. She gave a running commentary on the game throughout the procedure. At the end of the procedure, the hypnotherapist suggested that she could finish the game and open her eyes whenever she was ready.

Brianna is a 4-year-old HIV-infected child with some degree of pervasive developmental disorder (autism). For her monthly immunoglobulin infusions the staff members all used to gather, as it took four people to start her IV. Her foster mother would stare at an undefined space around her feet as Brianna thrashed about on the examination table. Sporadically and without any guidance, the nurses had attempted a variety of interventions to make the experience less traumatic for all involved. No success had ever been achieved during previous visits by explaining the procedure to Brianna or by having her foster mother hold her. The staff's attempts to distract her were unfocused and of too short a duration to permit the medical procedures to be completed. For example, a nurse might say, "Brianna, look over here. There's a bird on the window sill!" Even if she did look, which was rare, she immediately looked back to the source of her concern, the needle. It was a battlefield and the lines were drawn. No one was on Brianna's side. "For her own good" was not in the realm of her understanding. So the approach was to get it over with as quickly as possible. When the IV needle was inserted, more often than not on a second attempt (on a moving target), Brianna's eyes would be big with fear and confusion, her tears would have run back to her ears, and her forehead would be beaded with perspiration. The nurses would be wordless, finding nothing to say to help anyone in the room.

Since Brianna had limited cognitive and expressive abilities, the logical choice for intervention was bubble blowing. Sometimes the simple things work best. Her social worker was a consistent, trusted person who was not part of any painful procedures, and so assumed responsibility for the teaching of the new skill. The members of Brianna's foster family were a little skeptical as the principles of this "Lamaze for kids" was explained. They were encouraged to participate as valued members of the care team. At this writing, 2 months after the beginning of bubble blowing during the procedure, Brianna's IV is now started by *one* nurse while her foster mother blows the bubbles. Brianna's social worker is also present, to steady her in case she gets too excited as she tries to catch the bubbles or claps in delight. This is worlds away from the nursing staff's previous experience. It's a story that is often repeated now.

NURSING EXPERIENCE
WITH THE PAIN MANAGEMENT PROGRAM

In a busy ambulatory care center focused on children with HIV/AIDS, the atmosphere is often highly charged. Patients present with a host of concerns, including physical complaints, social difficulties, and even spiritual conflicts. The team approach to the care of these families (in pediatrics it is always *family* care; the child cannot be treated as a separate entity) has met with a great deal of success. The doctor, nurse practitioner, nurse case manager, social worker, psychologists, and clinic staff work together to achieve "state-of-the-art" assessment, intervention, and treatment of HIV-infected children. Formerly, pain management was one of the areas in our program where we lacked a sense that we were providing optimal care. Introducing nonpharmacological interventions for pain management helped address that deficit.

In a time of shrinking resources, these are cost-effective interventions. A minimal investment in in-service training and "trinkets" resulted in improved and more timely delivery of care in a safer environment. In our clinic setting it was easy to implement some of the techniques immediately (e.g., by encouraging families to bring along a favorite book or music tape for each visit). Although bubbles and wands are not very expensive, we have nevertheless found maintaining a constant supply in a busy outpatient department to be costlier than one might think. Local women's clubs and church organizations can serve as good resources for donations, once they are made aware of the difference that such supplies can make in a clinic.

The practice of hypnosis does require an investment in professional training, but the cost is more than returned in a positive outcome for child and staff alike. Hearing the term "hypnosis" alone tends to distance caregivers and families, who may file the accompanying advice into a slot between witchcraft and astrology. It helps demystify hypnosis to have caregivers envision hypnotic methods as interactive relaxation techniques, drawing on familiar abilities to use imagination and to focus outside of self.

We observed that diagnostic and therapeutic procedures often evoked fear and loss of control in the children. By routinely integrating hypnotic techniques into the clinic practice, we were able to help them conquer their fears and regain control.

Those who care for children have long used some of these techniques in an informal way, but integrating a formal pain management program into clinic routines addresses children's pain more systematically and consistently. There are also pluses on the professional side of the experience. The fact that parents and children are not preoccupied with fear of what will conclude the visit improves cooperation during physical examinations. Procedures that previously required many hands for the physical restraint of a child can be done more safely with fewer staff members when the child is able to cooperate. Clinicians and case managers work more efficiently, as there is less need for repeated procedures, in an improved atmosphere with less screaming, crying, and stress.

The safety factor cannot be too strongly emphasized. An uncooperative child is extremely challenging to a clinician who must draw blood or perform other invasive procedures. Hepatitis B and HIV transmission through needle stick injury are dangerous occupational hazards for health care workers. Any measure that can reduce the risk must be taken seriously. When a child's stress level is high in anticipation of pain, the parent or caregiver feels helpless and isolated, and the health care worker is anticipating a struggle, accidents are more likely to happen. When there is a sense of urgency and frustration—for instance, during a third attempt at venipuncture—then tension adversely affects performance. Using nonpharmacological interventions for pain management results in a significantly safer and more positive experience for child, family, and staff.

REFERENCES

Adler, T. (1990, September). Pain management tools shown to help children. *APA Monitor,* p. 11.

Anand, K. J. S., & Hickey, P. R. (1987a). Halothane–morphine compared with high dose sufentanil for anesthesia and post-operative analgesia in neonatal cardiac surgery. *New England Journal of Medicine, 326,* 1–9.

Anand, K. J. S., & Hickey, P. R. (1987b). Pain and its effects in the human neonate and fetus. *New England Journal of Medicine, 327,* 1321–1329.

Anand, K. J. S., Sippell, W. G., & Ansley-Green, A. (1987). Randomized trial of fentanyl anesthesia in preterm babies undergoing surgery: Effects on stress response. *Lancet, i,* 243–248.

Bager, J., & Wells, N. (1989). Assessment of pain in children. *Pediatric Clinics of North America, 36*(4), 837–854.

Beaver, P. K. (1987). Premature infants' response to touch and pain: Can nurses make a difference? *Neonatal Network, 6,* 13–17.

DePiano, F. A., & Salzberg, H. C. (Eds.). (1986). *Clinical application of hypnosis.* Norwood, NJ: Ablex.

Diamond, M. J. (1984). It takes two to tango: Some thoughts on the neglected importance of the hypnotist in an interactive hypnotherapeutic relationship. *American Journal of Clinical Hypnosis, 27*(1), 3–13.

Erickson, C. (1991a). Applications of cyberphysiologic techniques in pain management. *Pediatric Annals, 20*(3), 145–156.

Erickson, C. (1991b, September). *Using hypnosis in pain management for children.* Presentation at the Introductory Clinical Hypnosis Workshop, Society for Behavioral Pediatrics, Baltimore.

Gibson, H. B., & Heap, M. (1991). *Hypnosis in therapy.* Hillsdale, NJ: Erlbaum.

Keefe, F. J., Dunsmore, J., & Burnette, R. (1992). Behavioral and cognitive-behavioral approaches to chronic pain: Recent advances and future directions. *Journal of Clinical and Consulting Psychology, 60*(4), 528–536.

Kohen, D. (1991). *Hypnotherapeutic approaches to persistent somatic complaints.* Presentation at the Introductory Clinical Hypnosis Workshop, Society for Behavioral Pediatrics, Baltimore.

Kuttner, L. (1991). Helpful strategies in working with preschool children in pediatric practice. *Pediatric Annals, 20*(3), 120–127.

Olness, K. N., & Gardner, G. (1988). *Hypnosis and hypnotherapy with children* (2nd ed.). Philadelphia: Grune & Stratton.

Olness, K. N., & MacDonald, J. (1987). Headaches in children. *Pediatrics in Review, 8,* 307–311.

Soskis, D. A. (1986). *Teaching self-hypnosis.* New York: Norton.

Spiegel, H., & Spiegel, D. (1978). *Trance and treatment: Clinical uses of hypnosis.* New York: Basic Books.

Usberti, M. E. A. (1984). Usefulness of hypnosis for renal needle biopsy in children. *Kidney International, 26,* 351–352.

Zeltzer, L., Dash, J., & Holland, J. (1979). Hypnotically induced pain control in sickle cell anemia. *Pediatrics, 64,* 533–536.

Zeltzer, L., & Ellenberg, L. (1980). The psychological effects of illness in adolescents. Impact of illness in adolescents: Crucial issues and coping styles. Journal of Pediatrics, 97, 132–138.

10

Support Group for Children with HIV/AIDS

Katherine A. Gomez, RN, MA
Heidi J. Haiken, MSW, ACSW
Sandra Y. Lewis, PsyD

This chapter describes a support group for HIV-infected children held at the Children's Hospital AIDS Program (CHAP), a multidisciplinary treatment program that operates out of Children's Hospital of New Jersey. CHAP treats children up to 19 years of age who have HIV infection or full-blown AIDS. In the fall of 1988, the CHAP team recognized the need to provide a safe forum in which the increasing numbers of infected school-aged children could express their feelings and concerns about their illness. Secrecy and the resultant isolation were recognized as major issues for this age group. These children were emotionally separated both from their peers by their need to hide their diagnosis, and from their families by the fact that discussion of their illness was generally considered taboo. It is generally acknowledged that children with chronic illness—and particularly an illness as devastating as HIV/AIDS—are at greater risk of adjustment and behavioral problems than their healthy peers (Pless & Roghmann, 1971; Pless, Roghmann, & Haggerty, 1972).

At CHAP, some of the children attended a monthly clinic for infusions of gamma globulin, each of which was given over a 4-hour period. In coordination with the Community Mental Health Center of the

University of Medicine and Dentistry of New Jersey (Newark), a group support modality in connection with the monthly clinic was conceived and planned for children who were identified as at particular emotional risk as a result of their frequent hospitalizations, separations from supports, and the difficult nature of their treatments. Our conception of this intervention was based upon well-documented use of small groups with chronically ill children (Adams-Greenly, Shiminski-Maher, McGowan, & Meyers, 1986; Tinkelman, Brice, Yoshida, & Sadler, 1976; Williams & Baeker, 1983). To our knowledge, no group intervention had previously been used with HIV-infected children. The group, which has evolved through two phases over 3 years, shows the progression of our thinking as well as the evolution of the children's themes.

PHASE I: THE BEGINNING STAGES

To begin the group, Katherine Gomez (a psychology intern with a nursing background and special interest in working with chronically ill, latency-aged children) was enlisted as co-leader, along with Heidi Haiken (a CHAP social worker). The inclusion of a CHAP team member as co-leader provided the children with a familiar, consistent person with whom they could remain in contact, once the intern completed her work at the hospital and left at the end of the school year. The need for a "transitional" person was particularly indicated for these children, because they had experienced previous parental and sibling losses as a result of HIV/AIDS. We also felt that different professional perspectives would enrich the group experience, as well as contribute to our own professional development. Whereas Gomez, the psychology intern, provided psychological expertise and objectivity, Haiken, the social worker, had expertise in the psychosocial issues of HIV infection and knowledge of the children's medical care and their families' psychosocial histories.

Model

We used a structural family therapy model with two cotherapists serving as the executive subsystem (or parental roles) to provide a supportive environment for self-disclosure and formation of peer bonds. This model, which was used by Gershoni (1985) in his work with latency-aged children, created a family-like environment, with two female parent surrogates. This scenario paralleled a situation often seen in our patient population, where female extended family members take on the caretaking roles when the parents are absent or otherwise unavailable.

Each session was divided into three subdivisions. The first segment consisted of 30 minutes of discussion, in which each child was encouraged to participate by discussing any subject pertaining to his or her life and illness experience. Although we intended to use a nondirective approach, certain issues (such as a member's absence) were directly addressed, because they affected group process and morale, and often elicited feelings associated with previous losses and abandonments. We refrained from making interpretations of individual feelings. Instead, we tried to identify feelings that were common to what others felt in the group. In this way, the participants were encouraged to share their experiences with one another. This discussion period also provided the children with an opportunity to speak with adults without fear of reprimand or betrayal of trust.

The second group segment, also a 30-minute period, consisted of a simple lunch provided by the hospital to capture the nurturing, mutuality, and sharing functions of a family and to foster feelings of affiliation and group cohesiveness. The final 30-minute period was devoted to creative art activities, in order to bring closure to the session and to facilitate nonverbal or symbolic expression of covert feelings and enhancement of feelings of mastery. These activities served to bind anxiety for the children as well.

Goals and Objectives

The following were the goals and objectives of the support group: (1) to provide the children with a safe peer network and opportunities for open expression of feelings and consensual validation; (2) to enhance their feelings of control, mastery, and competence; (3) to increase understanding of their illness; (4) to foster healthy coping mechanisms and problem solving; and (5) to supplement CHAP's information base for future group formation and use in meeting the psychological needs of the latency-aged children it serves.

Group Composition

The group members were selected on the basis of age, developmental level, and capacity for verbal expression. Children with severe emotional and behavioral difficulties were not considered appropriate for this intervention, and many of them were referred for individual or family therapy. A critical criterion for inclusion in our group was a child's awareness of his or her diagnosis. Knowledge of diagnosis was essential to our objective to create a safe, accepting, and open forum for these children.

On several occasions, other children meeting the inclusion criteria were invited to attend group sessions. Generally, this occurred when there were only one or two members in clinic and the children wished to hold group. Opening the group to other eligible children was agreed upon by the members and ourselves, following discussion regarding their need for additional group sessions if the children were removed from our clinic schedule because of illness or hospitalization.

Recruitment

Parents or guardians were contacted individually by Haiken in the clinic to discuss the group's purpose as well as inclusion criteria. A follow-up letter was sent to these parents, giving the date of the pregroup parent/guardian meeting with the two leaders. In spite of the interest previously expressed in the group by the five caretakers, only two attended the initial meeting. All but one eligible child were given consent for involvement by their guardians. This child's caretaker reported discomfort with discussion of the diagnosis.

Evaluation Component

The group met for eight monthly 90-minute sessions in a conference room adjoining the clinic area. Group time was designed to be free of medical treatments and intrusions from outsiders. The Piers–Harris Children's Self-Concept Scales (Piers, 1984) was the only standardized instrument administered; scores obtained following the first and second sessions were all within the average range. Projective drawings were used during our early sessions, not only to break the ice but to allow us to enter the children's inner world—their conscious and unconscious perceptions of themselves and significant others (Hammer, 1981). We also used the House-Tree-Person, the Chromatic Draw-a-Person, and the Draw-a-Family techniques.

Early Themes

We gained insight into the impact of HIV/AIDS on the lives of these children from analysis of recurrent themes in projective drawings and group discussion. Feelings of loss, social isolation, and anger were significant and powerful. In group, the children presented in either an extremely needy manner or with a pseudomature, self-sufficient posture. In the initial session, they expressed their desire to have a slumber/pizza party at Gomez's home, and created elaborate fantasies of the types of foods she would provide.

The children felt much ambivalence toward the clinic, its staff, and their medical treatment. Although they expressed love, attachment, and gratitude toward the hospital staff, they disliked and resented the long clinic visits and various medical procedures necessary to their treatment. One boy compared himself to a porcupine, as he had experienced multiple venipuncture sticks on numerous occasions; another child stated that he felt like a sponge, wrung out and absorbing hurt. Despite their feelings of being guinea pigs, the children were reluctant to blame or admit anger toward caretakers, parents, and doctors, perhaps due to fear of abandonment and retaliation. Events in the children's histories seemed to support such fears and anxiety. But Tinkelman et al. (1976) also found this difficulty with expressing anger toward parents in their group of early adolescent asthmatics.

One topic addressed by the group was the children's feelings about family and community members who made negative comments about people with AIDS. Group members revealed the negative impact this had upon their feelings of self-worth. These feelings were also related to the stigma of HIV infection that is often promoted in the media, particularly on television. The children expressed concern that the message they heard was that people with AIDS are infected because they have done something bad and they are going to die. The group process allowed us to discuss this and promote self-esteem. We were then able to work on issues of guilt and blame.

Anger was expressed verbally and, more frequently, nonverbally in the children's drawings of car crashes, accidents, and violent scenes. Nonverbal hostility was at times directed at us, the group leaders, who were the most accessible and perhaps the least threatening authority figures. This displaced anger was subtle and was often manifested in a resistance to entering the group room, despite eager anticipation only minutes earlier. At times the children refused to participate in an activity they themselves had initiated.

Some described their dislike of being treated as if they were different by their families and teachers. Guilt over increased attention or differential treatment by parents and teachers was reported.

The children freely expressed their dislike of needles, particularly IV needle insertion. Waiting in the clinic and interruptions of our sessions by the nursing staff (for IV maintenance) were also troublesome to them. The things the children liked most about the clinic were seeing their friends, the group itself, the cookies we provided, and (for some) missing school to attend clinic. Although the children differed in their need to know and utilize specific details about their treatment, they all appeared to have a working knowledge of hospital jargon. It was common to hear the children suggest another member have his or her IV flushed or identify an IV infiltration. This reflected adaptive strategies, attempts at gaining control, and identification with the medical/nursing team. This was further suggested by the verbalized aspirations of several members of the group, who expressed a desire to enter the helping professions when they were grown.

Although the importance of this first phase of the group experience for the members and ourselves is difficult to quantify, feedback from the children's families and the CHAP staff following our final session supported our observations that the children had established a close, supportive network and a group identity that persisted despite the termination of this phase of the group a year and a half ago. All of the children agreed to return for group if it should be offered again in the future. Since that time, the group has been reinstated with some additional members. Another group has been begun for younger children who do not know their diagnosis, and groups for siblings have been established.

PHASE II: CURRENT THEMES

After a recess, the group was reinstated. Heidi Haiken continued with the group, and Sandra Lewis, a psychologist, joined as cotherapist. The major group themes have become death and dying; going to heaven; hospitalization; medical procedures; who knows about the children's diagnosis; loss of family members and loved ones; and losing weight. The theme for each group session evolves from the play activity chosen by the children. The children's imaginations and our willingness to become involved in their ideas allow for a wide range of creative play, which provides a safe outlet for exploration of their thoughts and feelings. Since the children can become emotionally overwhelmed, limit setting for the group includes no hitting or rough play, apologizing for hurting someone's feelings, no running around the halls, and the use of time out when necessary.

Hospital play—using such props as an IV pole, Band-Aids, masks, rubber gloves, a thermometer, a stethoscope, specimen cups, construction paper, crayons, and puppets—is a frequent scenario. During one session, the children recreated the death of a group member, using a Zaydee© doll to represent the child who died. The play began with his hospitalization due to an acute illness, with the children acting as his nurses and doctors. We (the group leaders) played the roles of his relatives. After recovering and being released from the hospital, the child became ill again and was rehospitalized. The nurses and doctors were unable to revive him and told the relatives, "He's dead. Get some new clothes for him. He can't be buried in this." The child was prepared, and a funeral was held by the relatives. Initially, the children hid under the table, but came out when the relatives asked whether the medical team was coming to the funeral. One of the medical staff announced that one of the doctors had been killed in a car accident. We all then attended the doctor's funeral. The doctor and the child who died were playing in heaven together, while the rest of the group remembered how much we liked them.

At other times, when we have explored the theme of death, some children have acted out: They have become overactive, interrupted funerals, or pushed group members or ourselves, claiming that the child was not dead. In one session, the children pretended that we (the group leaders) were mother and grandmother, that one of the children was a daughter, and that the Zaydee© doll was another daughter. As in previous sessions, the child represented by the doll got sick and her family took her to the hospital, where other group members were her doctors and nurses. One child, who attends group infrequently and is uncomfortable with the theme of death, began to act out. The family did not want the child put on a respirator, but this child (playing a doctor) put Zaydee© on the respirator against the family's wishes. The children were whispering to each other whether or not to let Zaydee© die. The doctor whispered to the other children to let us (playing the mother and grandmother) kill her and then told the mother to take the tubing off.

After the death, during funeral services, this same child picked up the doll and ran around the room saying, "She's not dead." At this point we stopped the play, instituted limit setting, had a time out, and discussed the children's responses to death. The children were able to sit down and talk about AIDS and their specific illnesses that might lead to their own death.

The issue of death has also provided discussions and play related to the children's concepts of death and their spiritual beliefs about life after death. "Heaven" is a familiar concept for many of the children. One child, who was an integral part of the group process, was hospitalized and subsequently died. Many of her group members were very upset that they had not had the opportunity to say goodbye. Many of the children began making cards for their deceased friend and her family that said "I love you" and "I will miss you." Many found this session very comforting. In a later session, the children created a pictorial story about their concept of heaven. One common theme was being reunited with friends and family members who had died.

An important aspect of group process is inconsistency in the children's acceptance of their HIV/AIDS diagnosis. Each child at some point has denied the diagnosis of HIV/AIDS, only to admit it at another time. Though the denial appears to be adaptive, there is no obvious pattern to its use. The children have become somewhat confrontational about each other's denial of diagnosis. If a child claims not to have AIDS, another child may say, "Yes, you do." At these times, we discuss that everyone (including doctors, nurses, social workers, and psychologists) would like AIDS to go away, but that people can live with the disease. Knowing when denial is adaptive and when it threatens the group's integrity is a critical feature of group treatment.

SPECIAL TREATMENT ISSUES

Neurological Deterioration

Central nervous system (CNS) complications and neurological deterioration in some of the children have proved to be difficult group issues. One child presented with neurological and cognitive difficulties from the very beginning. Although he was initially coherent and able to participate, over time we began to notice memory loss, nonsequiturs, tangential speech, and increasing distractibility and hyperactivity. Despite everyone's awareness of the situation, we and all of the children had ignored it in order to compensate for his difficulties. Finally, in a group session where one of the children made a sign behind this child's back to signal that he was "crazy," we realized that this issue had to be addressed. We realized that his difficulties had become a "family secret" that was not discussed.

In a supervisory session, we openly and honestly discussed everyone's collusion of denying this child's neurological deterioration. Conscious of not wanting to place him in a "scapegoat" position, we began by addressing his behavior in group in a direct but supportive way. Gradually, we and the children, relieved at being able to discuss these issues, were able to consciously work out strategies for "bringing him back" when he became distracted or confused.

Children with HIV/AIDS are living longer, but many are experiencing progressive CNS disease. Practitioners and therapists doing this work can find creative ways of addressing such painful issues. Otherwise, they may become "family secrets" that all group members collude to avoid.

Role of the Therapists and Countertransference

Our role as therapists in these groups has been an evolving one. Initially, as stated above, we had to be directive and provide structure for the activities and the time. Gradually, by the second phase of the group the children were accustomed to the group process and brought in their own themes simultaneously. Ironically, this second phase placed even more demands on us as group leaders. We had to work very deliberately on our own communication during and after group, so that we could facilitate the group process and cope effectively with the needs and questions of the children.

In this second phase, the children incorporated us very intimately into their play. Consequently, the countertransference issues became very intense for us. As might be expected, it was challenging for us to discuss death openly with the children. We quickly recognized, however, that the children were ready and willing for this discussion.

We realized early in this phase that many of our roles in the group process were parallel to parental roles in the children's families, and that the children were very sensitive to the interactions between us. We therefore devoted a great deal of time outside of group to processing the children's group. We also processed our own co-leader relationship.

The key issue here was our individual and collective development as therapists. Although it is very clear in any therapeutic intervention that the therapist is the instrument, we learned to use ourselves in constantly evolving creative ways in the group process. We learned to communicate openly with each other during the group process, and even to model for the children how to solve problems and reach a consensus of opinion on a problem in the group. This process created a "safe environment" in which the children—especially those whose families were in denial or experiencing confusion about the disease—could feel free to express their own concerns and needs. Children whose HIV/AIDS was kept a secret at home, or who couldn't discuss their fears and concerns, benefited greatly from the openness and safety of the group that we consciously worked to create.

The Role of Supervision

Supervision or consultation is an essential part of any therapeutic intervention. For group therapists working with children and families with HIV/AIDS, it is an especially vital lifeline. Given the complexity of the issues discussed and the newness of the group process, we felt the need for a "consultant" to whom we could address our concerns.

The supervisory process also helped to develop and solidify our therapeutic alliance in each phase of the group. Since many of the life-and-death issues raised by these children went far beyond the typical issues raised by children in group psychotherapy, we often found ourselves in a pioneering position. We recommend that readers who play such a role in their hospital or agency seek supervision from a trained mental health professional with group psychotherapy experience. If this is not possible, they might begin a peer–supervisory group with other staff members doing this work at their hospital or at others in the area. We strongly advise keeping careful notes of group process and, if possible, making regular audiotapes or videotapes. Children's artwork should be saved and dated. All of these methods will help group leaders to trace themes.

Finally, running a group for terminally ill children can be very draining. Group leaders need a safe place where they can process their own countertransference reactions and obtain the refueling necessary to prevent burnout.

SUMMARY

In our work at CHAP, we have learned a great deal. These brave children have taught us how to work through their fears and concerns by using our imaginations, our relationships with one another, and ourselves. We have learned to follow their lead in play, to approach emotionally painful topics with sensitivity, and to help facilitate their ability to resolve difficult issues.

By encouraging children in a safe, therapeutic environment to openly discuss themes of illness and death, as well as general concerns about the nature and course of HIV/AIDS, we believe that it is possible to help them focus on living their lives to the fullest.

REFERENCES

Adams-Greenly, M., Shiminski-Maher, T., McGowan, N., & Meyers, P. A. (1986). A group program for helping siblings of children with cancer. *Journal of Psychosocial Oncology, 4*(4), 55–67.

Gershoni, Y. (1985). *The use of structural family therapy and psychodramatic techniques in a children's group.* Unpublished manuscript.

Hammer, E. F. (1981). Projective drawings. In A. I. Rabin (Ed.), *Assessment with projective techniques: A concise introduction* (pp. 151–185). New York: Springer.

Piers, E. V. (1984). *Manual for Piers–Harris Children's Self-Concept Scales.* Los Angeles: Western Psychological Services.

Pless, I. B., & Roghmann, K. J. (1971). Chronic illness and its consequences: Some observations based on three epidemiological surveys. *Journal of Pediatrics, 79,* 351–359.

Pless, I. B., Roghmann, K. J., & Haggerty, R. J. (1972). Chronic illness, family functioning and psychological adjustment: A model for the allocation of preventive mental health services. *International Journal of Epidemiology, 1,* 271–277.

Tinkelman, D. G., Brice, J., Yoshida, G. N., & Sadler, J. E. (1976). The impact of chronic asthma on the developing child: Observations made in a group setting. *Annals of Allergy, 37*(3), 174–179.

Williams, K., & Baeker, M. (1983). Use of small group with chronically ill children. *Journal of School Health, 53,* 203–207.

11

· · · · · · · · · · · · ·

Caretakers'
Support Group

· · · · · · · · · · · · ·

Theresa Kreibick, PsyD

There is a small but growing body of literature supporting therapeutic group interventions with significant others and families of HIV/AIDS patients (Pearlin, Semple, & Turner, 1988; Greif & Porembski, 1988; Kelly & Sykes, 1989). Some additional group interventions have been documented that focus on helping family members and loved ones cope with grief following the death of persons with AIDS (Murphy & Perry, 1988).

This chapter outlines a group model for therapeutic intervention with nonprofessional caretakers of children with HIV/AIDS.

WHY A THERAPEUTIC INTERVENTION
WITH CARETAKERS?

Caretakers are the forgotten casualties of the AIDS epidemic. The term "caretakers" is a very broad one and includes a diversity of persons who have assumed responsibility for children with HIV/AIDS. Caretakers include mothers and fathers, who may or may not have HIV/AIDS themselves; grandmothers; older sisters; aunts, uncles, and cousins; and lastly, foster mothers who, despite no biological tie, have taken affected children into their homes. Often caretakers assume responsibility for the uninfected siblings as well.

The lives of these caretakers revolve around the medical crises of the children. Fevers, unexplained rashes, and a whole bevy of possible opportunistic infections tax their energy and resources, resulting in financial, emotional, and social strain.

Often caretakers are precisely the persons who, over the years, have held their families together and been the bulwark of strength, courage, and wisdom in hard times. Many have raised their own families and were earnestly looking forward to rest and relief from years of caring for young children and adolescents. Some older caretakers, when they face the possibility of raising a second family, are reluctant to admit anger. The caretakers are placed in a double bind. If they do not take in and raise these children, social agencies will take the children and the children will be lost to the family. On the other hand, caretakers, in committing themselves to raise another generation of children on the limited resources of a retirement income, are often financially forced to return to work. Caretakers also fear that they will not have the energy, patience, or continued good health to cope with raising young children. Caretakers with personal serious health problems worry constantly that health difficulties will interfere with their ability to care for the children.

> Hanna, an older woman participating in our group, had raised her own family, but had several adult children who died of AIDS. As a result, Hanna was left with 11 grandchildren to raise on her retirement income. At the time of her participation in the caretaker group, she was raising the last two of these grandchildren. Hanna was tired, but grateful that only two of the grandchildren were left to raise. She was increasingly concerned that she might not be able to finish what she had begun, even though she loved the children and had done her best with very limited resources.

Many times the caretakers are angry at the unfairness of having to raise a second or even a third family because of HIV/AIDS. They often hold the anger within themselves and are fearful to express their feelings within the family for fear of making things worse. Their children who contracted the virus and passed it on to the grandchildren are often dead or terminally ill. Even if the caretakers want to work through the anger directly, it is not possible to do so with the appropriate persons. The anger is often complicated by unresolved grief issues that are difficult to resolve openly within the family. A group intervention can become a safe place for caretakers to learn to deal with this unresolved anger and grief, and to channel the energy into productive action toward obtaining needed services for their families. Within our group, it appeared that caretakers who had weaker blood ties with the children they were raising could more easily harness the energy resulting from anger for positive action, such as bringing about change within the family relationships. Biological mothers or grandmothers had a more difficult time learning to express and deal with their anger and grief directly.

Usually, when a family experiences a major illness or death, friends, neighbors, and extended family provide buffers to help the family members deal with the stress in their time of need. The family's social support system gives encouragement, sympathy, and help with small tasks, such as cooking food and babysitting. This allows the family to cope better with the painful transition of death, or the stress due to serious illness. However, because of the strong social stigma associated with HIV/AIDS, families fear harassment if the diagnosis of HIV becomes public knowledge. Frequently (and as was often true within the support groups we conducted), only the caretaker will know of the HIV diagnosis, which then becomes a closely guarded secret. The caretaker feels very alone and overwhelmed by carrying this burden of knowledge. As a way of protecting the family, the caretaker withdraws from the social support system, for fear that disclosure will bring the family greater hurt and harm. Even if other family members know of the diagnosis, there is usually agreement among family members not to discuss it with outsiders. A group intervention can be a place where caretakers can receive support, nurturance, and normalization of their experiences in a safe environment that buffers some of their stress. Caretakers in the group can begin to process their emotions and grief without adding more stress to their families.

Many of the caretakers who participate in support groups of this type would never seek out, or agree to, individual therapy. The risks of opening wounds while alone with a therapist would simply have generated too much anxiety and fear. The group intervention provides the security of sharing experiences with other caretakers who have had similar or familiar difficulties. But for all caretakers who participate, the group intervention is of benefit because it provides a safe place for the healing process to begin.

WHY A GROUP THERAPEUTIC INTERVENTION?

It is precisely because these caregivers have lost their social support systems that the group model becomes an important modality for therapeutic intervention. To some degree, everyone in these groups experience this loss. Group members share with one another concerns they cannot disclose to their families, for fear they will increase the family members' sorrow and pain. Often a caregiver has functioned as the one who holds the family together. If the caregiver shares personal pain, family members may feel that the family is vulnerable to collapse. The group intervention provides the opportunity for caregivers to begin to trust other people outside of the family circle. Through the group process, healing begins to happen when caregivers begin to realize they are not alone, and when their experience of social isolation and alienation is normalized and, to some degree, becomes understood. A solidarity is established among group members that replaces or augments their missing or damaged social support systems. For many caregivers within our groups, the group meeting was the first time in many months that they had laughed or had the freedom to cry without feeling they were adding to the burdens of their families. The caretakers begin to experience an increased sense of control over their lives, and, in the process, become empowered to function more effectively within their current difficult life circumstances. One group member, reflecting on what she had learned within her group, stated:

"The burdens are too heavy to carry alone, and they wear you down. But when you talk with others, you share the burden and it is easier for you. You realize you are not alone. The burden becomes lighter. And sometimes you realize you are not the only one with problems."

WHAT TYPE OF GROUP?

The main purpose of the group is to empower participants to cope better with their difficult life situations. Process, more than content, is stressed, to give caretakers the opportunity to learn ways of dealing with anger, grief, and guilt. Caregivers also are able to learn new and improved coping skills for dealing with the loss of social support systems. As the group leader, I functioned more as a guide and gatekeeper than as an authority figure who possessed the most education or knowledge. The warm emotional environment of the group is designed to provide enough structure and emotional support to buffer members' fears that they will experience personal disintegration if they risk revealing their personal pain.

From the beginning, hope is instilled in caretakers by stressing their learned expertise in dealing with HIV/AIDS in their families. Members are treated as experts who have important knowledge to share with one another, and it is emphasized that group members can build on one another's strengths. Caretakers often share little funny daily events, which adds humor to the gathering and helps to put the members' difficulties in clearer perspective. Members are treated with respect, and contributions to the group are valued and praised. When a group member cries, others express care and concern, without probing for specific reasons for the person's tears. Group members know that sharing is welcome, not forced. Agendas for the sessions are controlled by the group participants.

ASSUMPTIONS IN BEGINNING THE GROUP

Since caretakers have lost much or all of their social support systems, the group, even if it becomes only a social gathering over sandwiches and orange juice, would be valuable for the members' emotional well-being. But a key goal, additionally, is to enhance the caretakers' coping skills so that they can provide a healthier emotional environment for the children.

Of course, not all caretakers would choose to or are able to participate in a group. Pain, fear of disclosure, and inability to share feelings are only some of the barriers to participation. If family losses are very recent, members are probably still too close to the pain of events to be able to risk the vulnerability of sharing with others. Sharing pain, for some, might be seen as weakness or a betrayal of family privacy. Others might fear rejection or negative reactions by the group facilitator (myself) because of a decision not to participate. Thus, special efforts are made, to stress that caretakers who choose not to come are welcome to do so later if they should change their minds, but care is also taken to communicate respect for their decision.

The value of support groups is also predicated on the ability of caretakers to be empathetic with one another. A process of positive identification would (it is hoped) occur among group participants, so that individual caretakers inspired by the heroic efforts of their peers would begin to recognize their own personal strengths and contributions. This new self-view could result in a more realistic view of the tremendous contribution individual caretakers make to help their families.

IMPACT OF MODE OF HIV TRANSMISSION
UPON FAMILY RELATIONSHIPS

Almost inevitably, the diagnosis of HIV within a family activates issues of guilt, anger, secrecy, and fear. These issues are especially power-

ful when the risk factors involved in the transmission of the virus are
sexual behaviors and/or substance abuse, especially injection drug use.

Most frequently, when a newborn child is diagnosed as having
HIV, the family is shocked to find that the virus is in the family. The
diagnosis serves to focus on secrets known only to a few members of
the family, or secrets that are known but not discussed openly within
the family. Frequently the infected adult has chosen not to disclose
the diagnosis of HIV/AIDS to her family. Sometimes, however, the family accidentally finds out and displaces their shock and anger onto medical personnel. In cases in which medical and mental health
professionals, because of legal restrictions, may not be able to inform
the family directly, a family intervention may enable the family to finally be able to talk openly with each other. They would then be able
to grieve about the diagnosis within the safety of the family intervention session. Family members frequently offer their support to the infected parent and child since the family may come to realize that drug
addiction might negatively impact on the consistency of care needed
in order for mother and child to stay healthy. The family intervention
provides families with opportunities to change long-standing family
communication patterns and unite in facing possible loss of social supports and in dealing with the stressors generated by the diagnosis of
HIV/AIDS in a family member.

Rage, a sense of betrayal, and deep depression often result when
a person learns that HIV has been transmitted to him or her by a relationship partner. In many cases, the diagnosis and subsequent
knowledge of the partner's behaviors can seriously damage or destroy
the relationship.

In the case of heterosexual transmission of the virus, as in that
of transmission via injection drug use, the first indication of the risk
for infection is often the diagnosis of HIV in a newborn child. If a
mother has contracted the virus from her male sexual partner, she may
have feelings of anger and rage toward him for having given a life-
threatening virus to her and her child, but she may also still have feelings of love for him. These conflicting feelings, and the associated guilt,
are confusing and stressful to her.

Frequently the woman's family members become very angry with
her partner when they learn of her diagnosis. Withdrawal of the family's emotional or financial support is a ploy frequently used to drive
a wedge between the woman and her partner. As a result, the woman
feels trapped, becomes depressed, and perceives her only options as
rejecting either her sexual partner or her family of origin. She may even
contemplate suicide.

In the case of a family where the risk factor for transmission of the virus is a past blood transfusion, guilt, anger, secrecy, and fear are also present, but for somewhat different reasons. The diagnosis of HIV/AIDS is a shock, since the family members trusted the life of their relative during a medical procedure to professionals. The professionals were not able to protect the relative from infection because the medical intervention happened at a time when the presence of HIV was not yet known, or it occurred during the early years of the AIDS crisis, when the blood supply was not known to be contaminated. The viral transmission may have even occurred through blood transfusion at a time when blood supplies were monitored, but a mistake was made in the screening process. In any case, the family perceives the medical establishment as the cause of the infection. There are usually strong feelings among the family members, who feel cheated or misled by the medical establishment.

EFFECTS OF SECRECY ON FAMILY MEMBERS

A caretaker is usually very aware of the social stigma associated with HIV/AIDS, and may experience feelings of personal vulnerability when the presence of HIV within the family becomes known. In the past, the caretaker may have depended upon his or her social support system—friends, neighbors, and extended family—to buffer and ameliorate the effects of daily stressful hassles and major life crises. With the diagnosis, the caretaker becomes fearful of retaliation and public embarrassment if it should become public knowledge. Concerns about rejection by close friends and acquaintances increase the fear of disclosure, sometimes to the point of slight paranoia.

As noted above, the diagnosis of HIV in a newborn is often the first time a family learns of the presence of the virus. The family becomes painfully aware of the risk factors that potentially caused the HIV infection: homosexuality or bisexuality, injection drug abuse, or heterosexual contact with an infected partner. In most families, the diagnosis tends to exacerbate existing family problems. There may be a long family history of denial or secrecy regarding family members' risk behaviors. The diagnosis may serve to reinforce existing secrecy boundaries or alliances already present within segments of the family. In any case, it will generate tremendous emotional pressures.

For some families, the diagnosis may spur a healthy boundary realignment. It may even become an opportunity for a family to join in a common mission to support the HIV-infected member. Shock is a common response. Conflicted feelings about the infected person and associated risk behaviors that challenge strongly held religious and/or moral values may also emerge. Often the conflict is between anger and disappointment about the behavior of the infected person and the need of other family members to comfort and help that person.

Often the caretaker becomes so fearful of disclosure that the diagnosis is not shared even with other family members living within the same household. The caretaker is upset and tries to hide his or her emotional turmoil from other family members, which only creates more strain for the family system.

When the infected family member becomes medically compromised, maintenance of secrecy becomes less possible. Family members often "stumble" upon the truth, sometimes in an abrupt and sometimes embarrassing manner. Uninformed family members may also feel angry at not being trusted, appreciated, and included in knowing the family secret. Often the disclosure comes so late that family members are denied the opportunity to prepare for loss and grief when the infected relative dies. Thus, the social stigma and secrecy issues associated with HIV/AIDS affect the entire family system, and effectively strip all members of their social support system.

GUILT RELATED TO THE TRANSMISSION OF HIV TO A CHILD

In cases in which the caretaker is a parent who has transmitted HIV to the child, guilt issues are very intense. The guilt is often associated with anger regarding past risky behaviors, which the parents felt were far behind them. With the diagnosis of the virus in the family, hopes of leaving the past behind are shattered. A cycle of anger and guilt has begun, sometimes with suicide viewed as the only escape. As the health of family members deteriorates the guilt and anger may become too great to handle and the parent may leave the family because of the parent's perceived failure to protect the child from his or her past.

In a case in which an HIV-infected woman discovers she has an infected child, frequently much anger is generated. As the child becomes more severely ill, the anger often becomes unconsciously directed outward and is projected onto medical personnel, who, despite their best efforts, are helpless to stop the decline of the child's health. Medical personnel often have difficulty understanding why the mother is so angry with them and noncompliant with their suggestions.

Another example involves a grandmother who secretly worried that she was the cause of all of her grandchild's suffering. She felt guilty and blamed herself for not having been stronger and challenged her adult child when she suspected injection drug use. The presence of her sick grandchild became a painful reminder to her of her own perceived failure as a parent. Alternatively, the grandmother viewed her afflicted grandchild as a second chance to correct the mistakes she felt she made in raising her own children. Such a scenario underscores the anguish of grandparents who perceive the sickness and suffering of their grandchildren to be a consequence of their failure to properly parent their own children.

In many such cases, a grandmother has little time to mourn the sudden death of her own child before having to assume responsibility for one or more grandchildren. The grandchildren are also immersed within the grief process after losing their parent(s). Often the grandmother/ caretaker is not able to help grandchildren with their grief because she has not even begun to deal with her own grief in losing her child.

ROLE OF THE GROUP FACILITATOR
WITH HOSPITAL STAFF

One of the first tasks of the facilitator in beginning a therapeutic group intervention is to earn the trust of the caretakers—a process that often takes time, and must be continued even after caretakers regularly attend group sessions. Initially, it can be helpful if the group facilitator forms an alliance with the clinic's medical personnel. In most cases, caretakers have already established a relationship, perhaps even a trusting one, with the medical doctors. These doctors were probably present at the time of diagnosis and the first family conference—one of the most difficult times for caretakers and families. During medical crises, the physicians were the persons who cared for their children. Thus, it is very important for medical doctors to openly support the group intervention with caretakers by attending the first few sessions, if possible.

The mental health professional can also assist medical personnel in dealing with medical compliance issues. Anxiety, depression, guilt, anger, fear, and the loss of social support systems all have a serious negative impact on the ability of caretakers and families to follow medical recommendations for the HIV-infected child. By dealing therapeutically with emotional issues, a mental health professional can bolster and support the caretakers. For a physician, this may translate directly into more consistent care of the child with HIV/AIDS, and better compliance with medical directives. In addition, when there is bad news, the physician has another ally whom the family trusts and with whom he or she can share communicating the message with the caretaker and other family members.

The facilitator also needs to establish good relationships with other members of the support staff in the pediatric AIDS clinic. Some staff education regarding the purpose and goals of the group intervention is needed. This may be accomplished informally by one-on-one conversations with adjunct staff members. However, a formal introduction to the intervention strategy, in which the help of the staff is explicitly solicited, is also needed. Adjunct staff members need to feel that the group can also be of help to them, rather than a duplication of their efforts, and is not something "secret" or "just talk." It is very important for the facilitator to defuse these images and to establish a personal relationship with the adjunct clinic staff. Otherwise, staff members may subvert the group intervention, either knowingly or unknowingly.

There should be a good communication flow between medical and adjunct clinic staff members and the facilitator. The facilitator needs to know well before the beginning of the weekly group when children are very ill or have died during the week. The death of a child touches not only the family of that child, but all caretakers who hear the news. Unresolved grief and loss issues are sure to be raised in the group, and the facilitator needs to know that it may be very difficult to assemble the group that week.

EXAMPLES OF ISSUES DISCUSSED

In the first sessions of one group, because clinical trials of zidovudine were just beginning, physicians directing the program, attended the first four weekly sessions, either together or separately. The agendas raised by caretakers in these first sessions addressed difficulties in deciding whether their children should begin taking zidovudine. Prior to the clinical trials the caretakers were accustomed to accepting medical recommendations from the physicians. With the beginning of the clinical trials, however, the physicians also assumed the role of researchers and could not advise caretakers how to make the decision regarding zidovudine for the children. The caretakers were overwhelmed by this role change and felt inadequate to make the decision regarding participation in the clinical trials. In the group, caretakers were able to verbalize their uncomfortable feelings. The group also provided the physicians with a forum for explaining why the role change had occurred.

One major issue frequently raised in the sessions was the loss of friends and social support systems. Caretakers frequently spoke of their loneliness before the group had started. The caretakers helped one another deal with the secrecy they felt they needed to protect themselves and their families. Some caretakers spoke with anger about the harassment they had endured at the hands of neighbors, former friends, and extended family members. They helped one another decide how, and how much, to tell school officials who needed to be informed that the children were taking zidovudine during school time.

Another major concern of the caretakers was how to tell the children about the nature of their illness. Some of the older children had learned of their HIV/AIDS status through being taunted in public by playmates in their neighborhood; this had been a very painful experience. Also, children who were 7 years of age or older began to ask about their illness. Their questions focused on why they, and not their siblings, needed to see the doctor all the time. Caretakers found that discussions on how to disclose the HIV/AIDS status to their children were very helpful to them in communicating this information.

Concerns for uninfected siblings of an HIV/AIDS child were also frequently raised as issues discussed within the group. Many of the siblings felt guilty because they did not have HIV and were very aware of their ill sibling's suffering. Sometimes they felt neglected and left out because the sick child appeared to be getting all the family's attention. Uninfected children also frequently became depressed by the illness and loss of a parent or a sibling. Methods for recognizing depression in a child and information on how to obtain services to help the depressed child were provided in the group.

Grief and issues of loss were often agenda items for group discussion. Each time a new loss occurred, the unresolved grief issues of past losses and separations were reawakened. As group members listened to one another, they received strength and courage from one another.

Laughter was especially helpful for the healing process, and the caretakers often delighted in sharing funny stories of better times with their children. Often, the laughter of the group helped balance the current stress or pain the caretakers were experiencing. If there was an issue caretakers felt they needed to share within the safety of the group, they would attend a group meeting even when it was not their clinic day.

DEPARTURE OF THE FACILITATOR
AND A FOLLOW-UP NOTE

If the facilitator has to leave her or his position, it is important that that departure be discussed. At least 3 months before leaving, the facilitator needs to speak about it during the weekly sessions: It is important that the departure be dealt with sensitively, so as not to add to the pain and grief associated with past losses suffered by the group's participants and to avoid their experiencing one more loss.

After the first year of weekly sessions with one support group and with the departure of the facilitator, during a "Family Night" program, some members asked of the director of the program whether they could be trained to intervene with other parents, grandparents, and foster parents. They wanted to serve as "buddies" for new families coming into the program.

REFERENCES

Greif, G. L., & Porembski, E. (1988). AIDS and significant others: Findings from a preliminary exploration of needs. *Health and Social Work, 13,* 259–265.
Kelly, J., & Sykes, P. (1989). Helping the helpers: A support group for family members of persons with AIDS. *Social Work, 34,* 239–242.
Murphy, S. P., & Perry, K. (1988). Hidden grievers. *Death Studies, 12,* 451–462.
Pearlin, L. I., Semple, S., & Turner, H. (1988). Stress of AIDS caregiving: A preliminary overview of the issues. *Death Studies, 12,* 501–547.

12

. . . .

Death and Dying/
Bereavement
and Mourning

. . . .

Nancy Boyd-Franklin, PhD
Elizabeth W. Drelich, MSW
Elena Schwolsky-Fitch, RN

Witnessing the death of a child, sibling, or parent is traumatic under
any circumstance (Walsh & McGoldrick, 1992), but when the loss is
a result of AIDS, the mourning process is that much more difficult
(Walker, 1991). In this chapter we highlight two issues that are critical for mourning and bereavement in HIV/AIDS families: (1) anticipatory loss, which is an inevitable consequence of a chronic (and
ultimately terminal) disease; and (2) survivor guilt, which is the anguish any relative (particularly a parent) feels when a family member
(particularly a child) dies an untimely death.

As HIV/AIDS patients live longer, bolstered by prophylactic treatments that arrest opportunistic infections, the patients and their families need to cope with anticipatory loss and the challenge of living with
a chronic terminal illness. The paradoxical dilemma for these families is how to maintain normality of life to at least some degree,
while preparing themselves emotionally for the painful inevitability
of death. If families can actively encourage and help their relatives
with HIV/AIDS to continue with work, school, and other ongoing activities, they are often more at peace when their relatives die, and

thus to some extent less likely to suffer from the anguish of survivor guilt.

This chapter focuses on bereavement and mourning in survivors in families of AIDS patients. However, some HIV-infected children and adults must cope with their own death- and dying-related issues while simultaneously mourning family members who have died. (See Chapters 8 and 10 for discussions of the issues for children who are dying. Chapter 14 explores the issues of bereavement and loss for professional caregivers.)

The mental health profession has begun to address the great need, among survivors of AIDS patients, for clinical and counseling support. The last section of this chapter addresses how to provide support for bereaved AIDS families, and offers examples of bereavement counseling interventions.

ANTICIPATORY LOSS

Anticipatory loss is an important issue for individuals and families coping with any terminal issues (Wolfelt, 1983). The complex nature of HIV/AIDS—course, symptomatology, and side effects—often elicits in family members a feeling of profound anticipatory loss. For this reason, the process of mourning may begin before the final stages of illness. This section discusses three aspects of HIV/AIDS that trigger the early onset of mourning: protracted illness, disfigurement, and neurological complications (Worden, 1991).

For families who witness the progressive mental and physical deterioration of an AIDS patient, the mourning period can begin early and is often painfully prolonged. AIDS, a harsh and relentless disease, may turn healthy, attractive young adults and children into virtual skeletons. Frequently, the gradual disfigurement and "wasting away" of patients cause family members to withdraw at this stage of the illness; as a result, many experience intense guilt once death has occurred. If this guilt is not discussed with anyone, it may continue to fester until it produces psychiatric symptoms such as depression. Such individuals should be referred for individual, family, or group therapy, or for bereavement counseling (Walker, 1991; Tiblier, Walker, & Rolland, 1989).

Neurological complications are often present in AIDS patients; as many as 80% suffer central nervous system damage. Depending on the area of the brain affected by the virus, behavior changes can reflect a deterioration as extreme as that experienced by Alzheimer's patients. Dementia, for example, can result in an early grieving response in the patient's family and friends (Worden, 1991, p. 114). Hanna and Mintz (Chapter 3) have discussed neuropsychological and cognitive deficits in children that are progressive and can exacerbate the grief reactions in parents and grandparents.

Families are frequently unprepared for the manifestations of neurological deterioration and dementia, which can include memory loss, loss of motor functioning, impaired gait, and inability to recognize family members. This can be painful and confuse children, who may feel that they somehow caused the deterioration. Educating relatives about physical and neurological deterioration will help them begin the process of preparatory mourning before death ensues.

It is vital for health and mental health professionals working with the relatives of AIDS patients to recognize the impact of severe or unexpected disease symptomatology, and thus to explore ways to work with the inevitable anxieties and need for mourning that such systems engender.

SURVIVOR GUILT

Once a patient has died, the bereavement process, like anticipatory mourning, goes through phases. Parkes (1972) writes of three types of reactions in survivors—(1) numbness, (2) yearning, and (3) disorganization and despair—which occur before the family begins to put its life back together. The response of survivor guilt is also commonplace, and, if unattended, can adversely affect the family's capacity to grieve.

As stated throughout this book, families stricken with HIV/AIDS experience multiple losses. Family members may not have time to mourn one death and loss before another occurs. HIV-infected children, having watched the deterioration of a family member, may grieve for that person while anticipating their own death. Often the burden of grieving and mourning falls on older extended family members, who must deal with a reversal of generational expectations: The loss of a child or grandchild is seen by some families as "against the laws of nature." There is often a great deal of survivor guilt associated with these losses for older family members. However, AIDS-related illnesses also affect both young adults and their children, who must deal with losses that occur at an unexpected time in their own life cycle.

Although guilt can play a major role in any form of bereavement and loss, it has particular implications for HIV/AIDS patients and their families. First, there is guilt over having infected others (including possibly a spouse or children), which may be fueled by family members through their own accusations. Second, when substance abuse is involved, grandparents who feel guilty and responsible for their children's deaths attempt to overcompensate with their grandchildren.

As with anticipatory loss, health providers need to recognize survivor guilt as being a frequent, sometimes inevitable aspect of the mourning process; thus, it should be addressed openly and directly whenever possible.

STAGES OF DENIAL, ANGER, DEPRESSION, AND ACCEPTANCE

AIDS patients and their families tend to undergo parallel processes of mourning. In our own work with surviving families, a model developed by Kübler-Ross (1969) in her seminal work with the dying has proved to be very useful. According to Kübler-Ross (1969), the five critical phases involved in mourning are denial, anger, bargaining, depression, and acceptance. This section focuses on denial, anger, and depression.

Denial—of the presence of disease, the severity of symptoms, or even the possibility of death—is a common response among relatives of HIV/AIDS patients. If family members are in denial at the time of diagnosis, it is likely that denial will persist during the asymptomatic stages of the disease. The patient and the family members require a great deal of understanding, patience, and support in this early phase. As a child or an adult becomes symptomatic, fear on the part of family, significant others, and even care providers may motivate a denial of the deterioration. In the case of a child, this denial can be intense and can involve a reluctance to disclose the illness to the child or other family members. It is important to note, however, that some aspects of denial can be healthy and protective, in that they allow patients to remain focused on life and the tasks of living (Detwiler, 1981; Tasker, 1992). But in general, when the patient's and family's energy is aimed at denying or avoiding the reality of the illness, the capacity to prepare adequately for the loved one's death is severely compromised.

The stage of anger or rage is critical for most patients and their families, but it is perhaps the most difficult part of the mourning process for everyone (including health care providers) to cope with. Many relatives' anger is initially directed at whoever or whatever—infected persons, infected needles, drugs, blood transfusion, medical procedure—is believed to be the source of the infection. It is doubly difficult if they themselves are the source. Nurses, doctors, therapists, and counselors need to anticipate this stage and discuss it openly with patients and their families as it occurs.

As the fact of death becomes real, sadness and loss are experienced. The patient (adult or child) may show vegetative signs of depression and may cry or weep often. For many grieving families, this is a time of great need and pain. A family counselor or therapist can facilitate communication by helping both the patient and family members understand where they are in the process. As the illness progresses toward a terminal stage, the family members should be especially encouraged to talk openly about their sadness among themselves or in support groups. Therapy can also be of benefit to the family during this difficult time.

Unfortunately, patients and family members often do not go through the process of mourning and bereavement at the same pace. Patients (children or adults) may be in the phase of acceptance of their disease and want to discuss the illness even as relatives are still in denial. Each new family member, upon learning the diagnosis, will go through mourning differently. The following case illustrates how differently the two parents of a child with AIDS dealt with their son's illness.

Case Example: Contrasting Stages within a Family

At 5 years of age Wendell Ingram came down with severe gum disease that required emergency surgery. Because the condition was so rare in a child of Wendell's age, the doctors who treated him took a detailed family history and recommended that Wendell and his parents be tested for HIV.

Although Mr. and Mrs. Ingram agreed to be tested, they repeatedly expressed their disbelief that either of them could be HIV-infected, despite Mrs. Ingram's former injection drug use. Mrs. Ingram, who had been clean and sober for 7 years, was convinced that if she had contracted HIV during her period of drug use she would have already exhibited signs of infection.

When the results showed that Mr. Ingram was negative but that both Wendell and Mrs. Ingram were positive, the family disputed the accuracy of the tests and insisted that they all be tested again. However, the results of the second test were the same.

Mr. Ingram, who was 15 years older than Mrs. Ingram, worked full time outside the home while Mrs. Ingram was a full-time homemaker. Wendell was their only child.

The parents agreed not to tell Wendell of his or his mother's diagnosis. At that time Wendell's only symptom had been the gum disease, and that had been successfully treated.

Although Mrs. Ingram was very involved in her son's treatment, Mr. Ingram avoided the medical staff and did not come to the clinic with Wendell. He would not even talk to his wife about their son's condition in the privacy of their home. The different ways in which the Ingrams were handling their son's disease was causing strain in their marriage.

Wendell attended the local public school and did very well until his medical status became more complicated. He started losing weight and energy. When his memory and ability to concentrate became compromised his grades began to suffer. His mother noticed him becoming more dependent upon her, and his emotions were more erratic. A series of psychological tests suggested that, over a year's time, his cognitive and graphomotor skills had significantly deteriorated.

Mrs. Ingram inquired about medical options that might be available to deal with her son's weight and energy loss. Even when an extreme medical treatment was recommended—a central line broviac that would provide total parenteral nutrition—Mr. Ingram continued not to get involved with the decision making.

Mrs. Ingram felt that the time had come to tell her son the truth, but her husband still resisted, claiming it would only increase his son's suffering.

Mr. Ingram's views prevailed, and Wendell was not informed of his diagnosis when the broviac was placed. Wendell seemed to accept the explanation he was offered: that he had problems with his blood and gaining weight and that the tube in his chest would allow his body and blood to get better by having food and medicine go directly into his bloodstream.

Mrs. Ingram felt the need to get as much information as she could for herself and Wendell before a crisis occurred, and she explored the alternatives of do not resuscitate (DNR) orders, living wills, and autopsies. As of now she is continuing to try to get her husband involved in the decision making and has achieved progress in this area. Although he is still firm in many of his opinions, he is listening to the other side and asking appropriate questions.

Mrs. Ingram, whose health status has remained stable and asymptomatic, has stated many times that she is living life one day at a time. She does not want her son's life to be overshadowed by a miserable death, but wants him to have as beautiful, fun-filled, and full a life as possible despite his illness. She is planning for the future with all the information she can gather.

BEREAVEMENT ISSUES IN CHILDREN

Health care providers do not always recognize that children and adults have very different responses to the death of a family member from

AIDS. As Wolfelt (1983) points out, children suffer more from "the loss of parental support than from the death experience itself" (p. 9). These child survivors are too often neglected when the rest of the family is busy coping with a loss.

Factors Influencing Children's Responses to Death

Wolfelt (1983) lists the following major factors influencing a child's response to death:

- the relationship with the person who has died—the "meaning" of the death
- the nature of the death—when, how and where the person died
- the child's own personality and previous experiences with death
- the child's chronological and developmental age
- the availability of family/social/community support and
- most importantly, the behavior, attitudes and responsiveness of parents and other significant adults in the child's environment. (p. 21)

Children may ask questions after the death as a way of connecting with their parents or other extended family caretakers. If children learn of the AIDS-related death of a parent, sibling, or family member through rumors, it then becomes a "toxic family secret" that the entire family colludes to avoid. For an adequate process of grief and mourning to occur, the energy invested in keeping this secret has to be gradually and gently released.

Children's Perceptions of Death
at Different Age Levels

Researchers who have explored children's perceptions of death at different age levels (Nagy, 1948; Anthony, 1971; Melear, 1972; Wolfelt, 1983) agree that children are ignorant of the meaning of the word "death" before the age of 3 or 4. From about ages 3 to 6, children believe that death is temporary and that a dead person will reappear. At 6 children begin to understand that death involves the cessation of biological functioning and is final. Children from ages 5 to 9 are often preoccupied with death rituals and will play them out over and over (Anthony, 1971).

Nagy (1948) and Anthony (1971) have shown that at about age 9 or 10 children begin to develop a philosophical understanding that death is inevitable for all of us (Nagy, 1948) and to acquire a realistic perception of the meaning of death.

Children's Psychological Adjustment to the Death of a Parent

A number of researchers have explored children's psychological adjustment to the terminal illness and death of a parent (Siegel et al., 1992; Wolfelt, 1983; Silverman & Worden, 1992). Particular attention has been paid to the psychological tasks that these children must undergo (Baker, Sedney, & Gross, 1992; Silverman, Nichman, & Worden, 1992). In addition, an increasing body of research is documenting the connection between parental death in childhood and vulnerability to depression and anxiety in adulthood (Mireault & Bond, 1992; Saler & Skolnick, 1992). Given these realities, it is very important that health and mental health providers be aware of the nature of children's grief reactions, as well as of preventive interventions that can help increase the likelihood of a positive mental health outcome for these children.

Childhood Grief Reactions and Preventive Interventions

Jackson (1965), Wass and Corr (1982), Vogel (1975), and Wolf (1973) have provided a number of guidelines that are helpful to parents and professionals in telling children about death and helping them to understand death. It is important, however, to be aware of the potential range of responses to death and loss that may be seen in HIV/AIDS children (see Chapters 8 and 10) as they begin to deal with anticipatory loss. HIV-infected children and their noninfected siblings may respond individually to the death of a parent, family member, or another sibling from AIDS.

Wolfelt (1983) has described a child's initial response to the death of a loved one as emotional shock, denial, disbelief, and numbness, and states that the major task of the adult caregiver—whether a family member or a health or mental health professional—is to "keep the grieving child in touch with a supportive, caring part of the world" (p. 33).

Adults, unaware that children do not comprehend the permanence of death until after age 6, may be shocked when they go right on playing after being told of a death. Active play is often their way of working it through. However, there are frequently also somatic manifestations of grief in children, such as insomnia or hypersomnia; appetite loss or excessive hunger; exhaustion; nervousness; headaches; stomach aches; difficulty in swallowing; shortness of breath; and rashes.

Another common reaction of children to death and bereavement is regressive behavior—unwillingness to be separated from parents or significant others, even to go out to play; the desire to be "babied," to be rocked or nursed, or to sleep in the same bed as a parent; talking in "baby talk"; asking others to do things the children could now do themselves; changes in behaviors relating to school (e.g., a refusal to work independently, demanding constant attention, or feigning illness to avoid school); and difficulty in acting appropriately with peers (Wolfelt, 1983). Parents and caregivers should also be aware that children who have lost family members to AIDS may begin expressing fears of losing others and may become unusually clingy, anxious, and fearful of going out.

Families overwhelmed by multigenerational HIV/AIDS may snap or yell at the children, telling them to "grow up." With a counselor's help, parents or grandparents can offer more support to the children involved. When adults meet the surviving children's needs of love and support, these regressive behaviors often stop.

Other common responses in children are panic about survival and worries about whether they will be taken care of, particularly when a parent has died of AIDS. If the children have had no opportunity to prepare for their parent's loss, panic will supersede the initial numbness and shock. Health and mental health professionals can intervene preventively with such a family by helping parents, grandparents, and extended family members to facilitate honest, open discussion of the parent's death and the plan for caretaking of the children—ideally in family counseling sessions prior to death, when the parent can be helped to say goodbye to his or her children and leave them in caring hands. In most situations, however, the sessions occur after a loss. In an atmosphere of secrecy, when children have not been included in the plans for their future caretaking, intense acting out can often occur. Many different treatment modalities can be utilized, including bereavement groups for children (Siegal, Mesagno, & Christ, 1990).

In many cases, children as young as 9 or 10 years of age, particularly in multigenerational inner-city families, assume the "parental child" role by caring for their own parent(s) and younger siblings during the final agonizing stages of AIDS or after a parent's death. Although these children may appear to be very functional, particularly in disorganized and chaotic families, they may begin to manifest acting-out behavior as they get older if appropriate adult generational control does not reassert itself. Because children are often very angry when parents or much-loved family members die, the resultant acting-out behavior (tantrums, fighting, defiance with parents and grandparents, academic problems, etc.) is a very common but little-understood way for them to express the pain of their grief over the death. Family bereavement counseling is advised, so that adults do not abdicate their parental role.

In fact, it was the acting-out behavior of noninfected children of parents who had died of AIDS or the siblings of HIV-infected children that first brought HIV/AIDS to the attention of mental health professionals at our Community Mental Health Center.

A multiple-family group for 10–12-year-old conduct-disordered children and their caretakers was started at a mental health facility. The family treatment model consisted of having the children seen by one team of therapists, and the caretakers by another team during the first half of each session. The two groups were then brought together for the last half of the session.

Initially, the parents and caretakers had difficulty pinpointing what was occurring in their families when their children first began to act out. After about 3 months of treatment, one of the caretakers disclosed that a family member had died of AIDS at approximately the time when the acting-out behavior had begun. Gradually, all of the parents and caretakers revealed that they had each had members of their extended families die AIDS-related deaths.

When the caretakers and the children were brought together, it became clear that these issues had never been discussed, and that adults and children alike had been carrying the burden of the secrecy. Many of these noninfected children also felt angry and ignored by the adults, who were preoccupied with caring for ill family members. Their acting-out, conduct-disordered behavior became more understandable as both adults and children discussed together for the first time the unresolved feelings of sadness, loss, and mourning. This therapeutic process occupied the work of the group for many months.

Foster parents or extended family members who take in children who have experienced multigenerational losses because of AIDS often report that the children refuse to get close to them. The fear of future loss in these children is often disguised as acting-out, hostile, rejecting, and oppositional behavior. Family therapy interventions (see Chapter 7) can help these surrogate parents understand the underlying dynamics of grief and fear of loss, and set limits on acting-out behavior, yet also respond to the children's plea for love, support, acceptance, and understanding.

Guilt and self-blame are common grief responses in children and adults alike. Young children often believe that they are responsible for a parent's death and engage in "magical thinking," whereby if they think something they can make it happen. With children, it is often good practice to ask the following question: "Kids who have had a parent [or sister or brother] die often tell me that they believe they did something to cause it. Do you believe that you did something?" (If the answer is yes, inquire what.)

Case Example: Magical Thinking

Sue was a 5-year-old child whose sibling Carol (age 6) had died of AIDS. Sue began acting out and throwing temper tantrums after her sister's death. When the question above was posed to her, Sue tearfully confessed that she felt that she had killed Carol by her anger.

Sue had been very angry because Carol had "gotten everything because she was sick." She got a special Christmas party and presents from Santa Claus at the hospital. She also got to go to Disney World (a gift from the Make-a-Wish Foundation) and Sue was not allowed to go. It was only during a therapy session that the therapist working with Sue was able to help her see that she had been angry at her sister and jealous of her, but that thoughts and anger and wishes could not kill someone.

Children often have difficulty expressing their feelings of sadness, emptiness, and withdrawal in words. Individual play therapy (see Chapter 8) can help children with HIV/AIDS work through their intense feelings in play, art, work, or writing. Chapter 10 describes the application of these techniques to group therapy to deal with death, dying, bereavement, and grief in children who are HIV-infected.

The Good Grief Program at Judge Baker Children's Center in Boston, founded by Dr. Sandra Fox, enables schools, camps, and community groups to help children deal with death and dying. The program's approach is based on the idea that "children can be taught skills that will enable them to deal with loss" (Foundation of Children with AIDS, 1990, p. 93). The grieving process, which often takes 2 to 3 years in adults, may take longer in children. Psychologists in this program have found that "bereavement comes in waves," echoing Bowen's (1976) concept of the "emotional shock waves" caused by a death.

Zambelli and DeRosa (1992) have described bereavement support groups for school-aged children. These can be very helpful as a preventive intervention during a period of loss.

OTHER ASPECTS OF BEREAVEMENT AND GRIEF COUNSELING WITH CHILDREN AND FAMILIES

Preparing for Anniversary Reactions

Many families are unprepared for the profound impact of the anniversary of a death. It is very painful when friends, coworkers, and extended family members are not sympathetic and expect them to "get on with life." A pediatric nurse, who has cared for HIV/AIDS children and families and who has herself experienced the loss of her husband to AIDS, eloquently describes the power of these anniversaries.

> As a pediatric nurse I had been working with children with AIDS since the earliest years of the epidemic. In one devastating moment, when my husband was diagnosed in 1988, AIDS went from being someone else's problem to being part of the fabric of my own life.
>
> After the diagnosis, we faced the issues this disease confronts a family with: the possibility of other infected family members, disclosure, bouts of acute life-threatening infections, discrimination, loss of income, and acceptance of the terminal stage of illness.
>
> As a nurse, I had worked with many families following the loss of a loved one, but I was totally unprepared for the confusing flood of emotions I experienced following my husband's death in May 1990. My mind kept wandering back to the last few hours of his life and the actual moments of his dying. I felt a great need to talk it through over and over again, to try to understand.
>
> During this time, friends would call to find out how I was or what I was doing. After a couple of weeks, most people seemed to assume that I would go back to work and get on with my life. I felt that they needed me to be "all right" so they could resume their normal routine without having to worry about me. Only the bereavement group I had joined and a few close friends gave me the support I needed to grieve in my own way without a timetable.
>
> I missed my husband intensely for months. I looked at old photo albums, staring at pictures of us together, remembering his voice, his hands, little quirks of his personality. Later, there was a period of time when I couldn't look at his pictures and I put them all away.
>
> It has now [November 1991] been 18 months since my husband's death, and I am still very aware of many "anniversaries" of our life together.
>
> The first anniversary of my husband's death has come and gone, and I am still surprised by unexpected grief that overtakes me on days that seem to have no particular significance until I remember: "Oh,

this is the weekend we drove up to the country and went bike rid-
ing." Major holidays loom ahead like raging rapids in a river—to be
negotiated with great care. I emerge on the other side of each one
with tremendous relief. Though the warm memories are beginning
to replace some of the pain now, something as simple as a schmaltzy
movie can open the floodgates.

Health and mental health care providers can learn a great deal from
these sensitive words: first, that grief reactions are very individual; second, that they can continue over time and can be triggered by unlikely "anniversaries"; and finally, that family members often need time
to process these reactions and to discuss the death of their loved one
many times before they can fully integrate the reality.

Addressing the Lack of Support
for Bereaved AIDS Families

Support for families through the bereavement period after the AIDS-
related death of a child or another family member is often lacking. Because of the stigma and secrecy surrounding AIDS, medical, nursing,
and social service professionals who treat AIDS patients provide the
primary caretakers or significant others with their main means of support. Often, informal networks of caregivers and family members form
during the visiting hours of clinics and hospitals. However, after the
death of a child or a family member with AIDS, the surviving caretakers or family members or children often find themselves cut off from
these supports, in part because of the survivors' own reactions and
in part because of service delivery overload within the health care
system.
   Surviving family members may be so overwhelmed by their grief
reactions that they cannot bear to enter the hospital after a death. Some
will avoid coming near those who knew the child or family member
who died, because the constant reminders are too painful. Other
caretakers and family members project their own feelings of power-
lessness and helplessness onto the doctors and nurses, and become angry at them for not being able to save their loved one. Still other family
members report that they didn't feel that they "belonged" any more
once the death occurred. Some caretakers withdraw because they sense
that other families are frightened by the death; it is a painful reminder
of the mortality issues for their own ill family members. Finally, pediatric and medical units are often conflicted about reporting deaths of
patients, for fear that it will cause other families to lose hope. This
attempt at protection is misguided, because families may become very

close during the course of the illness and experience unresolved grief reactions when they are not allowed to say goodbye to or mourn for a child or patient from another family.

In our experience, nurses, physicians, social workers, psychologists, and psychiatrists working in AIDS programs deal with large caseloads; this makes it difficult to follow up adequately on families of patients who have died. In addition, these nursing, medical, and mental health professionals may have trouble maintaining ongoing contact with some of the families of a child or patient to whom they were close (see Chapter 14) because of their own bereavement process. In other cases informal networks continue to function for years, as infected adults keep in touch and continue to look out for each other, sometimes calling care providers to report the worsening condition of adults who are not obtaining regular health care.

Programs for children and adults with AIDS must provide some mechanism for bereavement counseling and support for both families and staff (Wiener & Septimus, 1991). This often involves outreach during the early stages after the loss. The program could be modeled after hospice programs and should involve home visits to counter the feelings of abandonment experienced by survivors.

Among the most powerful interventions for families have been multiple-family bereavement groups led by health and mental health professionals. The groups meet in a setting removed from the hospital or clinic, such as a church or community center. Some groups are time-limited and provide approximately 3 months of postbereavement counseling. Others are ongoing, with families participating over time and new families replacing those who have left the group. Some bereavement groups work well on a once-per-week model; others might meet every other week. It is important that the frequency, time, and place of the meetings remain constant. Since meetings are open to any family member who has lost a relative to AIDS, different ages and generations within the families are represented.

Barouh (1992) discusses a model for a bereavement support group that has been developed to address the isolation often experienced by families after the death of an AIDS patient. The bereavement support group has evolved from our support group for the caretakers (Chapter 11 has described the prototype of this group). Both groups are held consecutively on the same evening and have the same facilitators, which fosters continuity and allowed bereaved family members to stay in contact with and obtain support from their former support group members.

The caretakers' support group focuses on the loved ones who are ill, while the bereavement group focuses on the caretakers themselves and their own reactions. Those who have participated in the support group usually enter the bereavement group a few weeks after the death of their loved ones, when the initial shock of the death has begun to be absorbed and many of the funeral rituals have ended.

The bereavement group becomes a focus for mourning and loss issues for members on many levels (Barouh, 1992). Parents and grandparents express survivor guilt at having outlived their children. Moreover, during the bereavement and mourning period, family members are able to address concerns about their loved ones' risk behaviors (homosexuality or bisexuality, drug use, etc.), which may have been unspoken while the patients were dying.

"Unfinished business" with the deceased, including feelings of guilt, anger, blame, and loss, are explored. It may be difficult for families with a strong religious or spiritual belief system to discuss their anger at the Supreme Being and/or at religion, but it is often very helpful for such families to recognize that other families have felt this and have come to terms with these conflicts.

Finally, the bereavement group often helps family members to cope with the issues of "getting on with their lives" after the death of a loved one. This is often difficult on many levels. Guilt intrudes when survivors question whether it is okay to have fun, enjoy life, or even make a new life. The process of caring for a terminally ill family member is an all-consuming and isolating undertaking. The process of reconnecting surviving family members to friends, family, work, and so forth is complicated with AIDS families, in that members often deal with more than one AIDS patient and must cope with anticipatory loss issues for the next infected family member; thus, they may be unable to move on with their own life issues.

Barouh (1992) eloquently states that although most surviving family members would acknowledge that working through bereavement and grief issues is painful, the "healing process" of sharing their "humor and tears" with the other bereavement group members makes it all worthwhile (p. 65).

REFERENCES

Anthony, S. (1971). *The discovery of death in childhood and after*. London: Allan Lan.
Baker, J., Sedney, M. A., & Gross, E. (1992). Psychological tasks for bereaved children. *American Journal of Orthopsychiatry, 62*(1), 105–116.
Barouh, G. (1992). *Support groups: The human face of the HIV/AIDS epidemic*. Huntington Station, NY: Long Island Association for AIDS Care.

Bowen, M. (1976). Family reaction to death. In P. J. Guerin (Ed.), *Family therapy: Theory and practice*. New York: Gardner Press.

Detwiler, D. A. (1981). The positive function of denial. *Journal of Pediatrics, 99*, 401–402.

Foundation of Children with AIDS. (1990, July/August). Bereavement [Special issue]. *Children with AIDS Newsletter, 2*(4).

Jackson, E. N. (1965). *Telling a child about death*. New York: Channel Press.

Kübler-Ross, E. (1969). *On death and dying*. New York: Macmillan.

Melear, J. D. (1972). Children's conceptions of death. *Journal of General Psychology, 123*(2), 359–360.

Mireault, G. C., & Bond, L. (1992). Parental death in childhood: Perceived vulnerability and adult depression anxiety. *American Journal of Orthopsychiatry, 62*(4), 517–524.

Nagy, M. (1948). The child's theories concerning death. *Journal of General Psychology, 73*, 2–37.

Parkes, C. M. (1972). *Bereavement: Studies of grief in life*. New York: International Universities Press.

Saler, L., & Skolnick, N. (1992). Childhood parental death and depression in adulthood: Roles of surviving parent and family environment. *American Journal of Orthopsychiatry, 62*(4), 504–516.

Siegel, K., Mesagno, F., & Christ, G. (1990). A prevention program for bereaved children. *American Journal of Orthopsychiatry, 60*(2), 168–175.

Siegel, K., Mesagno, F., Karus, D., Christ, G., Banks, K., & Moynihan, R. (1992). Psychological adjustment of children with a terminally ill parent. *Journal of the American Academy of Child and Adolescent Psychiatry, 31*(2), 327–333.

Silverman, P., Nichman, S., & Worden, J. W. (1992). Detachment revisited: The child's reconstruction of a dead parent. *American Journal of Orthopsychiatry, 62*(4), 494–503.

Silverman, P., & Worden, J. (1992). Children's reactions in the early months after the death of a parent. *American Journal of Orthopsychiatry, 62*(1), 93–104.

Tasker, M. (1992). *How can I tell you?: Secrecy and disclosure when a family member has AIDS*. Bethesda, MD: Association for the Care of Children's Health.

Tiblier, K., Walker, G., & Rolland, J. (1989). Therapeutic issues when working with families of persons with AIDS. In E. Macklin (Ed.), *AIDS and families* (pp. 81–127). Binghamton, NY: Harrington Park Press.

Vogel, L. (1975). *Helping a child understand death*. Philadelphia: Fortress.

Walker, G. (1991). *In the midst of winter*. New York: Norton.

Walsh, F., & McGoldrick, M. (1992). *Living beyond loss: Death in the family*. New York: Norton.

Wass, H., & Corr, C. (1982). *Helping children cope with death: Guidelines and resources*. New York: Hemisphere/McGraw.

Wiener, L., & Septimus, A. (1991). Psychosocial consideration and support for the child and family. In P. Pizzo & C. Wilfert (Eds.), *Pediatric AIDS* (pp. 577–594). Baltimore: Williams & Wilkins.

Wolf, A. (1973). *Helping your child understand death.* New York: Child Study.

Wolfelt, A. (1983). *Helping children with grief.* Muncie, IN: Accelerated Development.

Worden, J. W. (1991). *Grief counseling and grief therapy: A handbook for the mental health practitioner* (2nd ed.). New York: Springer.

Zambelli, G., & DeRosa, A. (1992). Bereavement support groups for school age children: Theory intervention and case example. *American Journal of Orthopsychiatry, 62*(4), 484–493.

SECTION V
......

SERVICE DELIVERERS AND SYSTEMS ISSUES

13

A Multisystems Approach to Service Delivery for HIV/AIDS Families

Nancy Boyd-Franklin, PhD
Mary G. Boland, MSN, RN

All complex health problems involve numerous treatment providers, clinical settings, and levels of interventions pertaining to different disease stages, from emergency hospitalization to home care. Pediatric HIV/AIDS—a chronic, multigenerational, ultimately terminal disease with many psychosocial stressors—in particular necessitates an approach to health and mental health service delivery that is flexible and takes into account the multiplicity of people and institutions involved in providing these services. Such a "multisystems approach" is at the heart of the Multisystems HIV/AIDS Model outlined in Chapter 1 and described throughout this book.

The goals of the multisystems approach described in this chapter are as follows: (1) to integrate medical and psychosocial care; (2) to support the family unit by providing backup mental health/therapeutic social services; and (3) to empower families to manage the numerous institutions and agencies involved, and to participate as much as possible in the treatment process and in the decisions made regarding their children and family members.

RELEVANCE OF A MULTISYSTEMS APPROACH FOR INNER-CITY POOR FAMILIES

Contrary to stereotypes, the reach of HIV/AIDS is demographically diverse—encompassing rural as well as urban areas, middle-class as well as poor families. Accordingly, the multisystems approach is useful for any family living with HIV/AIDS. However, it is essential for work with inner-city poor families; therefore, this chapter focuses primarily on those families.

Within the context of life for inner-city families, the daily hardships of poverty, homelessness, unemployment, crime, violence, drugs, teenage pregnancy, and high child mortality rates abound. Given this context, HIV/AIDS becomes one more overwhelming problem in a landscape of many. Poverty for many inner-city families is accompanied by the intrusion of numerous outside systems and agencies into their lives. Boyd-Franklin (1989) has explored the impact of schools, courts, child welfare agencies, housing agencies, welfare departments, police, and mental health care providers on these families. With HIV/AIDS, one must add to that list hospitals, health care systems, Medicaid, Medicare, visiting nurses, hospital and clinic social workers, and medical transportation systems. For many families, this vast array of agencies and individuals is overwhelming. The difficult task of managing all of these systems becomes a major additional stressor for these families.

The multisystems approach provides a means by which families and service providers can be empowered to cope with these issues. In order to utilize this model effectively, one must first understand the complexity of these many agencies and systems. The key aspects of the approach are as follows: (1) coordination of care and effective case management; (2) the use of a multidisciplinary team; and (3) involvement of the family in the decision-making process.

ASPECTS OF THE MULTISYSTEMS APPROACH

Coordination of Care and Effective Case Management

Boland, Czarniecki, and Haiken (1992) and Anderson (1990) have demonstrated that HIV-infected children require so many medical, mental health, and social services that the task of coordinating their care is a mammoth one. Barth, Pietrzak, and Ramler (1993) have pointed out that any child or family may have as many as 12 case managers within different clinics and agencies. The multisystems approach provides an opportunity for cooperative efforts on the part of the agencies involved to provide coordinated care. The case example at the end of this chapter gives a demonstration of how this can be accomplished.

A central issue for the different agencies and individuals involved in the care of HIV-infected children is the question of who is going to take the responsibility for the coordination of care and case management. This question is complicated by the fact that each agency, clinic, hospital, and so on has its own case management staff. In the ideal world, it would be preferable for one case manager to take charge of coordinating and communicating with other systems. The real world, however, is often characterized by duplication of effort and lack of clarity regarding the boundaries of responsibility. Therefore, it is very important to be aware of the need to call multisystems meetings with representatives from different programs in order to clarify roles and responsibilities (see the case example, below). At this meeting, the group can decide on an overall coordinator who will disseminate information to the other care providers and to the family or foster family caretakers.

These issues can exist within a program as well as between programs. In hospitals, for example, where a medical model exists, it is extremely important for providers from different disciplines to meet often for multidisciplinary team case conferences, in order to discuss successful interventions and to foster future coordination in situations where there has been boundary confusion or duplication of effort.

The Use of a Multidisciplinary Team

A recognition of the complex needs of HIV-infected children and families has stimulated the development of innovative programs designed to provide a multidisciplinary team approach, which offers comprehensive services and minimizes fragmentation. HIV infection requires a care delivery system capable of meeting physical, psychosocial, and family needs. Various approaches can be used, provided that family participation is viewed as an integral component of the process.

A number of studies have begun to address the multiple needs of these families. Falloon, Eddy, Werner, and Pizzo (1989) found that the vast majority (72–82%) of parents stated that they sought information pertaining to HIV infection and available treatment, as well as assistance with dealing with the disclosure of the diagnosis. Many families were concerned about disclosure to other systems, including neighbors, school, extended family, church, and community members.

Programs such as the Children's Hospital AIDS Program and the

Family Place in Newark have adopted a multidisciplinary team approach as a method of coordinating services within an agency. Recognizing that the chronicity of HIV infection requires a comprehensive approach to care, the Children's Hospital AIDS Program is organized to provide such services. The program, although based in a hospital, is not site specific. Continuity of care is maintained for the families by using multidisciplinary care providers, who recognize the family as a significant participant in the team. Services are delivered in a manner that seeks to reduce the time burden for families, who must see many different care providers, with case managers available to assure coordination. Significant time and energy is directed toward supporting parents and guardians to interact assertively with the multiple systems that impact their lives.

Seibert, Garcia, Kaplan, and Septimus (1989) describe three pediatric AIDS programs in New York, Miami, and Los Angeles. Developmental and educational services for the children, community outreach efforts, and attempts to meet the social and emotional needs of the children and the families are discussed, as well as counseling interventions and the inclusion of psychologists and social workers.

Falloon et al. (1989) describe the program at the National Institute of Mental Health, where a well-organized multidisciplinary team follows the pediatric cancer patient model. In addition to the medical and nursing staff, the team includes social workers, psychologists, dieticians, teachers, clergy, and occupational, physical, and recreational therapists. A social worker and primary nurse, who facilitate communication and compliance and who respond to needs, are assigned to each family upon initial contact. Important considerations include (1) structured and informal educational sessions to answer questions and provide information to promote optimal care of each child; (2) early psychosocial evaluation and intervention, including counseling of child and family; (3) appropriate referrals to agencies and services to deal with issues of child care, foster care, child custody, school arrangements, home health care, and finances; and (4) referral of family members to substance abuse programs as necessary.

The Developmental and Family Services Unit at the Rose F. Kennedy Center University Affiliated Program in New York City uses a multidisciplinary team to assess the developmental and psychosocial needs of HIV-infected children and their families. The team includes developmental pediatricians, social workers, psychologists, a medical ethicist, a psychiatrist, a psychoeducational specialist, and occupational, physical, and language therapists, each of whom performs a complete evaluation. At a multidisciplinary conference, an Individual Family Service Plan for each child and family is formulated. The needs of the children and the families have included referrals for special educational services; occupational, physical, speech, and psychoeducational therapies on a regular basis; advocacy and help in obtaining concrete services; and ongoing supportive psychotherapy and counseling to improve parental coping skills in handling children with developmental disabilities and chronic illness. Counseling for both biological and foster siblings has also been provided (Happios, Gross, & Lieberman, 1990).

Before we present a case example relevant to the multisystems approach, two other important systems must be discussed: the child welfare and foster care systems.

MULTISYSTEMS ISSUES WITHIN THE CHILD WELFARE AND FOSTER CARE SYSTEMS

Among the most complex multisystems issues that health care and mental health care providers encounter are those presented by the child welfare and foster care systems. Often, interventions with these systems have been delegated to social workers within the major systems. Other professionals (i.e., physicians, nurses, psychologists, and psychiatrists) frequently receive little training in the roles of these systems.

Given the increasing burdens and demands placed on all of the systems, which are being exacerbated by cuts in services resulting from the economic recession (both federal and state), the key areas of case management or coordination of services are often either redundant (i.e., replicated within each agency) or nonexistent. It is therefore important that health and mental health providers of all disciplines have a working knowledge of the complex multisystems issues involved in the child welfare and foster care systems. This section addresses the following key areas:

- Involvement of child welfare and child protective services with HIV/AIDS families
- Biological family care versus foster care
- Providing good-quality foster care interventions for HIV-infected children
- Transitional placements: Shelter and respite care
- Treatment issues for children in foster care
- The role of child welfare workers
- The role of therapists and mental health workers

Involvement of Child Welfare and Child Protective Services with HIV/AIDS Families

Many, although not all, inner-city families raising children with HIV infection are or have been involved with child welfare and/or child protective services. In some instances, this involvement predated the diagnosis of HIV. Some of these families have a multigenerational history of drug involvement. Often, if a parent (particularly a mother) is involved with drugs, the care of the children has been precarious for some time. If the parents have been reported to child protective or child welfare services for abuse or neglect, there may be a history of such involvement. In many families, placement with extended family members is informal, and the placement decision is made within the family. In other cases, the child protective services may make an extended family or kinship placement of a child or children; if such a placement is not available, foster care may be sought.

In some hospital systems, when a diagnosis of pediatric HIV infection is made, child welfare systems are automatically notified, especially if the child's mother is drug-addicted. (Since this is not true of all systems, workers should review procedures in their state.) Also, as parents who have AIDS and are caring for their own HIV-infected children reach the terminal stage of the illness, child welfare authorities often become involved in the permanency planning for the children.

Biological Family Care versus Foster Care

Because HIV/AIDS is a multigenerational family disease for many inner-city families, it often depletes key family resources through the death or medical incapacity of many of the adult family members. Often, overburdened relatives are unable to continue to care for children and grandchildren after a parent or other adult family member dies. This may be true for many reasons; one of the most important of these may be financial. For example, whereas foster parents receive between $900 and $1200 per month to care for a child who is HIV-infected, extended family members typically receive *no* financial assistance. Therefore, caring for one and often more than one infected child or grandchild can often become a burden on relatives who may already be living below the poverty level. One area of multisystems advocacy for these families might be to work to change child care laws so as to provide a more equitable financial allowance for extended family members who are supporting relatives' children. One grandmother who had already lost two adult children to AIDS reported that she and her husband were at one point caring for 11 of their grandchildren, with both of their Social Security checks as their sole income.

Although placement with family members or friends of the family is often seen as ideal, there are many situations in which this placement is not possible for a child. For example, there are situations in which both the grandparental and the parental generation have been devastated by AIDS, with most of the adults either dead or dying of the disease.

There are also situations in which grandparents or aunts/uncles have been called upon to raise their grandchildren or nieces/nephews during many years of their adult children's or siblings' drug abuse. Often these extended family members are in a rage at their relatives. When the drug-addicted adults and their children are diagnosed as HIV-infected, these revelations can sometimes become overwhelming for grandparents and other extended family members, increasing their rage and sometimes also their feelings of guilt. Matters may be further complicated by the fact that the children, sensing the instability in their lives and responding to their many losses, often begin acting out. Their caretakers then become even more overwhelmed and frustrated. In some situations, family therapy can be helpful in helping the caretakers to open up the "secrets" regarding HIV/AIDS with the children, as well as helping the family members to set limits.

In some cases, however, these interventions come too late, and caretakers such as grandparents are frustrated and angry. In these cases, therapists, physicians, nurses, and social workers, as well as child welfare workers must recognize that at times foster care may be necessary on a temporary or even a permanent basis. It is important that this not be conceptualized as an either–or situation (i.e., either foster care *or* extended family care), but as a possible combination in which a child may be in foster care but regular visits are arranged with extended family members. It is also important that the decision to utilize foster care not be conceptualized as a "failure," either by the family, by child welfare workers, or by medical or mental health professionals. Often these "helpers" become angry and frustrated with extended family members; they may therefore resist their requests for foster care placement and see this as their "giving up on the children." This process must be reframed so that contact with the biological family can be maintained if at all possible.

Providing Good-Quality Foster Care Interventions for HIV-Infected Children

Boland and her colleagues (Boland, Tasker, Evans, & Kereztes, 1987; Boland, Allen, Long, & Tasker, 1988) have outlined a number of key components to consider in the involvement of the foster care/child welfare system. A number of programs across the nation have addressed the needs of HIV-infected children requiring foster care. Anderson (1990) gives comprehensive overviews of a number of such programs, including the Leake and Watts Children's Home in New York City (Gurdin, 1990; Gurdin & Anderson, 1987); Kaleidoscope—Chicago's Star Program (Stehno, Dennis, & West, 1990); and the Children's Home Society of Florida (Coppersmith, 1990). All of these programs emphasize multisystems coordination of care and the need for a child welfare agency that is willing to facilitate the process (Anderson, 1990; Gurdin, 1990).

Although placement with the immediate or extended family is ideal, there are many instances where there is no one available to take a child or where family members are already so burdened that a child cannot be provided with good-quality care. Many of these HIV-infected children were "boarder babies" abandoned in hospitals. Therefore, the need to find skilled foster care has become critical. In order to answer this demand, these programs have initiated (1) recruitment and screening of foster parents; (2) training for foster parents in the care of HIV-infected children, as well as preparation for the stigma and fear of contagion these children often experience within their communities; (3) financial support and comprehensive coordination of medical care, transportation, nursing care, Medicaid coverage, Supplemental Security Income, respite services, and frequent home visits by the caseworker and the nurse. Some programs provide foster parents with ongoing counseling, education, and caretaker support groups. Gurdin (1990) lists the qualifications and qualities that are assessed in the home-finding process and assessment of potential foster families in the New York City program:

1. There should be no other non-seropositive foster children in the home and preferably no children under the age of six to reduce potential exposure to infections.
2. Family members must believe with absolute conviction that they cannot become infected with the AIDS virus by means of casual contact with a foster child in their home.
3. Family members must understand that the foster child may often be sick and require many medical visits, [that the child] may demonstrate developmental delays, failing to reach developmental milestones or regress[ing] from levels once achieved [, and that] in some cases, the child will die.
4. A responsible family member must be available in the home almost all of the time and employed foster parents must give evidence of a proven support system.

5. Caring for the child must be a top priority of the family such that schedules are rearranged to meet the child's needs.
6. The family must demonstrate an ability to respond to emergencies. (Gurdin, 1990, pp. 1, 11–12)

Transitional Placements: Shelter and Respite Care

Because of the shortage of foster homes for HIV-infected children, there is often a need for a transitional level of care for these children when hospitalization is no longer necessary and a foster home has not yet been found. In addition, because of the burden placed on caretakers of HIV-infected children, respite care is often necessary to give foster parents or caretaking relatives a respite from the demands of continual care. St. Clare's Home in New Jersey (Zealand, 1990) addresses both issues. When a child is placed at St. Clare's, planning is immediately begun for a long-term placement for the child, either with parents, with extended family members, or with a foster family. Zealand (1990) notes that a unique aspect of this program is that biological family members are encouraged to visit the child. Anderson (1990) describes a number of other such programs, including the Children's Home in Houston, Texas; Grandma's House in Washington, D.C.; and Farano Center for Children in Albany, New York.

As mentioned above, respite care is also a very necessary (and rarely provided) service for foster parents and family members caring for HIV-infected children. Zealand (1990), in describing the respite or temporary placement services at St. Clare's in New Jersey, gives the following examples of respite care needs: "[the] mother may be in ill health, the foster parent may need a vacation" (pp. 149–150). This respite care is also available on an emergency basis if the local child welfare agency discovers a situation in which HIV-infected children are at risk.

Treatment Issues for Children in Foster Care

Palacio and Weedy (1991) have documented a number of treatment issues for HIV/AIDS children in foster care. These can often complicate multisystems interventions and provide legal obstacles to the delivery of good-quality medical care. The most important of these is that the treatment of children with HIV/AIDS involves many medical interventions, including medications such as zidovudine and dideoxyinosine; however, the treatment of children in foster care raises many legal issues that are not relevant for children who are not wards of the state. For example, as Palacio and Weedy (1991) indicate, in foster care there are often three parties involved in the medical care of the child: the biological parents, the state and local governments (child welfare authorities) and the foster parents. This becomes complicated because while biological parents retain their legal right to consent to medical care and treatment . . . the ultimate responsibility for this care . . . lies with the state or local agency responsible for child welfare. (p. 569)

Foster parents, although they have daily responsibility for the child, have no legal right to make medical decisions. This can become a critical medical issue for a child with AIDS when emergency medical care is required or "do not resuscitate" decisions must be made. Since there are technically two groups of parties (i.e., biological parents and child welfare authorities) who have the legal right to consent to medical care, difficulties can arise when there are differences of opinion as to appropriate care. In some states (New York, for example), the commissioner of social services has final decision-making authority. Therefore, decisions about medication, participation in clinical trials, and prophylactic treatments all require the consent of several parties. This can take valuable time, particularly if the biological parents are unavailable or disagree with the medical recommendations.

The Role of Child Welfare Workers

Boland et al. (1987) have explored the role of child welfare workers. They have pointed out the various ways in which child welfare workers can influence and assist families who are willing to take and/or keep HIV-infected children. It is often very difficult for foster parents to manage the complex demands of the medical care, educational, and child welfare systems. Although many states now provide special training for foster parents who take HIV-infected children, this training is not universal. It often focuses on health precautions, but does not deal fully with the extensive other concerns. Boland et al. (1987) stress that many foster parents need help in understanding the rapidly changing field of medical knowledge and interventions regarding HIV/AIDS treatment. Caring for an HIV-infected child requires a great deal of coordination of medical, nursing, social work, transportation, and sometimes mental health services. Moreover, many foster families are very willing to take in an HIV-infected child, but they are often unprepared for the reaction of their own community and the stigma and harassment that can result. Child welfare workers can help foster parents deal with all of these issues.

Entry into school poses many other problems. Boland et al. (1987) point out that it is often difficult if not impossible to keep children's health information a secret. Many foster parents struggle with the question of how much to divulge to the school. Again, child welfare workers can be of help in this regard.

Many foster parents are very grateful for continuing opportunities to discuss their concerns. The need does not stop with the initial educational programs. Dialogue, education, question-and-answer periods, and support groups are a part of the ongoing support necessary for these foster parents to continue to function. It is also quite common that foster parents and grandparents become advocates for the children and become very angry at the parents of these children for infecting them. They must have opportunities to discuss these feelings, or they will be displaced onto the biological parents or onto the children themselves. Once again, child welfare workers can provide such opportunities and can furnish support.

Demands on Child Welfare Workers

It is no easy task to help foster families cope with all of these issues. However, child welfare workers are often in the position of having to accomplish this with very little training or support themselves. In the absence of family and extended family support, many child welfare caseworkers and medical staff often find that they become "surrogate" family members for a child (Boland et al., 1987). This is very demanding and can become a burden. Workers often need help and supervision on how to maintain an appropriate professional role and distance while being supportive.

Boland et al. (1987) have recommended the following steps for child welfare agencies in supporting their workers: (1) programs for educating managers and supervisors in ways to support their staffs; (2) formal training programs for staff members; (3) programs to identify staff members at all levels who are willing to work with HIV/AIDS patients and families; and (4) ongoing staff support groups. In addition, agencies should arrange to provide regular updates to their staffs on new developments and treatments related to medical care. Annin (1990) has developed and documented similar training strategies. The need for accurate, up-to-date medical and other information is particularly acute, as child welfare workers may have decision-making power regarding utilization of needed home-based services and placement decisions. For example, a foster parent may want to take her child home from the hospital to die. A well-intended but poorly educated worker may decide that this is too much work or too hard for the foster parent and may refuse to support her wishes.

These workers have a very demanding job—one that requires them to coordinate many levels of care for their child clients and foster families. This work often results in rapid burnout if the workers are not sufficiently supported.

The Role of Therapists and Mental Health Workers

Often, as a therapist begins working with an HIV/AIDS family, it becomes apparent that lack of coordination of care is a major psychosocial and mental health stressor for the family. It is important for such a therapist to be aware that these multisystems issues can and must be a major focus of the therapeutic interventions with the family system.

The following case vividly illustrates how to coordinate different levels of care and to promote cooperation and communication among different providers. It also demonstrates the role of the therapist in facilitating this process. Finally, it illustrates the complex involvement of the child; the grandparent; the absent parent; and the health (medical), social service, and mental health systems.

Case Example: The Multisystems Approach at Work

Kareem is a 7-year-old African-American boy who was diagnosed HIV-infected 4 years ago as a result of perinatal transmission from his mother, Kaleemah Potter, an injection drug abuser.

Kareem lived with his mother until his diagnosis at age 3. His mother reported that Kareem's father had died the year before (probably of AIDS). His mother frequently took Kareem to bars, crack houses, and heroin dens. She was often physically abusive to him and had been reported by neighbors to the state child welfare agency, who then removed him from his mother's care and placed him with his maternal grandmother, Mrs. Potter.

A year after the placement, his mother gave birth to a daughter, Sarita, who was also "taken in" by Mrs. Potter. Kareem was very upset by the baby's arrival and the sibling rivalry for the grandmother's attention became intense. During the same period Kaleemah would suddenly appear unannounced and then just as suddenly disappear. Kareem and his grandmother were aware that his mother was using drugs again and became very worried about her.

When Kaleemah did not visit the family on Mother's Day, after Kareem had made a special card and a drawing in school for her, Kareem became very angry. He kicked a kitchen chair so forcefully that it broke and was very oppositional toward his grandmother. During the next week in school, he acted out constantly, "talked back" to teachers, and fought with other kids. Finally, after a particularly angry fight with another child, he was suspended from school.

The school recommended family therapy and Mrs. Potter brought him in for treatment. The first two family sessions addressed Kareem's problems and helped to put the grandmother "back in charge" by giving her some tools for dealing with his behavioral problems.

By the third session, it was clear to the therapist that Kareem's grandmother was overwhelmed. Mrs. Potter revealed the loss of a major support, her own mother, 2 years earlier. Kareem's acting-out behavior was a major concern to her, because she wondered what would happen to her "Black male child" if he continued that behavior. Mrs. Potter was also overwhelmed by the number of different services and agencies involved: the school, the pediatric AIDS clinic, the community mental health center. In addition, she had petitioned the court for legal custody of Kareem and Sarita, feeling that the children's mother's inconsistent involvement in the children's lives and drug use rendered her unable to make vital decisions, including medical ones, for them.

As sessions continued, it became apparent to the family therapist that Mrs. Potter was also frightened and overwhelmed by HIV/AIDS. She had many questions about the disease that she had been afraid to ask the doctors. The therapist began doing some psychoeducational and reality testing work with her regarding HIV/AIDS as it related to both her daughter and her grandson. Mrs. Potter also expressed concerns about her granddaughter who had tested positive for HIV antibodies at birth, although the possibility still remained that she might seroconvert.

In the fifth session, the therapist helped Mrs. Potter to construct a genogram. It became clear that many of her key family and extended family had died or moved away, although she identified as support two "sisters" in her church, who were also neighbors. Additionally, her minister, who served as her spiritual adviser, was, at the beginning of treatment, the only person to whom she had confided the secret of the presence of HIV/AIDS in her family. (Later, when she was able to share this secret also with her two "church sisters," she found her burden easier to bear.)

By the seventh and eighth sessions, the therapist began helping Mrs. Potter develop a behavioral intervention for Kareem at home involving time out and a reward chart for good behavior. Mrs. Potter, also with the therapist's encouragement, was able to prioritize her concerns as: (1) improving Kareem's behavior in school as he had been suspended and the school had threatened to expel him; (2) managing Kareem's behavior at home; (3) gaining legal custody of

Kareem and his sister; (4) managing and coordinating the varied and sometimes conflicting messages from the different agencies involved with the family; and (5) understanding Kareem's HIV diagnosis and deciding the stage at which he should be told.

With the therapist's help, an ecomap (Hartman & Laird, 1983) was constructed which listed the agencies involved and their relationship to each of the issues Mrs. Potter had prioritized.

Because the school problem was perceived as most urgent, Mrs. Potter was encouraged to make an appointment at the school for herself and the therapist to meet with the principal, the counselor, and Kareem's teacher to discuss his behavior problems. The therapist role played with Mrs. Potter the key issues she wanted to present at the school meeting and helped to empower her to speak for herself. After a great deal of discussion, Mrs. Potter decided to share with the principal and the school staff Kareem's HIV diagnosis and her daughter's drug history and HIV status because she felt they could not fully understand his behavior without this knowledge. Despite much initial reluctance she decided that these individuals could be trusted with the secret.

On the day of the school meeting, the therapist served as a facilitator and worked with Mrs. Potter, the teacher, and the school authorities to develop a behavior management and time-out program for Kareem in school. Mrs. Potter was also able to ask for regular communication with the teacher about Kareem's progress. Mrs. Potter was a very effective advocate for her grandson.

As the school problems began to resolve themselves, Kareem's grandmother was able to focus her attention on other multisystems issues and decided that the issue of legal custody was her next priority. The therapist encouraged her to call a meeting at the therapist's office which included her case manager at the pediatric AIDS clinic, the legal aid lawyer helping her gain custody, a representative from child protective services, and of course her therapist. Together, they drafted a letter with Mrs. Potter, to be sent to the judge, that stressed her need to be able to make crucial medical, legal, and school decisions for Kareem. (It took approximately 6 months, but she was finally awarded full legal guardianship.)

The therapist and Mrs. Potter worked with Kareem to help him understand what was occurring and assured him that he would still be able to see his mother despite the guardianship order. Although attempts were made to include his mother in sessions, she did not show up.

As Kareem's behavior began to improve at home and in school, Mrs. Potter's concerns and questions about HIV/AIDS were then addressed. A number of sessions were held at the pediatric AIDS clinic with Mrs. Potter, Kareem's case manager, his physician, and the family therapist to clarify and answer Mrs. Potter's questions. When she reported that Kareem was raising questions at home, a series of meeting were held that included Mrs. Potter, Kareem, his nurse/case manager, and the family therapist. Slowly, over a series of sessions, Kareem's questions were answered and his diagnosis was revealed to him.

Finally, as a further support, Kareem was referred to a group for HIV-infected children, and Mrs. Potter was referred to a caretakers support group to help address her needs and increase her network.

The Potter family remained in treatment for a year. During that time, the therapist encouraged Mrs. Potter to call meetings with members of other agencies whenever she needed clarity and to ensure good case management. It is important to note that the therapist did not take on this task herself but empowered Mrs. Potter to advocate on her own behalf.

CONCLUSION

The multisystems approach described in this chapter provides a model for professionals working with all HIV/AIDS families. It is particularly relevant for working with inner-city, poor families, because of the added complexity of their psychosocial issues. It is extremely important for all professionals involved to recognize the central role of the empowerment of families in this process. As the case example indicates, the role of the professionals is to facilitate their mastery of the multisystems approach and to empower them to take an active role in coordinating their own care and in the decision making process.

One final note: Although coordination of care is an excellent treatment goal, it is one of the most vulnerable points in an often complex system of care. Whereas in an ideal world this task might be delegated to child welfare workers or to social workers on the medical unit, often these individuals are so overburdened by enormous caseloads that they cannot provide effective case management for all families. Therefore, readers of this chapter—whether their professional role is as therapists, nurses, physicians, psychologists, social workers, psychiatrists, or child welfare workers—may find themselves in a position in which a multisystems intervention is necessary and they must, by default, call the first meeting. As in the case example above, such a meeting can become an opportunity to appoint an interagency case manager, who becomes the central recipient of information regarding the child and family. Tasks and assignments can then be delegated to others, and coordination and follow-up are more likely to occur.

REFERENCES

Anderson, G. (Ed.). (1990). *Courage to care: Responding to the crisis of children with AIDS.* Washington, DC: Child Welfare League of America.

Annin, J. (1990). Training for HIV infection prevention in child welfare services. In G. Anderson (Ed.), *Courage to care: Responding to the crisis of children with AIDS.* Washington, DC: Child Welfare League of America.

Barth, R. P., Pietrzak, J., & Ramler, M. (1993). *Families living with drugs and HIV: Intervention and treatment strategies.* New York: Guilford Press.

Boyd-Franklin, N. (1989). *Black families in therapy: A multisystems approach.* New York: Guilford Press.

Boland, M., Allen, T., Long, G., & Tasker, M. (1988). Children with HIV infection: Collaborative responsibilities of the child welfare and medical communities. *Social Work, 33*(6), 504–509.

Boland, M., Czarniecki, L., & Haiken, H. (1992). Coordinated care for children in HIV infection. In M. Stuber (Ed.), *Children and AIDS.* Washington, DC: American Psychiatric Press.

Boland, M., Tasker, M., Evans, P., & Kereztes, J. (1987, Winter). Helping children with AIDS: The role of the child welfare worker. *Public Welfare,* pp. 23–28.

Coppersmith, S. (1990). Foster care for children to HIV infection: A special mission in a loving environment. In G. Anderson (Ed.), *Courage to care: Responding to the crisis of children with AIDS.* Washington, DC: Child Welfare League of America.

Falloon, J., Eddy, J., Werner, L., & Pizzo, P. (1989). Human immunodeficiency virus infection in children. *Journal of Pediatrics, 114,* 1–30.

Gurdin, P. (1990). Quality care for children: A specialized foster care program. In G. Anderson (Ed.), *Courage to care: Responding to the crisis of children with AIDS.* Washington, DC: Child Welfare League of America.

Gurdin, P., & Anderson, G. (1987). Quality care for ill children: AIDS specialized foster family homes. *Child Welfare, 66,* 291–302.

Happios, K., Gross, J., & Lieberman, J. (1990, August). *Technical report on developmental disabilities and HIV infection* (Report No. 6). Silver Spring, MD: American Association of University Affiliated Programs.

Hartman, A., & Laird, J. (1983). *Family-centered social work practice.* New York: Free Press.

Palacio, C., & Weedy, C. (1991). Treatment issues regarding children in foster care. In P. Pizzo & C. Wilfert (Eds.), *Pediatric AIDS.* Baltimore: Williams & Wilkins.

Seibert, J. M., Garcia, A., Kaplan, M., & Septimus, A. (1990). Three models of pediatric AIDS programs: Meeting the needs of children, families and communities. In J. M. Seibert & R. A. Olson (Eds.), *Children, adolescents and AIDS.* Lincoln: University of Nebraska Press.

Stehno, S., Dennis, K., & West, M. (1990). Kaleidoscope—Chicago's Star Program. In G. Anderson (Ed.), *Courage to care: Responding to the crisis of children with AIDS*. Washington, DC: Child Welfare League of America.

Zealand, T. (1990). St. Clare's Home: Shelter and transitional care for young children. In G. Anderson (Ed.), *Courage to care: Responding to the crisis of children with AIDS*. Washington, DC: Child Welfare League of America.

14

. . . .

Caring for the Professional Caregiver

. . . .

Nancy Boyd-Franklin, PhD
Mary G. Boland, MSN, RN

> The art of caregiving is the art of interdependence.
> It's a delicate [and] often precarious balance: being in-
> volved and keeping perspective: caring and yet being
> objective; spending time together and taking time to
> be alone; giving to ourselves and setting limits.
> —*Kairos House (1992)*

Health and mental health professionals throughout the country are coping with larger numbers of patients with HIV/AIDS. Medical workers
report feeling uncertainty, reluctance, and anxiety about performing
medical procedures with these patients. The emergence of tuberculosis in multiple-drug-resistant strains adds to these fears. Those who
perform venipuncture (i.e., draw blood) experience a continuing fear
of infection. Mental health care providers in medical settings are often
asked to provide consultation to medical staff members regarding these
anxieties.

But the medical risk inherent in the treatment of HIV/AIDS is only
one of many stressful aspects of this disease. The stigmatized nature
of HIV/AIDS also elicits complex psychological reactions in caregivers
of all professional disciplines. In the early 1980s, health and mental
health professionals were reluctant to acknowledge their work with

HIV/AIDS patients for fear of ostracism, not only for themselves but for their families. Moreover, some care providers continue to experience some discomfort or uncertainty dealing with additional issues that can accompany HIV infection, such as drug abuse, pregnancy, promiscuous sex, and homosexuality/bisexuality. Although reservations and concerns still persist, particularly in low-incidence communities or settings where there are minimal opportunities for worker training, much progress has been made. Increasingly, providers report positive feelings and a sense of satisfaction in their work.

Despite the recognition that work with HIV/AIDS patients is stressful, there has been surprisingly little research on identifying stressors and developing effective interventions to support these professional caregivers. In this chapter we provide an overview of the psychological reactions to this work, as well as supportive interventions that are designed to prevent and manage work-related stresses.

PSYCHOLOGICAL REACTIONS OF PROFESSIONAL CAREGIVERS

There has been a small but growing literature on the psychological reactions of professional caregivers to working with HIV/AIDS populations. Macks (1988a, 1988b), in describing countertransference reactions of female health care providers to women with HIV infection, identified seven possible reactions: (1) fear of contagion, (2) denial and magical thinking, (3) discomfort with sexuality and sexual behavior change, (4) combating helplessness and despair (5) anger and blaming the victim, (6) blurring of ethical and professional boundaries, and (7) fear of professional inadequacy. Flaskerud (1991) and Bolle (1989) have described psychosocial stressors on nurses and other health care workers as including fear of contagion and transmission, discomfort with homosexuality and drug use, intensive and complicated care, repetitive grief, facing one's own mortality, and conflict over goals of treatment. In this section, we explore these and other psychological and emotional reactions of professional staff members on AIDS units.

Being Surrogate Family Members

Caregivers' psychological reactions are complicated by the reality that they often serve as extended or surrogate family members for many HIV/AIDS patients and their families. Many medical, nursing, social service, and mental health professionals who work with HIV/AIDS have reported that they become a part of the support system for particular patients and their families, especially in cases where adult patients and parents of infected children are alienated or rejected by their own relatives. As persons with HIV live longer, caregivers will develop long-term relationships with children and families, similar to those experienced by caregivers of those with cystic fibrosis, cancer, and other chronic childhood illnesses.

Overidentification and Boundary Keeping

Although providing extended family support is important, it does present a number of very real difficulties for staff members. Sometimes it takes them out of their "professional role" and leads them to become more emotionally involved with a particular patient or family. This can lead to overidentification and difficulties in keeping the boundaries between patient and care provider clear.

Nurses, social workers, psychologists, family therapists, and physicians often have to struggle with the knowledge that *empowering* patients or families may be more beneficial or useful than *helping* them. In many situations, for example, it is more important to provide patients or adult caretakers with information to carry out a certain responsibility or task, rather than to do it for them. Many nursing, medical, and social service providers have had to struggle with the boundaries around their own roles. Macks (1988a, 1988b), as noted above, identified blurring of professional boundaries and fear of professional inadequacy as possible impediments to delivering effective care. Caregivers are all particularly vulnerable to the possibility of replicating their own family roles in the families with whom they work. For example, many service professionals identify with a disproportionate number of persons who are caretakers in their own families of origin. They may unknowingly usurp patients' or parents' rightful roles in their eagerness to help.

Care providers must struggle to provide a healthy balance between involvement and appropriate therapeutic objectivity if they intend to remain effective in this work. Overinvolvement can lead to an inability to set appropriate limits and say "no" to patients' demands, which in turn can lead to premature burnout.

Anger

Among the range of emotional reactions, anger is one of the most difficult for health, social service, and mental health professionals. Perhaps the most common manifestation of anger involves "blaming the victims," or assuming that "they did something to get it." Working with gay patients can be complicated by a provider's own prejudice. Injection drug users, particularly those who are actively using drugs at the time of treatment, often elicit a great deal of anger in staff members—especially when they continue to use drugs even after the diagnosis of HIV infection. Some abusers are manipulative and will lie about ongoing drug use. This can infuriate staff members, who feel that their work is being undone and that their patients may be increasing the risk of infection for others.

Other patients who elicit a great deal of anger from caregivers are those who continue to have many sexual partners without taking precautions or letting their partners know their HIV status. Often this anger on the part of staff members is a reflection of their own frustration in working with such patients. It may also be indicative of their own fear of infection from just such partners.

For providers working with children, the anger is often directed toward those who have infected the children—usually toward the mothers, and sometimes also toward the fathers if they are the ones who infected the mothers. The anger is even more profound in cases of transmission through sexual abuse of a child. Staff members thus replicate and voice the rage of extended family members toward these parents. Unfortunately, this perpetuates the cycle of anger and makes it difficult to work effectively with these patients.

As advocates for their patients, staff members may become very angry at families who, in their own grief and anger, reject their infected relatives. It is important that caregivers be helped to work this anger through. Once they have been given time and help to deal with the illness, family members will often re-engage with the patients. Sometimes the anger of the professionals can slow this reconciliation process or prevent it from occurring. This is also true of staff members who are working with adolescent patients or parents who may be drug abusers and are often very alienated from their families: The staff members, by unconsciously picking up and voicing that anger, can further contribute to that alienation.

The work of Kübler-Ross (1969) may be helpful in understanding how families' and professionals' reactions to an HIV/AIDS diagnosis may correspond to those of the patients—initial denial, then anger. Pain and anger are also common reactions when a previously asymptomatic, healthy-looking patient begins to become symptomatic.

Staff members immersed in daily care of large numbers of patients may be too overburdened to perceive how staff dissension is a natural consequence of the constant care demands and repeated experience of death and loss. In addition, caregivers may experience a tremendous amount of anger when, despite their best efforts, patients continue to die. If such anger is not talked about, it can be directed at patients, at their families, and at other staff members. The displacement of anger onto fellow staff members is a very common reaction and should be considered and discussed whenever tensions become high among staff members.

Since anger is one of the most difficult responses that providers experience, the program's administrators should make it acceptable for staff members to talk to coworkers, and also to develop an independent support system that can help them deal with their emotions.

Feelings of Personal and Professional Inadequacy

The AIDS epidemic, perhaps more than any other 20th-century medical condition, has had the capacity to elicit feelings of helplessness and inadequacy in health and mental health care providers of all disciplines. There are many reasons for these feelings. First, there is no known cure at this time. Second, caregivers often have to cope with the progression of illness and death of their patients. Third, medical and nursing professionals must perform procedures that inflict pain and further add to existing suffering. Fourth, care providers experience legitimate frustration in trying to get different systems to work together appropriately. In large metropolitan areas such as New York City, this can lead to an inability to monitor the delivery of even basic medical care. Fifth, the many problems (poverty, crime, homelessness, etc.) faced by inner-city AIDS families can overwhelm practitioners.

Even the most experienced care providers feel inadequate at times. Yet few in the health and mental health professions are fully aware of the pervasiveness of these feelings. Many HIV/AIDS workers are isolated from support systems and never have the opportunity to share their helplessness and even hopelessness.

A related response found in work with providers in different settings throughout the country is the "impostor syndrome"—feelings of inadequacy for one's job that can lead to potentially crippling personal and professional self-doubt. This is an extremely difficult feeling for professionals of whatever discipline to express and share with one another. In group discussions there is often tremendous relief when a staff member, particularly an experienced one, raises these feelings, as it encourages others to share them too.

Many interventions in the HIV/AIDS field are crisis-driven. Increasingly, the demands of patient care require new techniques and new ways to adapt existing interventions to the needs of patients and families. However, it is difficult for overworked front-line practitioners to keep abreast of new findings in medical procedures. The ever-expanding lexicon of terms and treatments can overwhelm both medical and nonmedical care providers. It is important for all providers to undergo continuing in-service training to keep up-to-date on recent developments.

Because of the crisis-oriented quality of AIDS treatment, staff members are forced to become "experts" quickly. Recognizing the need for ongoing training updates and giving staff members (particularly new ones) permission to ask questions and to say that we do not have all the answers can be a relief. Caregivers may find it necessary to acknowledge to patients and families that the field is constantly changing, and that the answers may be complex or even nonexistent.

A later section of this chapter focuses on the process of providing the support groups for staff members that are necessary for all levels of experience and different disciplines. Permission to acknowledge issues and share feelings honestly is not a panacea, but it can bring relief from the feeling of being the only one who experiences these feelings and issues.

Mourning and Bereavement

One of the most painful issues for all staff members in working with HIV/AIDS patients and their families is the continual experience of death, dying, and bereavement. Staff members often become very close to their patients and their families, and experience their own feelings of loss, sadness, grief, and anger when patients die. This can be particularly painful for those working with pediatric HIV/AIDS patients.

On a personal level, death and dying rekindle feelings of personal loss and memories of loved ones who have died. Since AIDS affects so many different ages and generations, it also stirs up issues of personal vulnerability and recognition of mortality.

For staff members in hospital or clinic settings, multiple, rapid losses of both patients and their family members may lead to feelings of being overwhelmed by grief. Since the crisis-oriented nature of HIV/AIDS care leaves little opportunity for caregivers to resolve the losses of patients, it is important for administrators to grant staff members permission to attend a patient's wake or funeral, as much for their own closure and need to say goodbye as to support the family.

When patients die unexpectedly or especially quickly, it is often helpful to have a special group session for staff members to deal with unresolved or painful feelings. It is also sometimes helpful for staff members and for other patients and their families in the program to participate together in a memorial service.

For care providers, the hardest dilemma may be how to keep hope alive for early-stage patients and their families while at the same time supporting patients who are near death or dying. One benefit of a team approach is that when one caregiver is overwhelmed with recent losses, another team member can relieve that person of the responsibility of working with a new patient and family who have just learned of the HIV diagnosis.

The experiences of patients who are dying can stir up feelings of inadequacy such as those discussed above. HIV/AIDS is still a relatively new disease, as are most AIDS-related interventions. Therefore, "mistakes," in which diagnoses are missed, particular treatment options are not taken quickly enough, or unusual symptoms are misdiagnosed, are inevitable occurrences as the medical field tries to catch up with the realities of this illness. Such difficulties complicate the coping abilities of dedicated medical and nursing professionals. In their own feelings of grief and guilt, they may "point the finger" and blame each other. In spite of very demanding schedules, time must be made available for these issues to be reframed and discussed. If these discussions emphasize "learning from mistakes," rather than accusations and blaming, each "mistake" becomes an opportunity to discover how to provide better patient care in the future.

The processes of bereavement and grief within a staff are complicated by individual staff members' experiencing grief at different times. Support groups can provide an opportunity for staff members to share these experiences. Also, more experienced caregivers may have developed their own strategies for coping with these issues, which they have never had the opportunity to share with newer staff members because of work demands. Often the front-line demands of AIDS work can make staff members unaware of or insensitive to one another's periods of loss.

Another experience related to death and dying experiences that must be noted here is that of "anniversary reactions." Often when a staff member (or a whole staff) has experienced a personal tragedy, a sense of loss can be reactivated by the anniversary of the original loss, by certain special holidays, or by a particular patient whose illness evokes a painful memory. Members of the staff may experience a feeling of being "down" or a feeling of grief "for no reason." Sometimes feelings of grief, loss, and abandonment can be manifested in anger at the families or in arguments among staff members. Open discussion of these anniversary reactions among staff members can bring these feelings into conscious awareness and allow them to be talked about.

Positive Feelings and Sense of Satisfaction

It is clear that working directly with HIV/AIDS patients elicits a complex range of emotions and behaviors in health and mental health care providers. Too frequently, the focus has been exclusively on the many complicated negative feelings and stresses of the work. Often overlooked are the positive feelings and sense of satisfaction experienced by many service providers.

For one thing, caregivers are now able to help patients live longer and can often have a positive influence on the quality of their patients' living and dying. For example, pediatric nurses and social workers help children continue to have birthday parties, holiday celebrations, and friendships, as well as to participate in support groups and summer camp experiences. These activities can help to keep hope alive and to give children and their families a sense of normality through participation in the joyful rituals of childhood. Many caregivers also find a sense of both challenge and accomplishment in the work—challenge as they face the unknown and are stimulated to devise solutions by applying their previous knowledge and experience; accomplishment when a routine act is experienced as significant by a child or family. Moreover, many professionals report that they are renewed by the strength and courage they witness in the children and families struggling to cope with the devastating illness. For some, this work defines what they wished to do when they entered the "helping" professions.

Yet, as the preceding discussion has made clear, this work is hard and stressful. Each provider brings his or her own personal and professional self, complete with strengths and weaknesses, to the work. The next section highlights the need to be alert for both personal and organizational problems that may occur.

RECOGNIZING POTENTIAL PROBLEMS

Identifying Burnout

Because work with HIV/AIDS patients and families can be so very stressful, it is important for caregivers to understand and recognize the signs of stress, so that they can seek support or help before actual burnout occurs.

First, it is very important for staff members, supervisors, and administrators to acknowledge the levels of stress openly and to recognize that staff members may cope with stress in different ways. For example, some may withdraw; some may "spill" constantly; some may become highly critical of or angry with one another; some may act as if stress doesn't exist. Once these different adaptations are identified, they can be addressed as individuals' reactions to a very difficult situation.

The demands of this work are so great and the needs of patients so many that, slowly and insidiously, the work may become the center of a staff member's life. It is essential for caregivers to be aware of the need to take time off regularly and to "have a life outside." Discussing the ways in which members "come down" or unwind from the stress of work can be helpful for the staff.

Little research has been done on the stress involved in HIV/AIDS work and the experience of burnout for HIV/AIDS health care providers. Professionals in the health and mental health fields must begin to explore whether, for example, there are times when individuals would benefit from planned respites or periodic reassignments from front-line work. There is frequently a reluctance to discuss these issues because the possibility of burnout is too threatening. In addition, considering whether there might be a time limit for doing this work may be seen as "disloyal." It is unfortunate when health and social service care providers deny themselves the opportunity and the permission to ask for a much-needed respite before burnout occurs.

Becoming Aware of Organizational Stressors

In the early years of the HIV/AIDS epidemic, individuals and organizations mobilized quickly to meet the growing demands for service. Existing organizations developed new types of programs and agencies, and organizations dedicated to HIV/AIDS care were started in both the profit and not-for-profit sectors. As individual managers and providers learned how to care for the HIV-infected, the massive volume of work often precluded any effort to meet the needs of the professional caregivers. Yet it soon became evident that the stresses experienced by individual caregivers affected their organizations adversely. Caregiver grief, once viewed as a personal issue, is now a legitimate concern of such organizations (Schoen, 1992). Unfortunately, however, when there is only one designated HIV/AIDS care provider within a system, no active and ongoing support may be available even on an informal basis.

Stress and burnout in the helping professions have been described (Pines & Aronson, 1988), but the unique qualities of HIV/AIDS and the ever-increasing number of cases make the need to recruit and retain experienced and compassionate caregivers within this subspecialty of health care more pressing. Individuals and organizations must be able to address their issues and concerns.

Developing an HIV/AIDS service program can be exciting: A small group of individuals bound by tremendous energy and commitment, and frequently led by a charismatic, risk-taking individual, come together to "help." This initial organization often lacks a formal structure or systems, as these individuals, guided by their own commitment to work, generally require minimal direction and supervision. Despite the difficulty of the work, the rewards are great, and a sense of camaraderie and group spirit provides the support necessary to deal with the stresses of the work.

However, when the numbers of patients increase, and funding makes it possible to expand the number and type of services provided, a formal organizational structure may have to be imposed that defines roles and sets limits. At this point, a difficult situation may arise. Original leaders, citing stress and burnout, may leave even before the transitional period is complete; they may be replaced by new managers with or without direct caregiving experience. When the organization undergoes expansion and refinement, professional caregivers who are now under stress as a result of administrative pressures instead of client work must be helped to understand that change offers the opportunity for growth and mastery and the improvement of client services. Successful programs offer support and security for providers while minimizing feelings of loss of control. Nonetheless, some staff turnover is inevitable at such times to allow the organization room for development. This is an evolutionary process that cannot be rushed. It must be guided by administrators who share a commitment to provide nurturing and support to clients, but recognize that caregivers need continuing nurturing as well.

Employee satisfaction is closely related to both organizational structure and management style. Because the direct caregivers witness suffering and death on a daily basis, their sense of competence and control is constantly challenged in ways that threaten their self-esteem and professional worth. Programs that support an interactional (rather than a command-and-control) style of management—one that encourages universal participation and involvement in decision making—are more likely to be successful in delivering service, retaining staff members, and remaining viable. Because both health and mental health settings traditionally ascribe stature and competence to credentials rather than to experience or merit, interactionally oriented programs may be viewed as mavericks. However, such programs report increased satisfaction on the part of both clients and staff members, decreased staff turnover, and minimized feelings of isolation and helplessness among staff.

Awareness and acknowledgment of AIDS-specific stressors on the part of administrators and supervisors are extremely important. The philosophy and tone for a particular hospital unit, clinic, or program are established by the administrative and clinical leadership. As discussed above, although mechanisms need to be created to recognize and counter staff stress and burnout, it is more important to anticipate the onset of stress and provide supports within the setting.

SUPPORTIVE INTERVENTIONS

The remainder of this chapter addresses two main areas of intervention that provide support for caregivers: (1) organizational and administrative (clear administrative policies; training and professional development as an antidote to staff burnout; and multidisciplinary teams); and (2) psychological (staff support groups; funerals, memorial services, and healing services; retreats; and access to outside mental health consultants).

Organizational and Administrative Support

The organizational response to stress must be proactive: developing multiple strategies to minimize the development of staff stress; providing mechanisms to acknowledge loss and grief; and offering flexible approaches that recognize the diversity of coping mechanisms among individual staff members. AIDS-specific agencies that utilize professionals and volunteers have been forced to develop formal organizational strategies to deal with issues related to stress and grief. The San Francisco-based Shanti project, an organization that provides emotional and practical support to people with HIV/AIDS, realized that occupational burnout exacted a heavy financial burden on them through high absenteeism and job turnover rates. This analysis led the organization to develop a staff care program, which incorporates an optional 4-day work week, encouragement to use full vacation time each year, support groups and grief circles, staff retreats, and staff participation in program development. A national telephone survey of seven large AIDS organizations sponsored by the Shanti project corroborated liberal leave and vacation policies, employee support groups, and management training as interventions that helped to prevent burnout (Soos, 1991).

The most commonly recommended and traditional approach to dealing with feelings in health care settings—the use of support groups—has met with varying success and is discussed in more detail below. By providing an organizationally sanctioned outlet for stress, a support group may send the message to staff members that the group is the only place where emotion is acceptable; caregivers may thus feel obligated to maintain a facade of competence for the rest of the work week. In addition, these group meetings may be used incorrectly as vehicles for administrative change when an accelerated rate of growth in HIV/AIDS programs creates the need for administrative adaptation.

Some organizations have found regular, specific "team-building" sessions an effective alternative to the more general support group. In an effort to strengthen staff morale, such sessions focus on the multiple dimensions of the entire team and its work, rather than localizing an area of weakness. At the core of any organizational intervention are the creation and maintenance of an organizational culture that supports the work and the caregivers. Since individual programs will develop stress management programs based on their particular circumstances, the process of the journey is as important as the outcome.

At the Children's Hospital AIDS Program, we have found through a process of trial and error that the ethnic and cultural diversity of our group requires a variety of options to meet the needs of different members. The impetus for the program comes from both the clinical care providers and the administrators, and the interventions range from the purely recreational to the therapeutic and can occur either at work or outside of work.

Clear Administrative Policies

In order to work effectively, HIV/AIDS unit staff members must be provided by their administrators with clear program goals and policies. This requires regularly scheduled staff meetings, as well as ad hoc meetings when new developments occur. Because of the ongoing stressors of the work, staff members need open-door access to managers and supervisors. There must also be formal channels to assure communication and address concerns and strains. Finally, there should be a formal, confidential program evaluation, as well as performance appraisals of individual staff on a regular basis.

Training and Professional Development as an Antidote to Staff Burnout

Boyd-Franklin (1989) has discussed training as an antidote to burnout for front-line service providers. Because of the constant demands for service delivery, providers often place too low a priority on ongoing training. This is unfortunate on many levels.

First, it is necessary that administrators and staff recognize the need—not only for those who are just beginning in this work, but also for those with many years of experience—to gain some distance from the constant work demands, to acknowledge strategies that have worked, and to explore new ones. Training for more experienced staff members can provide a framework for assessment of ongoing procedures, as well as much-needed opportunities for refueling and validation. Given the constant medical advances, there is also a need to provide continuing education and regular updates for caregivers.

Administrative support for the professional development of all staff members is also extremely important, as HIV/AIDS work has forced each discipline involved to redefine its professional roles. There is a continuing need for good training material and for the sharing of experiences. Staff members should be encouraged and allowed the opportunity to present their own work at professional/scientific conferences and to submit papers for journal publication. Interaction with colleagues through professional organizations is also very empowering, as it helps staff members to stand back and see the value of their own work and contributions to the field. The needs of managers, administrators, and supervisors for ongoing management training must not be overlooked. Often they are extremely competent in their particular discipline (nursing, medicine, social work, psychiatry, or psychology), but have had little or no training in organizational management.

Multidisciplinary Teams

Because of the demands of work with HIV/AIDS patients, it is important that staff members not become isolated or feel that they alone must meet all of the needs of a particular patient or family. Even the most experienced staff members need feedback and an opportunity to discuss difficult cases. For these reasons, multidisciplinary teams need to be established. As we have noted in Chapter 13, the services of many different disciplines are often required for a particular family. For example, a nurse, a pediatrician, a family practice physician, a social worker, a psychologist or psychiatrist, and inpatient and outpatient team representatives may all be involved with a particular patient or family. In this situation, roles blur. Because problems often occur when different professional disciplines have difficulty in clarifying and understanding one another's roles, "turf" issues need to be clarified.

It is important that these meetings or multidisciplinary rounds occur regularly, so that effective case management and division of labor can occur. Inevitably in this work, situations arise for which a particular physician, nurse, or social worker feels too close or involved to intervene. The team can provide other perspectives on difficult choices, and often can designate another team member to become involved.

Psychological Support

In addition to the organizational supports discussed above, administrators can also create psychological supports that provide professional caregivers with continuing opportunities for acknowledging loss. Informal peer support is extremely important, and staff members should be encouraged to recognize different styles of handling stress and loss. A simple intervention such as being available to talk to a colleague in a time of need can be very powerful. A shoulder to cry on or a hug received after the death of a patient can offer both comfort and support. Some units have instituted scrapbooks or bulletin boards that contain pictures of patients who have died. In addition to these caring interventions, there are four others that have proved very helpful in providing psychological support to HIV/AIDS caregivers: (1) support groups; (2) funerals, memorial services, and healing services; (3) retreats; and (4) access to outside mental health consultants.

Staff Support Groups

A support group where staff members can come together to discuss feelings about their work can be very effective within the hospital setting. In other situations, staff members have participated in support groups composed of professional HIV/AIDS caregivers outside of their own work situations.

Ideally, this group should meet weekly for approximately an hour and a half. Practical needs, however, may override the ideal and restrict this amount of time. Programs should not be discouraged if the stress of "one more meeting" makes a weekly support group impossible. Support groups can still be effective with bimonthly or even once-per-month meetings. It is crucial, however, that the support group meet in a regular time and place and that reminders be posted regularly for staff members. Consistent attendance needs to be stressed, but when service demands make this impossible, as many staff members as possible should be encouraged to attend.

The size of the group is frequently an issue. It is easier, of course, for smaller groups to meet together, and groups ranging from 6 to 12 individuals are ideal for comfort reasons. Once again, however, the demands of the service may not make this small a group possible.

The issue of who should attend is an important one for such a group. Sometimes support groups must be divided by discipline. In other units it works very well for nurses, social workers, physicians, supervisors, and administrators to attend. This issue needs to be considered carefully, because sometimes staff members may feel inhibited from sharing their true feelings when supervisors and administrators are present.

The rules about confidentiality must be clear. It is essential that group members be assured that their concerns will not be discussed outside the group, either by members or leaders. Staff members cannot be open about their feelings if they fear that their comments will be used against them in their evaluation process, so if supervisors do attend it is important for their role to be clarified.

Funerals, Memorial Services, and Healing Services

In the early days of the epidemic, many staff members on AIDS units struggled with the issue of attending the funerals of children and family members. It has been our experience in the Children's Hospital AIDS Program that this process can and should be encouraged, as it can be a very healing one for the staff and families. It provides the staff members with a prescribed time to mourn, cry, and express their grief openly.

A phenomenon on AIDS units that is often devastating for a devoted staff is a period in which many children (or their parents) die in rapid succession. At these times it has been very helpful to hold a memorial or healing service, whether it be for patients' families and staff members together or exclusively for the staff. Members can bring inspirational reading material or speak personally of a child they knew. Although most memorial and healing services are nonreligious, they may nonetheless be led by a member of the clergy. Such services are extremely important; they provide a ritual that helps to draw the staff members together and acknowledges their grief.

Retreats

Periodic retreats (which often combine psychological stress reduction, some work, and lots of play) are often crucial to team building. They can be held at a location away from the work setting and can be tailored to meet the needs of a staff at any given time. The mourning and grief rituals discussed above may also be components of retreats.

Some programs use retreats as an opportunity to stand back from the day-to-day stresses of the work, to review the past, and to plan program direction for the future. Since many new staff members who enter AIDS units experience them as "moving trains" that they must "jump on board" immediately, retreats can provide a rare opportunity for incorporating new members on a personal and professional level, in addition to sharing the history of the program and future goals.

Access to Outside Mental Health Consultants

The role of an outside mental health consultant (psychologist, social worker, psychiatrist, or family therapist) can be a crucial one in the ongoing survival of an AIDS staff. Often this person is in an ideal position to start support groups, plan retreats, and organize memorial services. Also, when such a person is brought in from the outside, staff members may feel more free to discuss personal/psychological concerns that arise from the stress of the work. This mental health consultant can be useful to the staff in providing training in stress management techniques, and can at times provide organizational consultation when conflicts within the staff or between staff members and administrators arise. Finally, the mental health consultant can serve both patients and staff as a resource for referrals for outside psychological assessment and therapy.

CONCLUSION

One final note: As this chapter has stressed, the human element in all of us must be acknowledged if we are to be effective in work with HIV/AIDS patients and their families. Most of us have been taught in the course of our professional training that we must be "objective," so these unexpressed feelings of grief, loss, sadness, and anger are overwhelming for us as individuals to bear. These are human emotions, and we put an unnecessary burden on ourselves if we expect ourselves to be "superhuman" and never allow for the expression of such emotions within the work setting. We must create a "safe" atmosphere in which we can share these feelings with one another and express grief and vulnerability through tears and sadness, if we are to continue to do important HIV/AIDS work.

REFERENCES

Bolle, J. (1988). Supporting the deliverers of care: Strategies to support nurses and prevent burnout in AIDS and holistic nursing practice. *Holistic Nursing Practice, 3*(4), 63–71.

Flaskerud, J. (1991). Psychosocial stresses on nurses and other health care givers. In J. Flaskerud & P. Ungvarski (Eds.), *HIV/AIDS: A guide to nursing care* (pp. 267–274). Philadelphia: W. B. Saunders.

Kairos House. (1992). *The art of caregiving.* San Francisco: Random House.

Kübler-Ross, E. (1969). *On death and dying.* New York: Macmillan.

Macks, J. (1988a, March). Countertransference reactions of female health care providers to women with HIV infections (Part One). *Focus: A Guide to AIDS Research and Counseling,* pp. 3–4.

Macks, J. (1988b, April). Countertransference reactions of female health care providers to women with HIV infections (Part Two). *Focus: A Guide to AIDS Research and Counseling,* pp. 3–4.

Pines, A., & Aronson, E. (1988). *Career burnout: Causes and cures.* New York: Free Press.

Schoen, K. (1992, June). Managing grief in AIDS organizations. *Focus: A Guide to AIDS Research and Counseling,* pp. 1–6.

Soos, J. (1991). *Caring for the AIDS caregiver: An evaluation of staff burnout at Shanti Project and a benefit–cost analysis of the "Staff Care Plan."* Unpublished master's thesis, University of California, Berkeley.

15

HIV/AIDS in the Schools

Ann Silver Pozen, PsyD

When the AIDS epidemic hit the United States, the majority of the nation's schools were unprepared for its impact. In the early 1980s, school officials were forced to make difficult policy decisions without legal guidelines and with only scarce and undefinitive medical research to assist them. The first students and school personnel with AIDS had to petition the courts to protect their right to an education and to preserve their jobs, respectively. Often with inadequate input from the medical community, the courts confronted the onerous task of determining the appropriate balance between the rights of people with HIV/AIDS and the right of the community to be protected from infection.

Eventually, with improved medical understanding of HIV/AIDS and with the courageous persistence of people with HIV/AIDS, the courts established legal precedents that have served to protect the rights of infected individuals. Now many HIV-infected children who are asymptomatic or mildly to moderately symptomatic attend school. With improved treatment to prolong life, the percentage of infected children surviving to school age is expected to increase.

As the AIDS epidemic continues to grow, the responsibilities of the schools are twofold. The first is to provide appropriate education to children with HIV/AIDS in an atmosphere that is supportive of their special needs and conducive to learning. This requires that the schools have a clearly defined written policy regarding the placement of these children that is sensitive to both the social and physical impact of HIV/AIDS, and that teachers and other school personnel be educated about HIV/AIDS and the effects on children.

The second responsibility of the schools is to provide a curriculum designed to prevent the spread of HIV infection. Such a curriculum must present not only basic information regarding HIV/AIDS, but also explicit information on risk reduction. In addition, the curriculum must serve to develop and foster risk-reducing behaviors.

As we enter the second decade of the AIDS epidemic in the United States, the schools are faced with an unprecedented challenge that threatens the lives of all of our children. It is crucial that this challenge be met effectively to ensure the future and welfare of all children—those who are already infected with HIV and those who have not yet been stricken by it.

HIV/AIDS AND SCHOOL POLICY

In the United States, 4,249 cases of AIDS in children under 13 years old were reported to the Centers for Disease Control (CDC) in 1992 (CDC, 1993). Although the vast majority of pediatric AIDS cases can be attributed to mother–infant transmission, the first cases of AIDS in the schools were predominantly among children who had been infected through treatment with clotting factor for hemophilia or who had received blood transfusions prior to 1985, when routine screening of the blood supply began (Smith, 1990).

Initial uncertainty among physicians regarding the transmissibility of HIV in the school setting resulted in school policies that gave priority to the protection of the uninfected over the rights of those with HIV/AIDS. Thus, in 1987, the Georgia Board of Education adopted a policy requiring HIV-infected school employees to inform school officials of their HIV-infected status. Failure to do so was to be considered grounds for termination of employment. In addition, to avoid dismissal, any employee suspected of being infected with HIV was required to present evidence of a negative HIV antibody test or to submit to HIV testing. Likewise, parents of children who were infected with HIV were required to inform the school. A student suspected of being infected was required to submit to testing or else "be treated as if he/she were an infected student" (Nayman & Poltrock, 1987, p. 1). Fortunately, the policy statement included a provision stipulating that it could be revised in accordance with current medical research and legal opinion. As the result of recent court decisions and the medical community's consensus on the limited transmissibility of HIV, Georgia's policy now conforms to those of most other states and districts. Individuals infected with HIV are no longer required to inform school officials, and any students or employees who do reveal their HIV-infected status are protected by state and local guidelines on confidentiality and by federal laws that prohibit discrimination and guarantee the right to an education.

Legal Protections for People with HIV/AIDS

Two acts of Congress have been interpreted by the courts to protect the rights of HIV-infected members of the school community. The Education of the Handicapped Act of 1975 mandates that all handicapped children receive a "free appropriate public education" or a special education designed to meet their specific needs. Children with HIV/AIDS who have a handicap mentioned in this act are also covered by the law, whether or not the handicap is the result of HIV infection.

In a case involving a Florida child with AIDS who had an IQ of 41, the court ruled that the child was entitled to be educated in a regular special education classroom, despite the fact that the child sucked her fingers and was not toilet-trained (Bradford, 1990; Smith, 1990). This decision was based on the child's eligibility under the Education of the Handicapped Act and on a revision in the American Academy of Pediatrics guidelines for HIV infection control in the schools (Task Force on Pediatric AIDS, 1988), which state that "HIV-infected children who are old enough to attend school can be admitted freely to all activities, to the extent that their own health permits" (p. 805). Earlier recommendations that children who lack control of their bodily secretions should be educated in a more restricted environment were deleted from the revised guidelines.

Those children with HIV/AIDS who do not require special education are protected by Section 504 of the Rehabilitation Act of 1973. This law, originally designed to protect handicapped people from discrimination, has been interpreted by the courts to apply to HIV-infected individuals in regard to education and employment. In a memorandum designed to provide guidance on the application of Section 504 to HIV-infected schoolchildren, the U.S. Department of Education concludes (Smith, 1990, p. 11):

1. The regulatory definition of a handicapped person will be applied to children with AIDS, who are virtually always "regarded as handicapped" within the meaning of this definition.
2. Unless currently presenting a risk of contagion due to the stage of the disease, a child with AIDS will remain in the regular classroom.

According to the memorandum, children with HIV/AIDS may not be excluded from their normal school placement solely on the basis of their illness.

Policy Development

Some of the school systems that faced initial lawsuits over the placement of HIV-infected children have subsequently formulated enlightened policies, which may serve as a model for other school systems. In 1984, school officials in Dade County, Florida, were notified of the HIV-infected status of three elementary-age sisters. Based on what the school board believed to be sound medical judgment, school officials arranged to place the girls in an isolated learning setting with a volunteer teacher. The American Civil Liberties Union sued the school board on behalf of the children's father, arguing that the girls should be admitted to a regular classroom (U.S. District Court Case No. 86-1513-CIV-DAVIS, May 1987). A settlement in the case resulted in the admittance of the two surviving sisters (one had died in the interim) to a regular classroom. In addition, the settlement required that the school system adopt a policy that included the following guidelines:

1. The school board would establish an advisory placement committee comprised of a teacher's union representative, a PTA representative, representatives of the health department and of the University of Miami's Jackson Memorial Hospital, and other school representatives to consider the placement of children identified as being infected with HIV.
2. Only the principal, teachers, and other school personnel working closely with students would be told of the illness of a student with AIDS.
3. The status of a child whose HIV infection had not progressed to AIDS would remain confidential and would not be revealed to the child's school.

The guidelines above continue to provide the basis for policy regarding students with HIV/AIDS in Dade County. Other school districts have adopted similar policies. However, controversy still remains concerning the issue of who needs to know when a child in school has HIV/AIDS.

Legal Issues Surrounding Confidentiality

The right to confidentiality concerning HIV status must be weighed against the right of the community to be protected from infection.

School policy on confidentiality must take into account the welfare of the infected child, protection of employees and students from infection, and potential liability. Although most school districts have a clearly defined policy that provides for confidentiality, the limits of confidentiality vary from district to district.

In New York City, when a child is identified to the school system as having AIDS, no one at the child's school is informed of the child's illness (Gerri Abelson [AIDS Education Project Director, New York City Board of Education], personal communication, 1990). In Dade County, Florida, as noted above, when a child is identified as having AIDS, the school principal and the child's teachers are routinely informed (Patrick Gray [Assistant Superintendent of Schools, Dade County, Florida], personal communication, 1990). In Newark, New Jersey, strict confidentiality is maintained, but parents of students with AIDS are encouraged to notify the school principal, the child's teacher, and the school nurse (Jeffrey Spector [AIDS Coordinator, Newark Public Schools], personal communication, 1990).

Current discriminatory attitudes toward people with HIV/AIDS and the unwarranted paranoia regarding contagion make the need for confidentiality undeniable. Children with HIV/AIDS have been barred from their classrooms and taunted by their classmates. Even their sisters and brothers have become the objects of ostracism. When the Rays of DeSoto County, Florida, notified school officials in 1986 that their three sons (who had hemophilia) were infected with HIV, school officials barred the children from attending school in their regular classrooms, offering instruction in an isolated classroom as an alternative. The parents sued the school system and won a preliminary injunction allowing the boys to attend school in their regular classrooms (Bradford, 1990). However, the community's hostility toward the Rays remained high: The boys and their uninfected sister were rejected at school, and the family was threatened with violence. Finally, when their home was burned down, they moved to another county. The Ray case demonstrates that without the protection of confidentiality, legal protections may be inadequate to preserve the rights and welfare of infected children.

The issue of confidentiality is complicated by several factors. First, even with policies designed to maintain the secrecy of a diagnosis of HIV/AIDS, confidentiality may be compromised inadvertently or deliberately. Medical records sent to the school by the child's physician may contain the diagnosis. Labeled bottles of medication, particularly zidovudine, administered by the school nurse may identify a child as having HIV/AIDS. Thus, even with the theoretical safeguards of a policy ensuring confidentiality, in reality secrecy may be difficult to maintain. Second, many children who are infected with HIV via mother–infant transmission come under the guardianship of someone other than their biological parents when their mothers die or are no longer able to care for them. Notifying the school that a child has HIV/AIDS can become the responsibility of the state foster placement agency, the foster parent, or a family member or friend with whom the child is living. This raises the question of whether the child's rights and best interests are being protected by the decision to inform. In Florida, for example, the state foster placement agency routinely informs the school when a child has AIDS, *regardless* of the school's need to know. Institutions involved with the care of these children must weigh the possibility that disclosing an HIV/AIDS diagnosis will lead to discrimination against the child against the likelihood that a child whose diagnosis is not known will not get the special educational attention that may be required.

Complete confidentiality in some circumstances may be detrimental to the welfare of the child with HIV/AIDS. The teacher who is unaware of a child's diagnosis may be less compassionate if poor school performance results from memory loss and poor concentration caused by the effects of HIV on the central nervous system. In contrast, a teacher who knows that a child has HIV/AIDS may serve as a source of help and emotional support to the child and to the overburdened parent or guardian.

Furthermore, recent findings suggest that fears that teachers will be biased against children known to have HIV/AIDS may be exaggerated (Walker & Hulecki, 1989). School districts have legitimate concerns about their potential liability in the event that HIV transmission occurs as the result of contact with an infected child. Although some school districts provide school personnel with training in body fluid precautions, a risk remains for anyone coming in contact with infected blood. For this reason, some schools routinely inform physical education teachers and school nurses, who more frequently come in contact with blood, when a child at their school is known to be infected with HIV.

Unfortunately, as long as discrimination against people with HIV/AIDS persists, confidentiality of a child's HIV-infected status must be maintained to the greatest extent possible. In a guide for the development of school policies regarding HIV infection, Fraser (1989) suggests:

> All persons should treat all information about HIV infection as highly confidential. All medical information and written documentation . . . should be kept by the superintendent in a locked file, with access granted only to those persons who have the written consent of . . . a student's parent or guardian. (p. 6)

It is hoped that continuing community education regarding HIV/AIDS will lead to the elimination of discrimination against people with HIV infection, and thereby preclude the need for such strenuous secrecy. The role of the community must be to reduce the burdens on the child with HIV/AIDS, not to add to them.

THE CHILD WITH HIV/AIDS

As has been previously noted, the child with HIV/AIDS is often a member of a "dying family" (Septimus, 1989). As of December 1992, 86% percent of all pediatric AIDS cases in the United States were the result of mother–infant transmission (CDC, 1993). This means that 86% of all children with HIV/AIDS have mothers who are infected with HIV or who have already died of AIDS. If a mother is still alive, she is frequently addicted to injection drugs, single, and poor. In addition, the majority of children with HIV/AIDS come from traditionally disenfranchised ethnic groups. As Hankins (1990) has noted, the result is that

> many parents [of children with AIDS are] emotionally and physically incapable of taking care of their sick child. These parents are perceived negatively as being disorganized and difficult to reach. In reality, often they are overwhelmed, lost in the complexity and the social and medical costs associated with the care of their child. (p. 447)

Those children whose mothers have already died may be living with extended family members, family friends, or foster care parents. Although many of these placements provide loving and competent care, the situation in others ranges from indifferent to neglectful or abusive. In addition, some child welfare agencies have a policy of not placing children infected with HIV in the same foster homes with uninfected children. As a result, a child with HIV/AIDS may be separated from healthy sisters and brothers, who would otherwise provide love, companionship, and a sense of identity.

The child with HIV/AIDS may suffer at school as well as at home. Although confidentiality is the rule in most schools, the diagnosis of HIV/AIDS can be revealed through other sources, leading to teasing and harassment by other children and blatant avoidance by school personnel.

In addition, children with HIV/AIDS may suffer from anxiety and depression in anticipation of serious illness and death. Such concerns frequently have an adverse effect on school performance. Even if a child is not aware of the diagnosis, other factors, such as neurological impairment or frequent absences because of illness or medical appointments, may affect the child's capacity to learn and do well in school. Physical exhaustion is also very common in these children and may result in poor concentration.

Many HIV-infected children come from disrupted or disorganized homes that provide little or no structure for the children to do homework and to develop learning skills. Frequently the classroom teacher is the only adult on whom a child can consistently rely for love and support. Indeed, the teacher often becomes the child's advocate in dealing with a variety of institutions, including the school, welfare agencies, the courts, and the medical community.

TEACHERS AND THE AIDS EPIDEMIC

Teachers of children with HIV/AIDS, as well as teachers who have the responsibility of teaching HIV/AIDS information and prevention curricula, require considerable education and training to deal with the emotionally charged issues created by the AIDS crisis.

Teachers of Children with HIV/AIDS

Preparation of classroom teachers for working with children with HIV/AIDS varies from district to district. In high-incidence areas, school systems have built on past experience to develop effective procedures for placing infected children in the schools.

The school system in Dade County, Florida, which has the second highest number of pediatric AIDS cases in the country (CDC, 1993), has developed a placement procedure for children with HIV/AIDS that facilitates a positive educational environment. First, an advisory placement committee decides whether a child requires special education or a specially designed program. The courts have ruled that whenever possible, a child with HIV/AIDS should be placed in his or her regular neighborhood school. This provision is designed to prevent the creation of a "leper colony" school (P. Gray, personal communication, 1990).

In Dade County, when a child has been identified as having HIV/AIDS, the school principal and the child's teacher are informed of the diagnosis (as noted earlier, no notification is made if the child's HIV infection has not progressed to AIDS). School policy provides that any teacher who refuses to teach a child with HIV/AIDS may request a transfer to another classroom. However, the school system tries to minimize the issue of teacher resistance, while at the same time maintaining confidentiality for the child.

When the school has been selected, the school system's AIDS Information and Education Program provides a special training seminar to all personnel in the school. The seminars have been so effective in creating a positive attitude in teachers that there has been no difficulty in placing these infected children. The Employee Assistance Program provides continuing support services to teachers of children with HIV/AIDS in the form of monthly support groups, ongoing training in HIV/AIDS, individual consultation, and grief counseling (Welty, 1990).

Teachers of children with HIV/AIDS suffer from multiple burdens. First of all, despite the minimal risk of HIV transmission in the school setting, even a sophisticated and well-informed teacher who is about to have a child with HIV/AIDS placed in the classroom may continue to have concerns regarding contagion. Moreover, the teacher may be anxious that expressing these concerns may make him or her appear resistant to the training regarding transmission of HIV. Fortunately, the fear of contagion generally abates rapidly as the teacher comes to know the infected child and they develop a relationship.

The majority of teachers of children with HIV/AIDS develop deep feelings of affection for these children and often become highly protective of them. Two factors in particular account for this. First, it is natural to feel protective of a terminally ill child; indeed, it is difficult to resist such feelings. The second factor derives from the unique sociology of pediatric HIV/AIDS. Many of these children are orphans or are living with mothers, frequently single, who are very ill themselves. Teachers of children with HIV/AIDS often find themselves becoming personally involved with the children's medical care and home situation, even to the extent of making medical appointments for the children, raising funds to provide toys at Christmas, giving food or money to the children's families, and visiting the children in the hospital.

Teachers may find themselves becoming advocates for these children in regard to the various institutions and agencies involved with the children's welfare. The experience of one teacher, referred to here as "Mr. A.," serves as a poignant example.

Case 1

Mr. A., who taught in a program for educable mentally handicapped children, was told by the school principal that a child with AIDS would be enrolled at the school and placed in his classroom. Grudgingly, Mr. A. received the little boy, who was living in a foster home, into his classroom. In a very short time, the lively and affectionate child had captured Mr. A.'s heart, and Mr. A. began to look forward to seeing him daily at school. It gradually became evident, though, that the boy's health was deteriorating. Mr. A.'s attempts to alert the foster mother were in vain. She would deny that the child was ill, or she would make weak excuses for not bringing him to the doctor. Mr. A. notified school officials, who in turn contacted the welfare agency that had placed the boy in his foster home, but these efforts were futile. Soon the little boy was so sick that he required hospitalization. Mr. A. visited him frequently and spent long hours by his bedside. The child died in the hospital.

Mr. A. was overcome with grief. During a grief counseling session arranged by the school system, the psychologist pointed out that Mr. A. had become the boy's psychological father and that the love between them was that of a father and son. Adding to the pain that Mr. A. was experiencing over the death of "his" child was the fact that no one had recognized the depth and importance of this relationship. Thus, he had received little comfort and support from his colleagues and family. The psychologist also pointed out that just as the boy had brought love and joy to the teacher, the teacher had provided a caring parental figure for the child—the only one that the child had had.

Case 2

In another case, a teacher working in a homebound teaching program (a program in which children who are too sick to attend school receive instruction from a visiting teacher) went to the home of one of his teenage students with AIDS. He found the student, who had recently had a colostomy, screaming in pain and threatening to cut her sutures with a pair of scissors. The mother had gone to the hospital to get some medicine that had been previously prescribed. The girl's two adult brothers were at home, but neither was able to cope with the situation.

The teacher called the school system's AIDS office for guidance and was told to call the county's emergency rescue service. He was reminded *not* to inform the rescue team that the girl had AIDS, as this would be a violation of confidentiality. When the rescue team arrived, the teacher accompanied the student first to a clinic and then to the hospital, where a bed was eventually found for her. He stayed with the girl until she was settled into her room. The entire ordeal took place over a period of many hours, and the teacher did not leave the hospital until 10:00 P.M. A year earlier, when he was first asked to teach a student with AIDS, this same teacher had not been sure that he wanted to be in the same room with the student.

Teaching a child with HIV/AIDS is a challenging experience. It is stressful to be emotionally attached to a child with a life-threatening condition. Moreover, teachers may often experience ostracism from their peers at a time when they most need support. Most importantly, they experience deep grief when a child dies. However, as these case histories illustrate, teaching a child with HIV/AIDS can provide a rare opportunity for personal growth.

Teachers Who Provide HIV/AIDS Education in the Schools

Thirty-three states and 80% of large school districts now mandate AIDS-preventive education (Putka, 1990). In January 1988, the CDC issued a set of comprehensive guidelines for HIV/AIDS education in the schools (CDC, 1988). The following recommendations were formulated after consultation with representatives of various health, educational, and religious organizations:

1. The principal purpose of education about AIDS is to prevent the spread of infection.
2. The specific scope and content of AIDS education in the schools should be locally determined and should be consistent with local and community values.
3. Education about AIDS may be most appropriate and effective when carried out within . . . a health education program that establishes a foundation for understanding the relationships between personal behavior and health.
4. A team of representatives including [all school administrative personnel, health care personnel, counselors, teachers, and support personnel] should receive general training about . . . the AIDS epidemic, the role of the school in providing education to prevent transmission of HIV, . . . and school policies for students and staff who may be infected.
5. All school personnel, especially those who teach about AIDS, periodically should receive continuing education about AIDS. . . .
6. In the elementary grades . . . education about AIDS should be provided by the regular classroom teacher. . . .
7. In the secondary grades . . . the health education teacher preferably should provide education about AIDS. (CDC, 1988, pp. 2–4)

To facilitate the implementation of HIV/AIDS education in the schools, the CDC has provided grant money to the states for in-service training and curriculum development. This money has been allocated to local school systems, which have developed programs appropriate for their particular local communities.

In-Service Training

The objective of in-service training is to provide accurate information to school personnel regarding all aspects of the HIV/AIDS epidemic, including epidemiology, modes of transmission, and legal and policy aspects of HIV/AIDS as it affects the schools.

Most school systems with in-service training programs provide intensive training workshops for teachers who will be responsible for teaching the HIV/AIDS education curriculum. Some school systems have developed a "trainer of trainers" model, in which a corps of teachers is selected and trained to prepare other teachers in their respective schools to teach the HIV/AIDS curriculum. Teachers and other school personnel who are not responsible for the HIV/AIDS curriculum may be given a less intensive training seminar. Workshops are generally given during regular school hours, and substitute teachers take over classroom responsibilities while the regular teachers are at the training sessions. Training updates are provided periodically to refresh the teachers' knowledge and to inform them of current research and policy.

Presentations should be structured to cover not only the factual and pedagogical aspects of HIV/AIDS education, but also the ethical, social, and psychological aspects. Those teachers who are responsible for the HIV/AIDS curriculum should be reminded that providing factual information to students is insufficient and that fostering the development of risk-reducing behavior is essential. The following information should be included in HIV/AIDS education workshops for teachers:

1. AIDS is caused by a virus (HIV). Teachers should understand how the virus destroys the immune system, as well as the effects of the virus on the central nervous system.
2. Screening tests for HIV detect the antibodies to HIV and not the virus itself. Individuals who are infected with the virus may transmit it to others even if seroconversion has not occurred.
3. HIV cannot be contracted from toilet seats, mosquito bites, eating utensils, donating blood, or the like. The virus is transmitted only through the blood, semen, vaginal secretions, breast milk, or donated organs of infected individuals.
4. AIDS is not just a disease of homosexuals and drug abusers. Everyone is at risk, and anyone can become infected.
5. There have been no reported cases of HIV transmission in the school setting. Saliva does not transmit the virus. There is no risk involved in hugging or drying the tears of a child with HIV/AIDS. Only the body fluids mentioned above pose any risk.

6. The proper use of latex condoms in conjunction with a spermicide containing nonoxynol-9 can reduce the risk of sexually transmitted HIV.

7. The risk of HIV transmission in the course of drug abuse can be avoided by never sharing needles. The risk can be reduced by washing the injection and preparation equipment with a solution of 1 part household bleach to 9 parts water. (The best prevention, of course, is avoiding injection drug use altogther.)

8. Homosexuality is a widespread sexual orientation. Many students and teachers are gay and are at risk for contracting HIV through homosexual activity. Discussions of homosexuality should be nonjudgmental and respectful.

9. Children with HIV/AIDS often suffer from the social problems associated with the condition. They may be orphaned or have very sick mothers who have sole responsibility for the children. They are also frequently poor and often come from socially disadvantaged backgrounds.

In addition to the factual information presented above, teachers should understand the policy of their local school system regarding HIV-infected students and personnel, federal and state laws applying to HIV-infected individuals, and the importance of maintaining confidentiality regarding HIV infection.

It should be recognized that those teachers who will be teaching the HIV/AIDS curriculum in their schools may experience embarrassment in discussing some aspects of AIDS prevention, particularly those involving the description of sexual acts and contraception. Teachers should be helped to accept their embarrassment as natural. However, it should be emphasized that frank and detailed discussion of sexual matters regarding AIDS prevention is necessary to protect the lives of their students.

Dealing with Teachers' Doubts

Although training sessions are generally well received, some teachers may remain skeptical, particularly with regard to HIV transmission. If these teachers express their anxiety and skepticism while retaining an open mind, the presenter can usually allay their fears by explaining current research and the rational basis of current policy. However, in almost any training seminar, at least one teacher will be resistant to the information presented and will express his or her skepticism in a hostile manner. Reacting in an argumentative way generally does not improve the situation. The best approach is to acknowledge, in a nonthreatening way, the teacher's unwillingness to accept the facts; to emphasize that this is the result of unrealistic anxiety; and to reinforce the importance of continuing with the training session for the benefit of those teachers who will use the information in order to perform their jobs effectively.

Teachers may explain their unrealistic skepticism in a variety of ways, ranging from primitive to pseudoscientific. One teacher may say, "My cousin is a nursing assistant and she won't go into the hospital room of a patient with AIDS without wearing a mask, gown, and gloves." A more sophisticated teacher may say, "I teach science, and scientists are taught that one can never prove a fact. Therefore, you can't prove that HIV isn't transmitted by shaking hands." It must be remembered that all such teachers are frightened and that their fear is a natural (though unrealistic) reaction to a scary illness. Unfortunately, with such resistant teachers, no amount of intellectual fact is likely to change their beliefs. The best approach is simply to say, "AIDS is a very frightening disease, and that makes it hard for some people to believe that HIV can be transmitted only in a very limited number of ways."

In general, most teachers find that in-service training increases their self-confidence regarding their knowledge about HIV/AIDS. As a result, they feel capable of informing others about HIV/AIDS and experience relief from unnecessary anxiety.

CURRICULUM DEVELOPMENT FOR HIV/AIDS EDUCATION

Most school districts with HIV/AIDS education curricula have incorporated the CDC (1988) guidelines into their pre-existing family life or health education curricula. However, HIV/AIDS education poses unique challenges that have caused much debate concerning what should be appropriately taught at each grade level. As a result, there is a great deal of variability among school systems, particularly among the lower grades. Clearly, even within the same school, children in the same grade will have different capacities for understanding the material, different levels of sophistication regarding sexual matters, and different levels of exposure to drug-related activities. In addition, there may be pressure from community and religious groups to restrict the information that is taught, particularly regarding sexual matters. This may be met with competing pressure from health agencies to provide essential, explicit prevention information as early as possible.

Frequently parents express concern regarding the HIV/AIDS curriculum. For this reason, the CDC (1988) guidelines recommend that the HIV/AIDS curriculum be developed in consultation with a panel of representatives of the community, to ensure that the curriculum is supported by the parents and community leaders. Many school systems send out information packets about HIV/AIDS and the curriculum. This preparation has served to reduce resistance to such curricula in the schools. In some school systems where parents are permitted to withdraw their children from class when the HIV/AIDS prevention curriculum is being taught, parents are required to attend a meeting where the content and purpose of the curriculum is explained. This serves to educate the parents about HIV/AIDS and to enlist their support for the curriculum.

Any HIV/AIDS curriculum must be taught in a manner that is likely to promote risk-reducing behavior. However, as studies have shown, having accurate information about HIV transmission does not necessarily change high-risk behavior (Weisman et al., 1989). This can be attributed to several factors. Ross, Caudle, and Taylor (1989) identified five areas of AIDS-related interpersonal activities in which high school students expressed tension or anxiety, including negotiating aspects of sexual behavior (such as abstinence and condom use), refusing to share syringes during drug-taking activity, and disclosing that one has a sexually transmitted disease. The authors suggest that reducing anxiety and increasing interpersonal assertiveness will lead to a reduction in high-risk behaviors. For this reason, many HIV/AIDS curricula include exercises in interpersonal assertiveness and role playing in simulated high-risk situations.

Failure of HIV/AIDS education to change high-risk behavior may also be attributable to other factors. Adolescents are notorious for believing in their own immortality; as a result, they may not take the need for precautions seriously. Individuals must also fear the disease in order for there to be a significant behavioral change (Wells, in press). For this reason, audiovisual materials may include interviews with young people who have AIDS, in order to emphasize to students that they are at risk. The Boston public schools have used peer instructors— students who are part of the training team—to teach students about HIV/AIDS. It is felt that teens may communicate more effectively with their peers and add to the program's credibility (McCormick, 1989).

Sexual behavior in adolescent girls is often interpreted as antisocial or "acting-out" behavior. However, when such behavior is understood in the context of a society that socializes females to yield to the demands and desires of those in authority, primarily men, sexual activity in adolescent girls can be seen to be simply the fulfillment of what these girls perceive to be their social role. This may also account for the fact that even among those adolescent girls who have accurate information regarding reducing the risk of HIV infection, there is a failure to use condoms (Weisman et al., 1989). An effective AIDS prevention curriculum must include an emphasis, particularly for girls, on one's right to resist the demands of others that one engage in dangerous behavior. Again, role playing in simulated high-risk situations, particularly for girls, can serve to reinforce self-protective assertive behavior.

It is important that educational materials about HIV/AIDS be culturally sensitive. Such materials must take into account the cultural beliefs and experiences of the target audience, and should be presented in language with which the audience can identify. Materials have been produced that specifically target inner-city African-American and Hispanic adolescents. The CDC (1990) has published a compendium of abstracts of HIV/AIDS education materials, including audiovisuals, curriculum guides, and pamphlets as well as other types of material.

Although the Surgeon General's report on AIDS (Koop, 1987) recommends that HIV/AIDS education be provided in the earliest possible grades, many school systems provide no such education in the elementary grades. The most difficult problem is deciding at what grade level to introduce detailed sexual information. Many school systems have been hesitant to present factual information regarding such subjects as condoms, oral and anal sex, and homosexuality. As a result, these issues are often not presented until the senior high school grades. Unfortunately, because of the realities of adolescent sexuality, this may be too late. In one study, it was found that 24% of 14-year-old boys reported already having experienced sexual intercourse (Zelnik & Kanter, 1980). The fact of preteen and early teen pregnancy confirms the need for HIV/AIDS education in the lower grades.

In the Irvington, New Jersey schools, the HIV/AIDS curriculum includes information regarding sexually transmitted diseases and homosexuality beginning in the fourth grade. There has been little objection to this on the part of parents or religious groups, because of a community advisory panel's involvement in approving the subject matter to be taught (McCormick, 1989). Obviously, it must be left up to the individual communities to decide what information is appropriate to provide at any given grade level. However, since the issue is one of life or death, we cannot afford to be too demure in presenting the risks of certain behaviors.

The following is an example of an effective HIV/AIDS prevention curriculum. It may serve as a guideline for the introduction of appropriate material at consecutive grade levels.

Kindergarten through Third Grade

The primary objectives of HIV/AIDS education at the early elementary level are twofold. The first is to reduce anxiety resulting from misconceptions about HIV transmission and manifestations of AIDS. Fassler, McQueen, Duncan, and Copeland (1990) found that elementary-age children expressed considerable anxiety about AIDS and that, unfortunately, television was their primary source of information about the disease. This underscores the importance of providing accurate information in the early school grades. The second objective of HIV/AIDS education in the early grades is to establish behavioral patterns that will lead to risk reduction.

1. *Anxiety reduction.* Children should be taught that people with AIDS can be treated as one would treat anyone else. They cannot "catch" the disease by shaking hands with someone who has AIDS, by playing with them, or by hugging them. Children can also be told that most children who have AIDS "caught" the virus that causes the disease from their mothers during pregnancy.

2. *Basic health information.* Children should be instructed that diseases such as AIDS are caused by microorganisms called viruses or bacteria. They should understand that our bodies can usually fight off these infections, but that sometimes we need medicine in order to kill the microorganisms. Students should be told that although we have medications that can help treat HIV infection, we do not yet have medication that will kill HIV in the body or cure AIDS. Students should be taught good health habits, including proper handwashing. They should be instructed not to touch other people's blood, and to wash with soap and water in the event that they do come in contact with blood.

3. *Drug abuse prevention.* Drug abuse prevention must play an important role in any AIDS prevention curriculum. Children should be taught to resist peer pressure to engage in the illicit use of drugs. They should also be taught not to touch discarded hypodermic needles or syringes.

4. *Self-respect and assertiveness.* Children should be taught that they have the right and the responsibility to protect their own well-being. Because sexual abuse is a potential source of HIV infection, children should be taught not to let anyone touch the "private parts" of their bodies, and to tell a parent or teacher if someone attempts to do so.

Teaching devices for the AIDS prevention curriculum in the early elementary grades may include visual material, coloring, role playing, and songs about good health habits.

Fourth and Fifth Grades

The most important objective for HIV/AIDS education in the later elementary grades is to prepare children for decisionmaking with regard to sexual behavior and drug abuse. Information learned in the earlier grades can be reinforced and expanded upon.

1. *Basic sex education.* Children can be taught the basics of sex education starting in the fourth grade. This is probably done most effectively when boys and girls are taught in separate classrooms. Instruction can begin with the basics of the anatomy and physiology of sexual reproduction. Children should be taught that HIV can be transmitted through intimate sexual activity.

2. *Drug abuse prevention.* More specific information can be presented regarding the transmission of HIV through drug abuse. Children can begin to learn how illegal drugs affect the body and how people become addicted to them.

3. *Anxiety reduction.* The modes in which HIV is *not* transmitted should be re-emphasized. Students should understand that HIV is not transmitted through casual contact, including touching, eating utensils, and bathroom facilities.

4. *Health education.* Basic information can be provided on how the immune system functions and how bacteria, viruses, and parasites cause disease. This can serve to lay the groundwork for explaining how HIV damages the immune system. Students can learn that the body produces antibodies to fight infections, and that the screening tests for HIV infection detect the presence of antibodies rather than the virus itself.

Sixth through Eighth Grades

The main objective of HIV/AIDS education at the middle school/junior high level is to provide clear and explicit information regarding the transmission of HIV.

1. *Sex education.* As in the earlier grades, sex education is best presented to boys and girls in separate classrooms; students may feel more comfortable asking questions about detailed sexual information in a same-gender context. The reasons for abstinence from sexual in-

tercourse should be emphasized, including the risk of contracting sexually transmitted diseases such as syphilis and HIV, the risk of pregnancy, and the need for emotional growth in order to be ready for satisfactory intimate relationships. Information about contraception, especially condoms and spermicides, should be provided. *Consumer Reports* (1989) has described, in detail, the proper use of condoms. Detailed information about the types of sexual activity that result in HIV transmission should be presented; this should include information about oral, anal, and vaginal sex. Homosexuality should be explained in a nonjudgmental manner.

2. *Drug abuse information.* Again, avoidance of drug abuse should be emphasized. However, given that some students may inject drugs anyway, information about reducing the risk of HIV transmission via dirty needles should also be provided, including avoiding the sharing of injection equipment and properly disinfecting used injection equipment.

3. *Health education.* Information regarding the progress of HIV infection, the types of opportunistic infections associated with AIDS, and current treatments can be presented. Students should understand that people infected with HIV may not become sick for a long time, that HIV disease may develop gradually with a variety of symptoms, and that AIDS is the endpoint of HIV disease. Students should also understand that even though an individual infected with HIV may show no symptoms, he or she can transmit the virus to others through sexual activity or needle sharing. Other modes of transmission, including needle sticks in health care workers and mother–infant transmission, can be discussed. Students should understand that the blood supply has been screened for HIV since 1985, and therefore that the risk of infection from blood transfusions is minimal.

4. *Self-assertiveness training.* Emphasis should be placed on a student's responsibility to protect himself or herself from HIV infection. Exercises in decisionmaking in high-risk situations should be presented, to enable students to practice their responses in a controlled situation and prepare them for real-life situations.

Although the emphasis of HIV/AIDS education at this level must be on risk reduction, students must also learn that people with HIV/AIDS should be treated like anyone else and are as deserving of compassion and support as anyone else with a serious illness.

Ninth through Twelfth Grades

Information learned in earlier grades should be reinforced at the senior high level. Students should have a comprehensive understanding of

HIV, including the modes of transmission, ways in which it is *not* transmitted, the function of the immune system, risk-reducing behavior, and other relevant information.

1. *Health information.* Risk reduction should be emphasized, particularly in the areas of sexual activity and drug abuse. Students should be made aware of anonymous HIV counseling and testing sites in their local area, including telephone numbers and addresses. Information regarding local drug treatment programs should also be provided.

2. *Social education.* Students should be encouraged to discuss the social and ethical questions that have arisen from the AIDS crisis. Questions such as the rights of the individual versus the welfare of the community and the purpose of the US Constitution can be discussed as a means of broadening the students' understanding of the issues involved.

3. *Self-assertiveness training.* Training in self-protective behavior should be continued, with emphasis on sexual behavior and drug abuse.

At all grade levels, it is recommended that students participate actively in the learning process through written exercises, special projects, and role playing. Teachers should keep in mind the CDC's statement that the primary goal of HIV/AIDS education is the prevention of HIV infection. Thus, emphasis should be placed on providing students with information regarding risk reduction and on strengthening behaviors to help them use that information effectively.

THE ROLE OF SCHOOL HEALTH CLINICS

Some school systems have health clinics that provide basic health services to students. Some of these clinics provide confidential testing and counseling on sexual matters, such as pregnancy and sexually transmitted diseases. Such clinics can provide an additional source of information about HIV risk reduction. Often the students who come to these clinics for counseling regarding sexual matters or for testing for pregnancy or sexually transmitted diseases are at the highest risk of acquiring HIV through sexual activity. The clinics thus provide an opportunity to reach those students and to support the implementation of the risk-reducing behavior learned in HIV/AIDS education classes. Students can be instructed about their risks and can also be given detailed information regarding the proper use of condoms with spermicide. The issue of whether these clinics should provide students with condoms, with or without parental consent, has been a source of much controversy. This issue should be resolved at the community level, with the input of health officials to explain the need to concerned parents and religious groups.

Those clinics that provide confidential drug counseling can also serve as sources for education regarding the risk of HIV infection and risk-reducing behavior. Unfortunately, because of the current lack of budgetary commitment to drug rehabilitation services, many of those seeking treatment for drug addiction find long waiting lists for entry into rehabilitation programs. As a result, the risk to drug-abusing students may not be reduced even though they are willing to undergo treatment.

SUMMARY

The AIDS epidemic in the United States presents a tremendous challenge to the nation's schools. With the steadily growing numbers of HIV-infected children entering school, the school systems must establish policies that protect both the rights of these children and the welfare of other members of the school community.

Children with HIV/AIDS suffer from burdens in addition to those imposed by their illness: They often come from traditionally disenfranchised ethnic groups, they are often orphaned, and they may suffer from social isolation and rejection. Often their teachers are the only adults upon whom they can consistently rely. The effects of HIV/AIDS may cause difficulties in learning, particularly in the areas of memory, attention, and motor skills.

Teachers must be prepared to receive children with HIV/AIDS into their classrooms. This requires that they be educated not only about the facts regarding HIV infection, but also about the unique sociology of pediatric HIV/AIDS. Teachers of children with HIV/AIDS have found their experience with these youngsters to be a source of emotional growth. Despite the sadness and the challenges, teaching these children helps them to discover inner strengths and capacities that may have previously gone unrecognized.

The nation's schools bear the responsibility for educating our children about the threat of HIV infection. Most parents have not received formal education about HIV/AIDS and do not have immediate access to current information. It is therefore essential that the schools provide HIV/AIDS education, especially regarding the prevention of HIV infection. It is important that the HIV/AIDS curriculum be supported by the local community, and it is therefore recommended that parents and community groups, as well as local health care agencies, provide input for curriculum development.

HIV/AIDS education can begin as early as kindergarten, in order to develop and establish behavioral patterns that will lead to risk reduction. Local school boards should decide at which grade levels specific information should be introduced. Since having accurate information about AIDS prevention does not guarantee a reduction in high-risk behavior, the HIV/AIDS curriculum should also foster the development of behavioral patterns, such as interpersonal self-assertiveness, that will enable students to effectively use the information they have learned.

School health clinics can serve as important adjuncts to the HIV/AIDS curriculum in educating students about HIV infection, especially those students who are at particularly high risk.

All of our children are at risk for being infected with HIV at some point in their lives. The only protection that we can currently provide for them is education about how to avoid high-risk behavior. We must therefore establish effective HIV/AIDS education in our schools. The lives and futures of our children depend on it.

REFERENCES

Bradford, V. (1990). *People in glass houses: Deciding the educational placement of children and adolescents with HIV/AIDS.* Unpublished manuscript.

Centers for Disease Control (CDC). (1988, January 29). Guidelines for effective school health education to prevent the spread of AIDS. *Morbidity and Mortality Weekly Report,* pp. 1–14.

Centers for Disease Control (CDC). (1990). *HIV and AIDS: A cumulation of the AIDS school health database.* Atlanta: Author.

Centers for Disease Control (CDC). (1993, February). *HIV/AIDS surveillance report: Year-end edition.* Atlanta: Author.

Consumer Reports. (1989, March). Can you rely on condoms? pp. 135–141.

Fassler, D., McQueen, K., Duncan, P., & Copeland, L. (1990). Children's perceptions of AIDS. *Journal of the American Academy of Child and Adolescent Psychiatry, 29,* 459–462.

Fraser, K. (1989). *Someone at school has AIDS: A guide to developing policies for students and school staff members who are infected with HIV.* Alexandria, VA: National Association of State Boards of Education.

Hankins, C. A. (1990). Issues involving women, children, and AIDS primarily in the developed world. *Journal of Acquired Immune Deficiency Syndromes, 3,* 443–448.

Koop, C. E. (1987). *Surgeon General's report on acquired immune deficiency syndrome.* Washington, DC: U.S. Government Printing Office.

McCormick, K. (1989). *Reducing the risk: A school leader's guide to AIDS education.* Alexandria, VA: National School Boards Association.

Nayman, L., & Poltrock, L. (1987, June 30). *Compulsory AIDS testing of* teachers, school support personnel, and students. Memorandum to the American Federation of Teachers Executive Council.

Putka, G. (1990, June 12). Uncharted course. *Wall Street Journal,* p. 1.

Ross, M. W., Caudle, C., & Taylor, J. (1989). A preliminary study of social issues in AIDS prevention among adolescents. *Journal of School Health, 59,* 308–311.

Septimus, A. (1989). Psychological aspects of caring for families of infants infected with human immunodeficiency virus. *Seminars in Perinatology, 13,* 49–54.

Smith, W. L. (1990, April 5). *Guidance on application of Section 504 to children in elementary and secondary schools.* Memorandum to U.S. Department of Education, Office of Civil Rights senior staff.

Task Force on Pediatric AIDS. (1988). Pediatric guidelines for infection control of human immunodeficiency virus (acquired immunodeficiency virus) in hospitals, medical offices, schools, and other settings. *Pediatrics, 82,* 801–807.

Walker, D. W., & Hulecki, M. B. (1989). Is AIDS a biasing factor in teacher judgment? *Exceptional Children, 55,* 342–345.

Weisman, C. S., Nathanson, C. A., Ensminger, M., Teitelbaum, M. A., Robinson, J. C., & Plichta, S. (1989). AIDS knowledge, perceived risk and prevention among adolescent clients of a family planning clinic. *Family Planning Perspectives, 21,* 213–217.

Wells, J. A. (in press). Fear of AIDS and condom use. In G. L. Albrecht (Ed.), *Advances in medical sociology* (Vol. IV). Greenwich, CT: JAI Press.

Welty, A. S. (1990, April 25). *District practices relative to the placement of students with HIV/AIDS.* Memorandum to Paul Bell, Superintendent of Schools, Dade County, FL.

Zelnik, M., & Kanter, J. F. (1980). Sexual activity, contraceptive use, and pregnancy among metropolitan-area teenagers: 1971–1979. *Family Planning Perspectives, 12,* 230–237.

16

Professional, Ethical,
and Moral Issues

Nancy Boyd-Franklin, PhD
Hazel Staloff, JD
Patricia M. Brady, EdD

As the epidemic of HIV infection and AIDS has spread in the United
States, ethical dilemmas have been addressed, and the personal and
group morality of professionals challenged. This chapter presents a discussion of the moral and ethical issues involved for professional
caregivers—issues so complex that most of the professional associations involved give vague, nondirectional guidelines to practitioners.
Since regulations vary widely, professionals are cautioned to become
familiar with those in their own state that deal with discrimination,
access to health-related services, confidentiality, and specialty entitlements (such as education and public benefits). It is also incumbent upon
clinicians to keep current with the literature in this area, as it is an
ever-changing landscape.

The AIDS epidemic brings with it a unique social history. From
the initial discovery of HIV/AIDS within urban gay communities—a
phenomenon exacerbated by the hysteria of early media reports
(Temoshok, Sweet, & Zich, 1987)—through its inexorable spread to
injection drug users and their sexual partners, AIDS has been identified by mainstream society as a behaviorally related disease that affects others. Although the disease is no longer restricted to groups that
have been traditionally marginalized in this country, the psychologi-

cal reactions of society remain stubbornly resistant to catching up with reality.

Health and mental health care providers are not immune from the discomfort and denial that surround HIV/AIDS. Some professionals, struggling with their own humanity, show great resistance to HIV/AIDS knowledge. Is this an unspoken attempt to shield themselves from having to deal with HIV-infected people? Is there an ethical obligation to gain knowledge and to do such work, and under what circumstances might this vary?

In trying to define limits, ethical codes often include standards that are mutually antagonistic. For example, the weighing of individuals' privacy against public health needs reflects the professional dilemma of whether to maintain confidentiality or respond to a duty to report a person's HIV status. How does one balance the freedom of an individual against potential harm to others? Is the presence of HIV a dangerous situation and when? The ethical ramifications of such issues, along with those in research, clinical trials, and access to care, are discussed.

CONFIDENTIALITY VERSUS DUTY TO PROTECT AND TO REPORT

Among the ethical issues in regard to HIV/AIDS, the major controversy has centered on the discrepancy between the right to confidentiality of individuals with HIV/AIDS on the one hand, and the duty to protect the welfare of the community and society at large on the other (Fost, 1991; Harding, Gray, & Neal, 1993; Knapp & VandeCreek, 1992; Pizzo & Wilfert, 1991; Grady, 1992). Confidentiality is a particularly salient variable for professionals involved in psychotherapy or counseling with HIV/AIDS patients, because it is so central to the development and maintenance of the therapeutic bond. Although these issues may have existed with other infectious diseases, the consequences of disclosure of HIV status are uniquely injurious (Grady, 1992). They include the real possibility of social stigma, discrimination, and isolation, as well as loss of job, housing, insurance, and the right to attend school, among other things (Brown, 1987; Cooke, 1990; Eisenberg, 1986; Milliken & Greenblatt, 1988). Therefore, the issue of disclosure is fraught with difficulty for many HIV-infected individuals and their family members.

However, the failure to disclose, while protecting the individual, may threaten great potential harm to others. In recent years, arguments have been made for allowing breach of confidentiality in extreme cases where public safety or the protection of other individuals is a significant risk (Girardi, Keese, Traver, & Cooksey, 1988). These authors cite the *Tarasoff* case (*Tarasoff v. Regents of the University of California*, 1976), in which a California court ruled a that a psychotherapist had a duty to warn the intended victim of threatened violence when a patient stated that he intended to kill his girlfriend. The facts in the *Tarasoff* case, however, are very different from situations involving HIV/AIDS. Therefore, it should not be viewed as providing license for clinicians to breach confidentiality.

The application of *Tarasoff* to the treatment of patients with HIV/AIDS has produced a great deal of debate (Harding et al., 1993; Knapp & VandeCreek, 1992), because the analogy is not direct. Wood, Marks, and Dilley (1990) and Harding et al. (1993) have indicated that the following factors would have to be present before a therapist would be held liable for failure to protect an intended victim:

> (1) The counselor must know the patient is HIV infected; (2) the parties engage in unsafe behavior on a regular basis; (3) such behavior is actually unsafe; (4) the client intends to continue such behavior even after counseling by the therapist; (5) HIV transmission will be the likely result. (Harding et al., 1993, p. 300)

Several commentators have argued for maintaining confidentiality (Healey, 1987; Wood et al., 1990; Harding et al., 1993).

If, in a given situation, all other models of intervention have failed and a clinician feels that a significant risk of transmission exists, a controversy arises as to who should inform them (Grady, 1992). HIV-infected persons can be helped to inform their own partners, and there have been reports that psychotherapy may be effective in helping HIV-infected persons to disclose their status to others who may be in danger (Knapp & VandeCreek, 1992; Perry, 1989). However, when this does not occur, the President's Commission on the HIV Epidemic (1988) has recommended the development of state and local confidential partner notification programs, wherein infected persons unable or unwilling to notify their partners would be reported to the public health authorities, who would take responsibility for such notification (Grady, 1992).

Confidentiality Issues Specific to Adolescents

In regard to disclosure to sexual partners or individuals at risk for exposure through needle sharing, adolescents present many of the same confidentiality issues as adults. However, other complex ethical and legal questions also occur in treating this age group (Futterman & Hein, 1991). Ginzburg (1991) indicates that "many states permit minors to receive treatment for sexually transmitted diseases, substance abuse and hepatitis and counseling for family planning without parental consent or knowledge." Since states do not require that parents be notified if an adolescent seeks testing and care for HIV infection, technically the physician has no right to inform the parents (Ginzburg, 1991). This issue can also become extremely complex in psychotherapy. The treating physician or therapist should discuss the "advisability of the patient's informing his or her parents but the final decision rests with the patient" (Ginzburg, 1991, p. 762). This can create very complicated treatment realities. Although the numbers of HIV-infected adolescents are still small, ethical dilemmas of this type will arise as more cases are diagnosed.

Positions of Professional Organizations on Confidentiality

Harding et al. (1993), in their comprehensive review, have summarized the positions of major professional organizations regarding HIV/AIDS confidentiality and duty to warn. Neither the American Association for Counseling and Development (AACD, now the American Counseling Association) (AACD Governing Council, 1988) nor the American Psychological Association (1991) gives specific, clear guidelines for service providers regarding duty to warn with HIV-infected clients (Harding et al., 1993).

The American Psychological Association (1991) policy on legislation regarding confidentiality and the prevention of HIV transmission is that confidentiality is to be preserved, and a "legal duty to protect third parties from infection should not be imposed" (p. 1).

This policy was developed to provide guidance to the legislative process. It states:

> If, however, specific legislation is considered, then it should permit disclosure only when (a) the provider knows of an identifiable third party who the provider has compelling reason to believe is at significant risk for infection; (b) the provider has a reasonable belief that the third party has no reason to suspect that he or she is at risk; (c) the client/patient has been urged to inform the third party and has either refused or is considered unreliable in his/her willingness to notify the third party. (American Psychological Association, 1991, p. 1)

The National Association of Social Workers (NASW) leaves agencies
the responsibility to establish guidelines for their workers:

> In the absence of standard statutory or regulatory guidelines, practition-
> ers and agencies may perceive a responsibility to warn third parties of
> their potential for infection if their spouses, other sexual partners or part-
> ners in intravenous drug use are HIV infected and the partners refuse to
> warn them. Agencies have a responsibility to establish clear guidelines
> for workers whose clients place others at risk for infection. (NASW
> Delegate Assembly, 1990, p. 5)

The ethical issues in the area of confidentiality versus duty to warn
and protecting the interests of society are complex and constantly
evolving. It is incumbent upon health and mental health care providers
to contact their professional organizations on a regular basis for
guidance on these issues.

The American Psychiatric Association's policy on confidentiality
and duty to warn in HIV/AIDS is clearer:

> If a patient refuses to agree to change his or her behavior or to notify
> the person(s) at risk . . . it is ethically permissible for the physician to noti-
> fy an identifiable person who the physician believes is in danger of con-
> tracting the virus. (American Psychiatric Association Ad Hoc Committee
> on AIDS Policy, 1988, p. 541)

The American Medical Association (AMA) issues a stronger statement
still:

> Ideally, a physician should attempt to persuade the infected party to cease
> endangering the third party; if persuasion fails, the authorities should be
> notified and if the authorities take no action, the physician should notify
> and counsel the endangered third party. (AMA Council on Ethical and
> Judicial Affairs, 1988, p. 1361)

The American Nurses Association (ANA) allows for a breach of confidentiality under stringent criteria:

> [ANA] endorses the concept of an ethical responsibility to disclose other-
> wise confidential information about probable HIV exposure when the pa-
> tient fails to uphold his/her duty to protect others by preventing
> transmission of the infecting agent *but* only when specific criteria have
> been met and documented. (ANA, 1992, p. 15)

DUTY TO TREAT

Medical, nursing, and other health care providers are presented with the risk of contracting occupationally acquired HIV infection, and although studies have shown that the risk of acquiring HIV from a single needle stick exposure or mucocutaneous splash is very low (Henderson et al., 1990; Grady, 1992), perceptions and fears rather than reality are often operative in the response to HIV infection and risk in the health care professions (Freedman, 1988). Thus, some nurses and other health care providers (Grady, 1992) have refused to care for persons known to be HIV-infected (Cooke, 1990; Eisenberg, 1986; Lo, 1990a, 1990b). Even mental health professionals—who have virtually no risk of contracting HIV infection in their clinical work—remain fearful. Grady (1992), however, cautions against overlooking the large numbers of professional caregivers who provide excellent care to these clients, and points out that most professional organizations recommend the use of universal precautions to protect staff members (Centers for Disease Control [CDC], 1987; Creighton, 1986).

In the HIV/AIDS literature, the debate over the duty of professionals to provide services to those requesting them is second only to the debate over confidentiality. The prevailing view (Bisbing, 1988; Ginzburg, 1988; Morrison, 1989) of national medical, psychiatric, and nursing associations is that one cannot refuse to treat patients whose needs are within one's professional competence, although the psychological community operates under a less clear standard.

In a nonemergency situation, the medical professional may refuse to treat an individual who has not been his or her patient, as long as there is no discrimination in the decision (Bisbing, 1988). But mental health clinicians' diagnostic, therapeutic, consultative, and educational roles are unlikely to expose them to HIV infection. Indeed, it is unethical and illegal for mental health and social service professionals to engage with clients in the kinds of behaviors that are known to transmit HIV.

Morrison (1989) suggests that a psychologist who is uncomfortable dealing with HIV-infected clients may be well advised to refer them to colleagues, and Melton (1988) warns that such discomfort may render the psychologist ethically unable to treat an HIV-infected person. However, having chosen a profession, the individual accepts the obligations and risks that are part of that practice (Emanuel, 1988; Young, 1986). Melton (1988) also suggests that a professional has a "duty to become capable" (p. 945), which encompasses obtaining ade-

quate knowledge and consulting with experienced colleagues in order
to provide treatment to HIV-infected clients.

INFORMED CONSENT TO TREATMENT

"Informed consent to treatment" exists when a competent patient
makes decisions about treatment methods, diagnostic tests, and care,
based upon disclosure of all relevant information (Grady, 1992).
However, the uncertainty of many HIV/AIDS treatments, their experimental nature, and the lack of full knowledge and information
about this disease all create difficulty in obtaining such informed consent (Grady, 1992). Price et al. (1988), Ostrow and Gayle (1986), Cooke
(1990), and Veatch and Fry (1987) have also discussed the high incidence of neuropsychiatric disease (such as dementia) that occurs with
HIV infection; this may impair a patient's ability to make crucial decisions regarding treatment. In the case of a parent who is mentally in-
competent because of advanced neurological disease, decisions as to
custody and care of surviving children after the parent's death become
extremely complex matters (Fost, 1991; Pizzo & Wilfert, 1991; Cooper, Knight, & Leonard, 1991).

Consent can also become complicated in situations in which infants or children require specific treatments and their parents are either
unavailable or unreachable because of their own illness or because of
prolonged drug use. Such dilemmas are particularly acute in the case
of emergency treatments requiring parental consent (Fost, 1991; Pizzo & Wilfert, 1991; Ginzburg, 1991).

Yet another area of difficulty with informed consent to treatment
has to do with life-sustaining therapy. Grady (1992) has indicated that
"because AIDS is ultimately a fatal disease, decisions about life sus-
taining therapy commonly arise" (p. 435). Treatment, "do not resuscitate" decisions, and decisions to refuse life-sustaining therapies are
often complicated with HIV/AIDS because of the high incidence of neuropsychiatric deterioration. Grady (1992) states clearly that "decisions
about life-sustaining therapy should always be individualized. Blanket
policies such as no intensive care for people with AIDS not only are
unfair but also deprive people of their rights to make decisions about
treatment to care" (p. 436; see also Cooke, 1990; Veatch & Fry, 1987).

These ethical dilemmas may become even more complex when
medical treatment team members may reach different decisions from
family members or from intensive care unit staff, or when there is more
than one caretaker for children of an infected parent. In addition, as
more children live longer with HIV/AIDS and as more adolescents are

diagnosed, their opinions and preferences need to be taken into account. Open communication among all of the parties discussed above may also be complicated by "secrets," as well as by the confidentiality dilemmas discussed above.

RESEARCH AND CLINICAL TRIALS

Informed Consent, Research, and Clinical Trials

The issue of informed consent for participation of HIV-infected children in research and in clinical trials has been much debated. Ginzburg (1991), Pizzo and Wilfert (1991), and Fost (1991) have addressed these concerns.

As clinical trials of experimental drugs have been introduced, there is a concern that patients living below the poverty level, and others lacking and/or with very limited insurance coverage, will feel coerced and unable to give consent totally freely (Grady, 1992; Pizzo & Wilfert, 1991). Ginzburg (1991) raises the concern that since many HIV-infected children live in impoverished areas, decisions affecting state and federal Medicaid funding will have an impact on their care. Ginzburg (1991) states that

> parents may be forced to accept "voluntary" participation in research protocols for themselves and their children as the only avenue by which to gain access to tertiary medical care. In some instances, informed consent ultimately may be found to be invalid if it has involved this type of coercion. (p. 759)

Equally complicated are situations involving children who have been placed in foster care or with members of the extended family. Palacio and Weedy (1991) indicate that children in foster care are under the care of the state, and that legal custody lies with the child protective agency rather than with either the biological parents or the foster parents. In many states, the local commissioners of social services are responsible for making decisions about and giving consent for medical care. Palacio and Weedy (1991) have raised ethical concerns regarding the need to ensure that children who are wards of the state do not become "targets" for studies involving experimental drugs. These concerns are exacerbated in minority communities, where there is great suspicion about involving children in drug studies. Complicated ethical and legal issues can also arise regarding the needs of foster children when biological and foster parents disagree with a decision by the child protective agency or with the medical authorities' decisions about treatment.

264

Research and Clinical Trials of Zidovudine during Pregnancy for the Prevention of HIV Transmission

Administration of Zidovudine (AZT) during Pregnancy

From April 1991 through December 1993 the AIDS Clinical Trials Group (ACTG) Protocol No. 076—a study funded by the National Institute of Allergy and Infectious Disease and the National Institute of Child Health and Human Development—was conducted with 477 pregnant, HIV-infected women. ACTG 076 was a double-blind, placebo-controlled, randomized clinical trial of zidovudine (AZT) to test its prevention of HIV transmission from infected mothers to their infants. Those who received zidovudine started their treatment at 14–34 weeks gestation, received it throughout pregnancy, and were administered zidovudine intravenously during labor. The newborns were given the drug for their first six weeks of life.

Of the 477 pregnant women enrolled in the study, 409 gave birth to 415 infants. HIV status is now known for 363 of the children divided almost equally between the two groups (180 in the zidovudine group and 183 in the placebo group). The results of the study, reported in the *New England Journal of Medicine* (Connor et al., 1994), were striking. There was a two-thirds reduction in HIV transmission: from 25.5% in the placebo group to 8.3% in the group of infants born to mothers receiving zidovudine (Connor et al., 1994).

Ethical Debate on Mandatory Testing

In anticipation of the controversy that the results of the ACTG 076 study would generate, the *New England Journal of Medicine* article detailing the findings was accompanied by two editorials that explored the ethical issues arising from the stunning results (Rogers & Jaffe, 1994; Bayer, 1994). The first editorial (Rogers & Jaffe, 1994) raised a number of concerns regarding the applicability and generalizability of the Connor et al. (1994) study: (1) The actual mechanism by which zidovudine reduces the risk of maternal–infant transmission is not clear; (2) it is still not certain as to the proportion of maternal–infant transmission of HIV that occurs in utero, during labor and delivery, and after birth through breast feeding; (3) since the sample was composed only of mildly symptomatic HIV-infected women, the efficacy of this treatment is unknown for women in a more advanced stage of the disease (Rogers & Jaffe, 1994).

The results of the ACTG 076 study provoked an immediate response (Kolata, 1994; Bayer, 1994; CDC, 1994). Bayer (1994), an ethicist and professor of public health at the Columbia University School of Public Health, concerned about the risk of exposing uninfected children to zidovudine, has questioned whether this risk is acceptable for the 70-80% of children born to HIV-infected mothers who will not be HIV-infected themselves.

The results of the Connor et al. (1994) study has renewed and reinvigorated the debate over mandatory AIDS testing for pregnant women (Kolata, 1994). Bayer (1994) is wary of the threat the findings pose to the privacy rights of women who are suspected of being at risk for HIV—a population that is largely poor and from ethnic and racial minority groups. He urges that pregnant women be persuaded to be tested for HIV, and that those who are found to be infected be urged to undergo zidovudine treatment "after being fully informed of the benefits and the uncertain, remote prospects of long term negative consequences" (p. 1225).

Bayer (1994) presents a very strong argument for informed consent of pregnant women and against mandatory testing as he views "mandatory treatment of competent adults . . . virtually never acceptable" (Bayer, 1994, p. 1224).

On the other side of the debate are those who believe the balance between the privacy rights of the mother and the right of her unborn child to live should fall in favor of the child. In a recent *New York Times* article (Kolata, 1994), Dr. Philip Pizzo, Chief of Pediatrics at the National Cancer Institute, maintains that without mandatory testing of pregnant women the spread of the epidemic in children will continue unabated. With such testing, Dr. Pizzo argues, the rate of HIV-infected babies born in the United States—which the Department of Public Health estimates to be between 1,000 to 2,000 annually—could be cut by two-thirds (Kolata, 1994).

The debate over mandatory testing shows no sign of resolution for now, and it illustrates the grave ethical issues HIV/AIDS has wrought for health care providers.

ACCESS TO CARE

Many HIV-infected individuals have been refused treatment by individual caregivers and by health care facilities such as health maintenance organizations (Cooke, 1990; Eisenberg, 1986). Also, since large numbers of HIV-infected patients are poor and from ethnic minority groups, they are likely to have experienced a lifelong struggle with inferior health care (Mitchell & Heagarty, 1991)—a condition that predates the AIDS epidemic.

Problems of urban and rural poverty (homelessness, drug use, etc.) may complicate receiving Medicaid or other forms of public assistance (Grady, 1992). The escalating costs of medical care for persons with HIV/AIDS are straining health care resources in high-prevalence areas (Green & Arno, 1990; Grady, 1992). Many persons with HIV/AIDS are often uninsured or underinsured, and therefore do not receive equal access to care (Green & Arno, 1990; Grady, 1992). Many poor patients who are undocumented or illegal immigrants not only have no insurance coverage, but face deportation when their HIV status becomes known (see Chapter 4).

Medicaid reimbursement payments are frequently inadequate for the treatment of persons with HIV/AIDS (Grady, 1992; Green & Arno, 1990; Thompson, 1988). Moreover, there is a requirement that an individual must be disabled for 24 months before meeting eligibility guidelines for benefits (Makadon et al., 1988; Thompson, 1988; Grady, 1992). Even patients with private health insurance coverage face major hurdles when expensive treatments—such as zidovudine, which costs approximately $5,000 per year—are not fully reimbursed.

These ethical dilemmas can also affect access to mental health care for HIV/AIDS patients, many of whom eventually lose their jobs and their insurance coverage (Grady, 1992). Chapter 17 discusses how the law has attempted to resolve the complex challenges HIV/AIDS has presented to U.S. society.

REFERENCES

American Association for Counseling and Development (AACD) Governing Council. (1988, July). *AACD position statement on acquired immune deficiency syndrome.* Paper presented at a symposium conducted by the AACD Governing Council.

American Medical Association (AMA) Council on Ethical and Judicial Affairs. (1988). Ethical issues involved in the growing AIDS crisis. *Journal of the American Medical Association, 259,* 1360–1361.

American Nurses Association (ANA). (1992). *Compendium of HIV/AIDS positions, policies and documents.* Washington, DC: Author.

American Psychiatric Association Ad Hoc Committee on AIDS Policy. (1988). AIDS policy: Confidentiality and disclosure. *American Journal of Psychiatry, 145,* 541–542.

American Psychological Association. (1991). *Legal liability related to confidentiality and the prevention of HIV transmission.* Washington, DC: APA Council of Representatives.

Bayer, R. (1994). Ethical challenges posed by zidovudine treatment to reduce vertical transmission of HIV [Editorial]. *New England Journal of Medicine, 331*(18), 1223–1225.

Bisbing, S. B. (1988). Psychiatric patients and AIDS: Evolving law and liability. *Psychiatric Annals, 18*(10), 582–586.

Brown, M. (1987). AIDS and ethics: Concerns and considerations. *Oncology Nursing Forum, 14*(1), 69–73.

Centers for Disease Control (CDC). (1987). Recommendations for prevention of HIV transmission in health care settings. *Morbidity and Mortality Weekly Report, 36*(Suppl. 2s), 3S–17S.

Centers for Disease Control and Prevention (CDC). (1994). Recommendations of the U.S. Public Health Service Task Force on the use of zidovudine to reduce perinatal transmission of human immunodeficiency virus. *Morbidity Mortality Weekly Report, 43*(RR-11), 11–20.

Connor, E., Sperling, R., Gelber, R., Kiselen, P., Scott, G., Sullivan, M. J., Van Dyke, R., Bey, M., Shearer, W., Jacobson, R., Jimenez, E., O'Neill, E., Bazin, B., Delfraissy, J. F., Culnane, M., Coombs, R., Elkins, M., Moye, J., Stratton, P., & Balsley, J. (1994). Reduction of maternal–infant transmission of human immunodeficiency virus type 1 with zidovudine treatment. *New England Journal of Medicine, 331*(18), 1173–1180.

Cooke, M. (1990). Ethical issues related to AIDS. In P. T. Cohen, M. Sande, & P. A. Volberding (Eds.). *The AIDS knowledge base* (pp. 1214.1–1214.8). Waltham, MA: Medical Publishing Group.

Cooper, E., Knight, J., & Leonard, E. (1991). Development of new drugs for the treatment of pediatric AIDS: Scientific and regulatory issues. In P. Pizzo & C. Wilfert (Eds.), *Pediatric AIDS: The challenge of HIV infection in infants, children and adolescents.* Baltimore: Williams & Wilkins.

Creighton, H. (1986). Legal aspects of AIDS: Part II. *Nursing Management, 17*(12), 14–16.

Eisenberg, L. (1986). The genesis of fear: AIDS and the public response to science. *Law, Medicine and Health Care, 14*(5–6), 243–249.

Emanuel, E. J. (1988). Do physicians have an obligation to treat patients with AIDS? *New England Journal of Medicine, 318*(25), 1686–1690.

Fost, N. (1991). Ethical issues in pediatric AIDS. In P. Pizzo & C. Wilfert (Eds.), *Pediatric AIDS: The challenge of HIV infection in infants, children and adolescents* (pp. 595–604). Baltimore: Williams & Wilkins.

Freedman, B. (1988). Health professions, codes and the right to refuse to treat HIV infectious patients. *Hastings Center Report, 18*(2, Suppl.), 20–25.

Futterman, D., & Hein, K. (1991). Medical management of adolescents. In P. Pizzo & C. Wilfert (Eds.), *Pediatric AIDS: The challenge of HIV infection in infants, children and adolescents* (pp. 546–560). Baltimore: Williams & Wilkins.

Ginzburg, H. M. (1988). HIV related diseases and the future of the delivery of psychiatric care. *Psychiatric Annals, 18*(10), 563–570.

Ginzburg, H. M. (1991). Legal issues in the medical care of HIV-infected children. In P. Pizzo & C. Wilfert (Eds.), *Pediatric AIDS: The challenge of HIV infection in infants, children and adolescents* (pp. 756–764). Baltimore: Williams & Wilkins.

Girardi, J. A., Keese, R. M., Traver, L. B., & Cooksey, D. R. (1988). Psychotherapist responsibility in notifying individuals at risk for exposure to HIV. *Journal of Sex Research, 25*(1), 1–27.

Grady, C. (1992). Ethical aspects. In J. Flaskerud & P. Unguarski (Eds.), *HIV/AIDS: A guide to nursing care* (2nd ed.). Philadelphia: W. B. Saunders.

Green, J., & Arno, P. (1990). The Medicaidization of AIDS. *Journal of the American Medical Association, 264*(1), 1261–1266.

Harding, A., Gray, L., & Neal, M. (1993). Confidentiality limits with clients who have HIV: A review of ethical and legal guidelines and professional policies. *Journal of Counseling and Development, 71,* 297–305.

Healey, J. M. (1987). Confidentiality and AIDS. *Law, Medicine and Public Policy, 51*(11), 757.

Henderson, D., Fahey, B., Willy, M., et al. (1990). Risk for occupational transmission of HIV-1 associated with clinical exposures. *Annals of Internal Medicine, 113*(10), 740–746.

Knapp, S., & VandeCreek, L. (1992). Public policy issues in applying the "duty to protect" to HIV-positive patients. In R. Weitz (Ed.), *Psychotherapy in independent practice.* New York: Haworth Press.

Kolata, G. (1994, November 3). Discovery that AIDS can be prevented in babies raises debate on mandatory testing. *The New York Times.*

Lo, B. (1990a). Clinical ethics and HIV-related illnesses: Issues in therapeutic and health services research. *Medical Care Review, 47*(1), 15–32.

Lo, B. (1990b). Ethical dilemmas in HIV infection. *Journal of the Pediatric Medical Association, 80*(1), 26–30.

Makadon, H., Seage, G., Thorpe, K., et al., & the Harvard Study Group on AIDS—Financing Subgroup. (1988, March). *Testimony before the President's Commission on the HIV epidemic.*

Melton, G. B. (1988). Ethical and legal issues in AIDS-related practice. *American Psychologist, 43*(11), 941–957.

Milliken, N., & Greenblatt, R. (1988). Ethical issues of the AIDS epidemic. In J. Monagle & D. Thomasma (Eds.), *Medical ethics: A guide for health professionals.* Rockville, MD: Aspen.

Mitchell, J., & Heagarty, M. (1991). Special considerations for minorities. In P. Pizzo & C. Wilfert (Eds.), *Pediatric AIDS: The challenge of HIV infection in infants, children and adolescents* (pp. 704–713). Baltimore, MD: Williams & Wilkins.

Morrison, C. F. (1989). AIDS: Ethical implications for psychological intervention. *Professional Psychology: Research and Practice, 20*(3), 166–171.

National Association of Social Workers (NASW) Delegate Assembly. (1990). *Acquired immune deficiency syndrome/human immunodeficiency virus: A social work response* (Policy statement). Silver Spring, MD: NASW.

Ostrow, D., & Gayle, T. (1986). Psychosocial and ethical issues of AIDS health care programs. *Quality Review Bulletin, 12*(8), 284–294.

Palacio, C., & Weedy, C. (1991). Treatment issues regarding children in foster care. In P. Pizzo & C. Wilfert (Eds.), *Pediatric AIDS: The challenge of HIV infection in infants, children and adolescents* (pp. 569–576). Baltimore: Williams & Wilkins.

Perry, S. (1989). Warning third parties at risk of AIDS: APA's policy is a barrier to treatment. *Hospital and Community Psychiatry, 40*(2), 158–161.

Pizzo, P., & Wilfert, C. (Eds.). (1991). *Pediatric AIDS: The challenge of HIV infection in infants, children and adolescents.* Baltimore: Williams & Wilkins.

President's Commission on the HIV Epidemic. (1988). *Report of the President's Commission on the HIV Epidemic.* Washington, DC: U.S. Government Printing Office.

Price, R., Brew, B., Sidtis, J., et al. (1988). The brain in AIDS: Central nervous system HIV-1 infection and AIDS dementia complex. *Science, 239,* 586–591.

Rogers, M., & Jaffe, H. (1994). Reducing the risk of maternal–infant transmission of HIV: A door is open [Editorial]. *New England Journal of Medicine, 331*(18), 1222–1223.

Tarasoff v. Regents of the University of California, 17 Cal. 3d 424, 551 P.2d 334, 181 Cal. Rptr. 14 (1976).

Temoshok, L., Sweet, D. M., & Zich, J. (1987). The three city comparison of the public's knowledge and attitudes about AIDS. *Psychology and Health, 1*(1), 43–60.

Thompson, J. (1988, January). Cost as an obstacle to care. *Testimony before the Presidential Commission on the HIV Epidemic.*

Veatch, R., & Fry, S. (1987). *Case studies in nursing ethics.* Philadelphia: J.B. Lippincott.

Wood, G. J., Marks, R., & Dilley, J. W. (1990). *AIDS law for mental health professionals: A handbook for judicious practice.* San Francisco: AIDS Health Project.

Young, E. W. (1986). AIDS: Emerging moral questions. *Journal of American College Health, 34*(5), 240–242.

17

Legal Issues

David C. Harvey, MSW, LCSW

In this, the second decade of the HIV/AIDS epidemic, the mental health field is confronted with complex legal questions concerning the delivery of HIV-related mental health services. By keeping abreast of recent HIV-related legal cases and issues, as well as professional guidelines that address such things as conflicts in the delivery of services or in providing access to biomedical research programs, the mental health clinician will not only enhance the therapeutic relationship, but may be able to remedy the specific legal concerns of his or her clients. For example, important components of counseling and support services include helping clients to cope with stigma and discrimination, assisting them with informed medical decision making, and being knowledgeable about entitlement and benefit issues. It is also important for clinicians to have established relationships with local legal and advocacy service providers when referrals are warranted.

Legal issues related to HIV/AIDS have prompted more litigation and court cases than any other disease in the history of the United States (American Civil Liberties Union [ACLU] AIDS Project, 1990). These cases have had a significant impact on the delivery of health and mental health services to those with HIV/AIDS. The legal overview of HIV/AIDS-related issues is intended for the mental health clinician as an introduction to disability law and recent significant cases in the areas of discrimination, informed consent, confidentiality, family law, and related issues of entitlements.

This chapter provides background information specific to identified concerns related to HIV/AIDS; the reader is advised to seek professional legal guidance if a specific legal question should develop.

DISCRIMINATION

People affected by HIV/AIDS have encountered profound stigma and discrimination in the United States. One study of reported AIDS discrimination cases found 13,000 reported complaints by people of all races, genders, ethnicities, and sexual orientations. In addition, complaints were recorded not only by persons diagnosed with AIDS but also by persons who are caring for persons with AIDS, or persons simply perceived as having AIDS (ACLU AIDS Project, 1990). The study also found that discrimination was most often experienced in areas of insurance, entitlements, and housing, and in rural health care services, especially among dental and nursing home providers. In some cases specifically involving the care of children with HIV/AIDS, providers have denied services based on the diagnosis of a fatal illness and the assumption that the children will not live long with AIDS. Such assumptions have been made despite recent gains in pediatric HIV/AIDS care and treatment, which mean that children and adults now live much longer with the disease.

Other studies have documented discriminatory practices that low-income persons living with HIV/AIDS have encountered in accessing health care services—services that, as health care reform is considered at the state level, are increasingly being provided through health maintenance organizations. Since large numbers of HIV-infected patients are low-income and from minority groups, they are likely to have experienced a life-long struggle in accessing good quality, affordable health care (Mitchell & Heagarty, 1991), a condition that preceded the HIV/AIDS epidemic.

Issues of urban and rural poverty, such as homelessness or drug use, may also complicate issues of receiving Medicaid and other forms of public assistance (Grady, 1992). The escalating costs of medical care for persons with AIDS are straining health care resources in high-prevalence areas (Green & Arno, 1990; Iglehart, 1987; Grady, 1992). Many persons with AIDS are uninsured or underinsured, and thus—as studies point out—experience discrimination in receiving access to health and social services provided in the private sector (Green & Arno, 1990; Grady, 1992).

It can be difficult to resolve issues of discrimination, in part because of clients' reluctance to experience further stigma through the judicial system, or to face the prospect of long and arduous litigation. In addition, resources to redress complaints are limited at some government agencies; legal and advocacy service providers may be backlogged, or there may be a shortage of attorneys willing to work on cases. Prior to the passage of the Americans with Disabilities Act of

1990, statutes at the federal and state levels offered fragmented and poorly coordinated legal protections. Because of variances in definitions of disability, in which entities were subject to the laws, and in the remedies available, it was often difficult to remedy claims of HIV-related discrimination.

Unfortunately, instances of discrimination will persist as long as ignorance and fear of people with HIV/AIDS continue. Stigma and discrimination are significant mental health concerns, and clinicians should be adept at recognizing the psychosocial issues experienced by clients who experience a range of HIV-related stigma or discriminatory actions by others.

Legal Principles in Remedying Discrimination

In the early years of the HIV/AIDS epidemic, legal developments centered on whether HIV infection could be considered a "disability" or "handicap" under definitions set forth in federal and state statutes, and if so, such statutes could provide remedies to the discrimination that HIV-infected people encountered. In one of the most important rulings related to people with HIV/AIDS, the U.S. Supreme Court noted in *Board of Education of Nassau County, Florida v. Arline* (1987) that an infectious condition cannot be separated from the disease itself but rather is a manifestation of the disease, and is therefore considered a disabling condition under Section 504 of the Rehabilitation Act. This ruling was interpreted to include the disabling conditions of HIV infection and AIDS, and helped to establish the framework in which people with HIV/AIDS can obtain federal and state legal remedies against discrimination and eligibility for federal and state entitlements. The following sections review four important statutes that provide legal remedies for claims of discrimination and services to benefit persons with disabilities.

The Rehabilitation Act

The Rehabilitation Act (1973) is the first federal statute that protects the rights of persons with disabilities or those who are perceived to have disabilities. Various sections of this act require affirmative action to hire persons with disabilities, and the provision of vocational and other rehabilitative services for persons with disabilities. Section 504, the antidiscrimination section, prohibits any programs that receive federal funds from discriminating on the basis of handicap in employment, benefits, services, and other areas. These programs include the major federal initiatives (such as Medicaid, Medicare, and Head Start), community services block grants, child welfare services, mental health services block grants, and any other federally supported program. The Civil

Rights Restoration Act (1987) included an amendment to Section 504 stipulating that an entire institution or agency is subject to the statute if any part of the institution receives federal assistance.

Consistent with the *Arline* decision in 1987, the U.S. Department of Justice (1988) later ruled that persons with *asymptomatic* HIV infection are also covered under the antidiscrimination provisions of Section 504. Because HIV causes abnormalities in the immune system, and because Section 504 covers persons who are "perceived" as disabled, persons with asymptomatic HIV infection and those who are perceived with the disease are also included as having a disability.

The act also refers to the legal concept of "otherwise qualified." This concept is important to understand in relation to discriminatory practices in admission to programs, schools, or other service settings for persons with HIV/AIDS. The act explicitly prohibits discrimination against persons with disabilities who are otherwise qualified to participate in the program. A program can only limit participation through admission guidelines that are sufficiently related to the purpose or objective of the program, and evaluated by the same procedures and standards used for all other health problems. Even after this evaluation, the act further prohibits discrimination if an individual may participate with "reasonable accommodations." Reasonable accommodations include any adaptation, modification, or service that may allow program participation without changing the "fundamental" or "essential" nature of the program. These concepts are important to note, especially regarding school admission policies related to children with HIV infection.

In extreme circumstances, programs may deny admission (usually not, however, in relation to a client's HIV status) following a further analysis or assessment of risk of transmission, outlined by the U.S. Supreme Court in the *Arline* decision. This analysis was proposed by the AMA and based on four principles; a summary of these principles, which were outlined by the American Bar Association (ABA, 1989) is as follows:

1. The nature of the risk (how the disease is transmitted).
2. The duration of the risk (how long the carrier is infectious).
3. The severity of the risk (what is the potential harm to third parties).
4. The probability the disease will be transmitted and will cause varying degrees of harm.

Of particular note is the fact that admission of children with HIV infection to schools and other service settings is normally warranted (see Chapter 15), since the above-described procedures and assessment of risk do not usually screen out children with HIV/AIDS.

The Individuals with Disabilities Education Act

The Individuals with Disabilities Education Act (1990), formerly the Education for All Handicapped Children Act (P.L. 94-142), requires states to provide free and appropriate education for children with disabilities, regardless of severity; individualized assessment of each child's needs; and an appeals process for parents. It also states that children must be educated in the "least restrictive environment." The act contains a more restrictive definition of disability; specified as disabled are mentally retarded, hearing-impaired, speech-impaired, visually handicapped, seriously emotionally disturbed, orthopedically impaired, and other health-impaired children, as well as children with specific learning disabilities. A child must also require special education and related services as a result of having one of the listed impairments. Most children with symptomatic HIV infection will meet this definition of disability and will be qualified for special education services. Children with asymptomatic HIV infection are still eligible to attend school and are protected under Section 504 of the Rehabilitation Act, discussed previously.

The Fair Housing Amendments Act

In 1988, Congress enacted the Fair Housing Amendments Act, which protects disabled people (including those with HIV/AIDS) from discrimination in housing. This act adds persons with disabilities to the list of protected classes; it prohibits discrimination in the sale or rental of property, conditions of sale or rental, housing loans and other financial assistance, and brokerage and appraisal services. This statute adopts Section 504's definition of disability.

The Americans with Disabilities Act

The Americans with Disabilities Act (1990) expands antidiscrimination protection for persons with disabilities in both the public and private sectors in the areas of employment, public accommodations, state and local government services, and telecommunications. The act extends the prohibition of discrimination in federally assisted programs established by Section 504 of the Rehabilitation Act of 1973 to all activities of state and local governments, including those that do not receive federal financial assistance, and incorporates specific prohibitions of discrimination on the basis of disability. The act borrows Section 504's definition of disability and subsequent legal frameworks of assessment of risks, and enables persons to file charges of discrimination in federal court. In the short time since passage of this act, it has been used to remedy specific HIV/AIDS discrimination cases throughout the United States.

INFORMED CONSENT

Well established within the medical and mental health professions are principles of informed consent. Following investigations and public inquiry in the 1970s related to institutional civil rights abuses, and also following new developments in psychopharmacology, disability attorneys, public advocates, and state policy planners placed an increased emphasis on informed consent procedures.

Central to principles of informed consent is the right to self-determination. In extreme situations where persons may lack decision-making capacity, the right to self-determination must often be weighed in competency hearings and in the courts. Mental health clinicians may be called upon to help clinically assess whether HIV/AIDS patients' decision-making capacity mitigates against their providing informed consent for medical treatment, drug trials, or other services, either for themselves or for their HIV-infected children. Adolescents are neither children or adults, whose rights are more clearly delineated; because of their ambiguous legal and age status, they pose special dilemmas in informed consent procedures and legal guidelines. To effectively monitor and understand the dilemmas clients may face in the other areas of the service system, the clinician should be knowledgeable about informed consent issues.

Legal Principles in Informed Consent

Generally, the law protects individuals in making their own medical decisions and requires that persons be legally competent to make reasoned decisions. Competency is a legal status and is not based on a single determination. Rather, it is based on three factors: age, mental capacity, and the legal decision at hand. According to most statutes, incompetency is determined by assessing the following: capacity to care for oneself; capacity for rational decision making; and physical or mental impairment that affects decision-making capacity. Generally, children are considered unable to make medical treatment decisions for themselves, and parents or legal guardians have the right to make decisions for them. Increasingly, states are enacting laws that recognize the right of older adolescents or "emancipated" adolescents to consent to treatment (ABA, 1991).

Informed consent necessitates that options and explanations be provided and explained competently. It must be given voluntarily and either orally or in writing, based on adequate information. In addition, the quantity and quality of information that must be provided may be governed by local community practices and state statutes. For example, some states require that clients understand the nature of the HIV test; to whom the test result could be disclosed; how the result will be used; and the risks and benefits resulting from the test (ABA, 1990).

Informed Consent for Foster Children

In situations where children with HIV/AIDS do not reside with their biological parents, foster parents may not have legal authority to give informed consent, further complicating the process. In these cases, child protection agencies have the legal authority to give consent, but usually in coordination with the biological parents. Another common occurrence is that the parents of infected children may not be competent to give informed consent if they themselves are too ill with HIV/AIDS. In the case of an emergency, health care providers can administer treatment because consent is implied by the urgency of the facts. In many state statutes, the term ''emergency'' is defined broadly (National Pediatric HIV Resource Center, 1992).

CONFIDENTIALITY

Confidentiality regarding the HIV status of an individual continues to be a controversial area of the law; it has been the subject of state and federal litigation, as well as state legislation governing record keeping and disclosures of HIV-related information. ''Confidentiality'' is a concept that is derived from common law, the U.S. Constitution, state and federal statutes, facility licensure laws, and codes of professional ethics, as well as the protection of civil rights. Policies and practices related to client and worker confidentiality are integral parts of the provision of services to persons affected by HIV/AIDS, including infants and children.

Legal Principles in Confidentiality

The underlying principle of confidentiality is the right to privacy, based on both legal and ethical considerations dating from the earliest days of the medical profession (ABA, 1991). Since public health and physician–patient treatment issues depend on the voluntary disclosure of information in order for patients to be effectively diagnosed and treated, failure to maintain the privacy of information could threaten the cooperation of persons with HIV/AIDS. In addition, given the widespread stigma and discrimination associated with having HIV/AIDS, concerns surrounding confidentiality have become more urgent.

Federal and state laws contain numerous provisions regarding confidentiality of client information in all types of public and private agencies, as well as professional codes of ethics (Kermani & Weiss, 1989). Most of these measures predate the HIV/AIDS crisis. The emergence of HIV/AIDS, however, has highlighted the inadequacy of existing laws and policies, and many state legislatures have passed measures specifically addressing HIV confidentiality (Intergovernmental Health Policy Project, 1988). Many of these new mandates deal only with health care facilities and providers and do not address other types of services, causing confusion on the part of some service providers. As a general rule, under existing laws and codes of ethics, no information in a patient's record may be disclosed to anyone other than the patient or authorized representative (often parents or legal guardians in the case of a minor) without the informed consent of the patient (ABA, 1991). Providers should be knowledgeable about informed consent procedures and should ensure that policies in this area are consistent with state-specific HIV/AIDS laws, other regulations, and codes of professional ethics.

Disclosure

Patient information within single institutions and health care facilities may be shared among professionals who specifically provide direct treatment for the patients. This type of disclosure is usually permitted under the implied consent provisions of a general release of information signed by patients or legal guardians upon admission. However, there may be situations involving other professionals who come into contact with the patient but are not providing direct care and do not have a need to know information concerning the patients' HIV status. This is probably the case in ordinary school settings, where courts have upheld the right of children with HIV/AIDS to attend school because most of these children do not pose any significant risk of transmission to others (American Academy of Pediatrics [AAP] Task Force on Pediatric AIDS, 1989; Fraser, 1989). In Head Start and other preschool programs, the status of children with HIV infection will not be known in most situations, and their confidentiality should be protected.

Some states have specific statutes governing the management of HIV infection in school settings, as well as procedures for maintaining confidentiality. Generally, the HIV status of a child can only be disclosed by medical personnel to school officials with the expressly authorized informed consent of parents or legal guardians (National Pediatric HIV Resource Center, 1992), although several states, including Illinois and South Carolina, are considering or have just passed statutes mandating the reporting of children's HIV status to school principals. These statutes are highly controversial and may conflict with other federal and state guidelines and with codes of professional ethics.

The duty to maintain patient information in confidence is not absolute. Health care providers are required in all states to report the diagnosis of HIV/AIDS, and in some states to report the names of infected individuals, for record-keeping and surveillance purposes. Most state reporting requirements include strict confidentiality provisions restricting the further dissemination of information. In addition, much has been written about "duty-to-protect" principles. As of this writing, there are no specific state statutes that require health care providers to warn third parties who may be potentially at risk of HIV transmission from a client (National Pediatric HIV Resource Center, 1992). However, prior legal decisions and court rulings are being used to justify "duty-to-warn" procedures in some extreme cases.

The framework for examining duty-to-protect issues includes the following: (1) defining the nature of the relationship between providers and clients; (2) evaluating the potential harm to a third party; (3) determining the foreseeability of the risk; and (4) evaluating the public interest in deterring the activity in question (Harvey & Decker, 1990; Eth, 1988; Girardi et al., 1988). The law is fairly clear about the responsibility of physicians to warn, but is not clear regarding that of other professionals (ABA, 1989). In the case of children, some parents have argued that on the basis of potential risk they have the right to know whether their children are attending school with a child who has HIV infection. Because the risk of transmission in school settings is now well established to be minimal, strong arguments exist for protecting the confidentiality of children with HIV infection by not disclosing their HIV status.

Generally, the physician's duty to warn is limited to identifiable potential victims—persons known to be at significant risk because of sexual exposure or sharing of needles in injection drug use. In certain other circumstances, violent behavior that could result in exchange of blood or forced sexual intercourse may be cited as an additional factor in determining whether a significant risk exists (ABA, 1989). The Centers for Disease Control and Prevention (CDC) and other professional organizations have commented on this issue through policy guidelines. Providers should consult literature published by the American Psychological Association, the American Hospital Association, the AMA, and the CDC.

Negligence and Potential Liability

Some service providers are concerned about the risk of liability if steps are not taken to warn third parties about a client who may pose a perceived risk of transmission, as well as other risks associated with caring for clients with HIV infection. Specifically, general principles of law will be applied to such findings of liability that may be brought against an agency or facility on claims of negligent transmission between clients or workers in the following situations: (1) An agency has failed to provide a safe environment; (2) negligent worker or client exposure to HIV has occurred; (3) the facility has failed to maintain confidentiality within the guidelines of the law and ethics; and (4) the facility has failed to protect or warn a third party in an extreme situation (Harvey & Decker, 1990).

When facilities institute state-of-the-art policies (such as universal precautions and infection control standards as defined by the CDC, the Occupational Safety and Health Administration, and other sources), and facilities have in place policies on informed consent and confidentiality as well as procedures for intervention in extreme high-risk situations, findings of liability may be reduced.

To minimize findings of liability for negligent exposure to HIV, protective actions to uphold the rights of clients and workers should include (1) infection control policies and procedures for implementation; (2) sexual behavior policies and procedures for counseling and intervening with employees and clients; (3) record-keeping policies and procedures on confidentiality; (4) HIV testing policies and informed consent procedures; and (5) creation of a professional advisory committee (whose multidisciplinary members include disability attorneys, physicians, social workers, etc.), to advise on policy development and ongoing issues (Harvey & Decker, 1990).

State School Notification Statutes

As noted above, some state legislatures have passed laws that require public health authorities to notify school principals or administrators about children's HIV status. Although some statutes require public health officials to obtain the informed consent of parents or guardians in order to notify school principals, other statutes simply mandate the notification of school administrators when the local health department receives HIV test results (Intergovernmental Health Policy Project, 1988). Some statutes indicate that this notification is warranted to guarantee appropriate educational and health services, although it appears that HIV infection is singled out for special notification requirements as compared with other childhood health conditions.

In Illinois, amendments to the AIDS Confidentiality Act of 1987 (Public Acts 85-677 and 85-674) permit state health department officials to disclose a child's HIV infection status to the district superintendent of schools for the district in which the child is enrolled, and to persons who are required, pursuant to federal or state law, to decide on placement or educational programs for the child. The Chicago Women and HIV Consortium (n.d.) reports that it opposes the mandatory reporting by name of children and young adults (ages 3–21), for reasons that include the following beliefs: that reporting is discriminatory to a child and family and can result in HIV-infected parents' being identified; that reporting is detrimental to health if parents decide not to have their child tested and diagnosed because of fears of reporting; that reporting of a child by name breaches confidentiality between a care provider and a family; that reporting does not negate the need to establish universal precautions in all school settings; and that reporting of adolescents by name diminishes the ability to obtain confidential or anonymous HIV testing of high-risk youths.

The AAP (1989) has issued guidelines for all child care settings. These recommend implementation of universal precautions, and suggest that child care personnel need not be informed of a child's HIV status to protect the health of caregivers or other children because the risk of transmission is so low. Parents may choose to inform school officials about the child's diagnosis so that medical assistance is provided, but it should be solely the parents' decision.

FAMILY LAW

Emerging as new concerns within the law are issues involving parents with HIV/AIDS and custody, visitation, and guardianship of their children. Cooper (1992) writes that few analyses have been completed of future planning for children who survive parents who die from AIDS. At least one national project[1] has begun policy analysis on the need for standby guardianship laws and other needs of the expected 80,000

[1]The Orphan Project: The HIV Epidemic and New York City's Children, 121 Avenue of the Americas, New York, NY 10013. Phone number: (212) 925-5290.

children and adolescents who will be left orphaned by mothers dying from AIDS by the year 2000 (Michaels & Levin, 1992). Other concerns involve parents who may be divorced, with one parent at risk of losing custody or visitation after a legal challenge by a former spouse on the basis of HIV status.

Increasingly, as more women with children become infected with HIV and develop AIDS, service providers are confronted with arranging for legal services to address parents' wishes as to who should take care of their children or be the legal guardians after the parents die. In New York State, the Surrogate's Court Procedure Act of 1992 was amended for standby guardianship, which allows parents who are ill to make permanent plans for their children's future without giving up their legal rights. At least one bill has been introduced in Congress concerning standby guardianship laws under the Social Security Act (U.S. House of Representatives, 1993).

Legal Principles in Family Law

Cooper (1992) cites the Uniform Marriage and Divorce Act as the primary approach to custody and visitation disputes in the United States. The act identifies a framework for courts to analyze these issues, based on such factors as the wishes of child and parents; the interaction and interrelationship of the child with parents and significant others; the child's adjustment to home, school, and community; and the health and mental health of the individuals involved. The last factor is frequently used in a custody or visitation challenge by a spouse; this often necessitates the education of the court about irrational fears or misinformation about HIV and its transmission. Cooper (1992) goes on to cite several court cases, which generally hold that HIV infection alone is not sufficient grounds for denying custody or visitation if a parent is able to care for a child, and that the risk of HIV transmission from parent to child is not a sufficient basis for making custody or visitation decisions.

Although some parents with HIV/AIDS establish future custody plans for their children, many do not (Nicholas & Abrams, 1992). When a single parent or both parents die from AIDS, questions emerge as to who should acquire legal guardianship. Many times other family members of deceased parents, such as their own parents or siblings, will take care of children left behind. In other situations, parents may not wish other family members or former spouses to care for their children (Nicholas & Abrams, 1992). Although guardianship laws vary from state to state, procedures to appoint a guardian are usually designated in a will that is drafted with the assistance of an attorney. Specific legal authority is given to the appointed guardian to provide consent for a child's medical care, and that person will be recognized by government entities to receive benefits and entitlements. Other legal arrangements involve adoption, foster care, or kinship foster care provided by a relative (AAP Task Force, 1989). Parents, however, lose significant legal rights when a child is placed in foster care, because the child becomes a ward of the state. Each option needs to be carefully considered by parents with the assistance of an attorney or advocate, which can help the parents decide on a flexible arrangement that may not negatively influence entitlement or other benefits that children may be receiving.

ENTITLEMENTS

Several federal and state programs provide funds for healthcare, services for the disabled, and income maintenance. HIV infection alone will not guarantee access to these programs, but as disability occurs with the progression of HIV/AIDS, eligibility criteria may be met. These issues are reviewed here in the context of developmental disability services, special education, and Social Security.

Not outlined here are Aid to Families with Dependent Children (the major federal–state welfare program based solely on low-income status), and Medicaid. Although the majority of families affected by HIV/AIDS will be eligible for Medicaid-reimbursed services, this area of public benefits is complex to analyze in relation to reimbursement for comprehensive HIV/AIDS services; moreover, it is not strictly a legal issue, but one of public policy. The reader is urged to consult other sources of information on Medicaid issues.

Developmental Disability Programs

The Developmental Disability and Bill of Rights Act (1972) provides funds to states and universities for direct services, education and training, and legal advocacy services. Developmental disability is defined under the act as a substantial functional limitation in three or more areas of life activity that requires lifelong support. Most children with HIV/AIDS will eventually meet the criteria for eligibility, depending on local resources. However, the act does not fund large-scale direct service programs. The definition of developmental disability is related to other federal and state disability services. Children with HIV/AIDS and their families may be eligible for legal advocacy services through the state protection and advocacy program for persons with developmental disabilities, funded under the federal act to provide free legal and advocacy services.

The Individuals with Disabilities Education Act

As previously discussed, all students with "handicaps" are eligible under the Individuals with Disabilities Education Act for a free education tailored to appropriate needs. Children with HIV/AIDS who are symptomatic will be eligible for special education services. The case of *Martinez v. School Board of Hillsborough County, Florida* (1988) helped establish legal precedents for assessing and guaranteeing special education services for children with HIV/AIDS. Of special note is Part H of the Education Act, passed by Congress in 1986, which requires that states electing to accept funds under this portion of the act provide services to infants, toddlers, and preschool programs for early intervention services for ages 0 through 2, and special education and related services for ages 3 to 5. Since children with symptomatic HIV or full-blown AIDS may experience developmental delays and intellectual deficits, early intervention may be beneficial. These services are currently being implemented by states; however, a major gap in this portion of the act relates to the provision of services for children with HIV who are "at risk" of substantial "developmental delay." The act does not define developmental delay and leaves it to states to define. Most states have adopted restrictive definitions that require a definitive diagnosis of impairment, which may have a negative impact on infants when HIV infection is not confirmed. However, in 1990, as reported by the National Association of State Special Education Directors, 14 states were adopting a broader definition that might include infants with HIV infection. Early intervention services listed under the act include health services, language and speech development, psychosocial support, and self-help skills.

Income Maintenance

Supplemental Security Income (SSI) under Social Security is a major federal–state cash benefit for which many women and children with HIV/AIDS may be eligible, based on disability, financial eligibility, and citizenship. In most states, eligibility for SSI means automatic eligibility for benefits under Medicaid (the major federal–state reimbursement program for health services for low-income persons). SSI eligibility is determined according to medical disability, as well as the following factors:

1. The applicant is unable to engage in substantial gainful activity by reason of physical or mental impairment that may result in death or has lasted for 12 months.
2. Impairment in a child must also be of a type listed by the Social Security Administration; if impairment does not fall within the listing, the child is entitled to an individual functional assessment to see whether comparable severity exists.

In June 1993, the Social Security Administration published revised regulations regarding medical eligibility for adults and children with HIV/AIDS; these include more HIV-related impairments and are easier to understand. Many manifestations of HIV infection now require no functional limitations test, allowing those affected to qualify on medical criteria alone. The functional test has been reduced in its stringency, requiring a demonstration of marked limitation in only one of three areas. Documentation of the presence of HIV may be supported by laboratory evidence or by other generally acceptable methods consistent with the prevailing state of knowledge and clinical practice. Medical criteria specific to women and children have been incorporated, and Social Security field offices can now give immediate compensation payments to persons with HIV, not just persons with a diagnosis of full-blown AIDS.

Specifically, the listing of impairments for adults now includes pelvic inflammatory disease, carcinoma of the cervix, diarrhea, neurological manifestations of HIV infection, dermatological conditions, and pulmonary tuberculosis resistant to treatment.An individual may still be eligible for benefits without meeting these criteria if the person has repeated manifestations of HIV disease that occur frequently or for long duration, or the person meets one of three functional restriction tests. The listing of impairments for children now includes failure to thrive, cardiomyopathy, and pelvic inflammatory disease. Methods for documenting HIV infection in children under 24 months of age have also been expanded.

SUMMARY OF LEGAL ISSUES

Discrimination

• Rights and entitlements may not be denied solely on the basis of a person's HIV status.
• Federal and most state laws prohibiting discrimination against persons with disabilities apply to HIV infection.

• Most persons with HIV infection are "otherwise qualified" to participate in public programs and activities, including school.

• Even when a person with HIV infection may pose a significant risk of transmission, federal and state laws may obligate providers of services to provide "reasonable accommodations" to reduce the risk to acceptable levels.

Informed Consent

• In the absence of special circumstances, informed consent must be obtained prior to providing medical treatment.

• The legal guardian of a child has the authority to consent to treatment for a child.

• Adolescents pose specific problems in regard to consent, and service providers may be confronted with conflicting laws. State laws are increasingly in favor of conferring right to consent to medical care on older or "mature" adolescents and "emancipated" minors.

• Informed consent is required for HIV testing under many state laws and is recommended by the CDC. Justification includes the potentially devastating personal and social impact on the person and family, and therefore is warranted as distinct from general consent to treatment for other procedures and routine tests.

Confidentiality

• Confidentiality involves principles of right to privacy, based on legal and ethical considerations.

• Since public health and physician–patient treatment issues depend on the voluntary disclosure of information in order for patients to be effectively diagnosed and treated, failure to maintain patients' privacy could threaten the cooperation of persons with HIV/AIDS.

• Under existing laws and codes of professional ethics, no information in a patient's record may be disclosed to anyone other than the patient or authorized representative (often parents or legal guardians in the case of a minor) without the informed consent of the patient.

• Generally, the physician's duty to warn is limited to identifiable potential victims—persons known to be at significant risk because of sexual exposure or sharing of needles in injection drug use. In certain other circumstances, violent behavior that could result in exchange of blood or forced sexual intercourse may be cited as an additional factor in determining whether a significant risk exists. The law is less clear on other professionals' responsibility related to duty to warn.

• General principles of law will be applied to charges of liability brought against an agency or individual on claims of negligent transmission between clients or workers in the following situations: (1) An agency has failed to provide a safe environment; (2) negligent worker or client exposure to HIV has occurred; (3) the facility has failed to maintain confidentiality within the guidelines of the law and ethics; and (4) the facility has failed to protect or warn a third party in an extreme situation.

Family Law

• Few analyses have been completed of future planning for children who survive parents who die from AIDS. Specific legal concerns involve parents who may be divorced, with one parent at risk of losing custody or visitation after a legal challenge by a former spouse on the grounds that HIV/AIDS impairs the infected parent's ability to care for the children. Other concerns involve advance planning and guardianship for children of a parent who is dying of AIDS.

• HIV infection alone is not sufficient grounds for denying custody or visitation rights if a parent is able to care for a child. The risk of HIV transmission from parent to child is not a sufficient basis for making a custody or visitation decision.

• Guardianship laws vary from state to state. Generally, procedures to appoint a guardian are usually designated in a will that is drafted with the assistance of an attorney.

• Standby guardianship laws allow parents who are ill to make permanent plans for their children's future without giving up their legal rights, and may be one effective option for parents with HIV/AIDS.

Entitlements

• Several federal and state health, social service, and income maintenance programs are particularly relevant for families with HIV/AIDS because of their low-income status. Determining eligibility for these programs may require the assistance of attorneys or advocates trained in entitlement issues.

• Developmental disability services and early intervention services under the Individuals with Disabilities Education Act may restrict eligibility for services on the basis of state and local resources, as well as local definitions of disability.

• Eligibility criteria are still evolving in the HIV/AIDS field for maternal and pediatric HIV/AIDS, although the Social Security Administration has recently revised eligibility standards for adults and children with HIV/AIDS to enable more persons infected with HIV to qualify for benefits.

REFERENCES

AIDS Confidentiality Act of 1987 (Illinois), Public Acts 85-677 and 85-674.
American Academy of Pediatrics (AAP) Task Force on Pediatric AIDS. (1989). Infants and children with acquired immunodeficiency syndrome: placement in adoption and foster care. *Pediatrics, 83,* 610–612.
American Bar Association (ABA). (1989). *AIDS and persons with developmental disabilities: The legal perspective.* Washington, DC: Author.
American Bar Association (ABA). (1991). *AIDS/HIV and confidentiality: model policy and procedures.* Washington, DC: Author.
American Civil Liberties Union [ACLU] AIDS Project. (1990). *Epidemic of fear.* New York: American Civil Liberties Union.
Americans with Disabilities Act of 1990, P.L. 101-336, 42 U.S.C. 12101.
Board of Education of Nassau County, Florida v. Arline, 480 U.S. 273, 282 (1987).
Brown, M. (1987). AIDS and ethics: Concerns and considerations. *Oncology Nursing Forum, 14*(1), 69–73.
Chicago Women and HIV Consortium. (n.d.). Unpublished guidelines, available through Cook County Hospital Women and Infant HIV Program, 1835 West Harrison Street, Chicago, IL 60612, (312) 633-5080.
Civil Rights Restoration Act of 1987, P.L. 100-259, 29 U.S.C. 701.
Cooke, M. (1990). Ethical issues related to AIDS. In P. T. Cohen, M. Sande, & P. A. Volberding (Eds.), *The AIDS knowledge base* (pp. 1214.1–1214.8). Waltham, MA: Medical Publishing Group.
Cooper, E. (1992). HIV infected parents and the law: Issues of custody, visitation and guardianship. In N. Hunter & W. Rubenstein (Eds.), *AIDS agenda* (pp. 70–117). New York: American Civil Liberties Union.
Developmental Disability and Bill of Rights Act of 1972, P.L. 88-164, 42 U.S.C. 6000.
Eisenberg, L. (1986). The genesis of fear: AIDS and the public response to science. *Law, Medicine and Health Care, 14*(5–6), 243–249.
Eth, S. (1988). The sexually active, HIV infected patient: Confidentiality versus the duty to protect. *Psychiatric Annals, 18*(10), 571–576.
Fair Housing Amendments Act of 1988, P.L. 100-430, 102 Stat. 1619, 42 U.S.C. 3604.
Fraser, K. (1989). *Someone at school has AIDS: A guide to developing policies for students and school staff members who are infected with HIV.* Alexandria, VA: National Association of State Boards of Education.
Girardi, J. A., Keese, R. M., Traver, L. B., & Cooksey, D. R. (1988). Psychotherapist responsibility in notifying individuals at risk for exposure to HIV. *Journal of Sex Research, 25*(1), 1–27.

Grady, C. (1992). Ethical aspects. In J. Flaskerud & P. Unguarski (Eds.), *HIV/AIDS: A guide to nursing care* (2nd ed.). Philadelphia: W. B. Saunders.

Green, J., & Arno, P. (1990). The Medicaidization of AIDS. *Journal of the American Medical Association, 264*(1), 1261–1266.

Harvey, D., & Decker, C. (1990). *HIV liability and disability services providers: An introduction to tort principles* (AIDS technical report No. 2). Washington, DC: National Association of Protection and Advocacy Systems.

Individuals with Disabilities Education Act of 1990, P.L. 94-142, 20 U.S.C. 1232.

Intergovernmental Health Policy Project, AIDS Policy Center. (1988). *AIDS: Communicable and sexually transmitted diseases, public health records, and AIDS specific laws.* Washington, DC: George Washington University.

Kermani, E. J., & Weiss, B. A. (1989). AIDS and confidentiality: Legal concept and its application in psychotherapy. *American Journal of Psychotherapy, 18*(1), 25–31.

Martinez v. School Board of Hillsborough County, Florida, 861 F.2d 1502, 1506 (11th Cir. 1988).

Michaels, D., & Levin, C. (1992). Estimates of the number of motherless youth orphaned by AIDS in the United States. *Journal of the American Medical Association, 268*(24), 3456–3461.

Mitchell, J., & Heagarty, M. (1991). Special considerations for minorities. In P. Pizzo & C. Wilfert (Eds.), *Pediatric AIDS: The challenge of HIV infection in infants, children and adolescents* (pp. 704–713). Baltimore, MD: Williams & Wilkins.

National Pediatric HIV Resource Center. (1992). *HIV/AIDS legal issues: A handbook for service providers.* Washington, DC: Feldesman, Leifer, Fidell & Bank.

Nicholas, S., & Abrams, E. (1992). The silent legacy of AIDS: Children who survive their parents and siblings [Editorial]. *Journal of the American Medical Association, 268*(24), 3478–3479.

Rehabilitation Act of 1973, P.L. 93-112, 29 U.S.C. 701.

Social Security Administration. (1993, June).

Surrogate's Court Procedure Act of 1992 (New York State).

Uniform Marriage and Divorce Act. (1973).

U.S. Department of Justice (1988, September 27). Application of Section 504 of the Rehabilitation Act to HIV-infected individuals. Washington, DC: Author.

U.S. House of Representatives. (1993). Proposed bill to amend Part E of Title IV of the Social Security Act (H.R. 1354). Washington, DC: Author.

SECTION VI

RESEARCH AND PUBLIC POLICY

18

· · · · · · · · · · · ·

Psychosocial Research Concerning Children, Families, and HIV/AIDS

A Challenge for Investigators

· · · · · · · · · · · · ·

Laurie N. Sherwen, PhD, FAAN
Susan Tross, PhD

THE NEED FOR PSYCHOSOCIAL RESEARCH

Few infectious diseases have produced an impact on society as dramatic as HIV/AIDS. HIV infection in children was first described in 1983, and since then has grown into the fifth leading cause of death for all children (Buehler et al., 1989). It is also one of the major causes of mental retardation and other handicapping conditions in children (Boland, 1989). According to the Centers for Disease Control and Prevention (CDC), women and children represent the fastest-growing segment of the infected population (Gwinn et al., 1991).

The prognosis for children diagnosed with HIV/AIDS has been grim. However, as the quality of supportive care improves and as new drug therapies are developed, the length of survival for HIV-infected children is rapidly increasing. Improved therapeutic modalities, specifically antiretroviral agents, have created a population of disabled, chronically ill children whom society will need to integrate into the community and help live "normal lives"—not just physically, but socially and psychologically as well.

Although behavioral research concerning children and families with chronic illnesses is a starting point for understanding the many psychosocial dimensions of living with HIV/AIDS, there are many differences between HIV/AIDS and other chronic illnesses. It has been illustrated throughout this book that HIV/AIDS is a multigenerational disease—whole nuclear families can become sick with the same disease and die. Other factors differentiate HIV/AIDS as well: the preponderance of cases among minority families; the stigma and consequent need for confidentiality.

Although HIV/AIDS cannot currently be cured, there have been extremely rapid advances in clinical knowledge and experimental treatments, such as drug trials; there is also a dramatic potential for prevention. In the meantime, intense services are needed to maintain child and family functioning, particularly as there is a disproportionate reliance on public financing and health care institutions for care (Meyer & Weitzman, 1991).

Finally, the pathology of HIV infection in children is also unique among chronic diseases, since as a multisystem disease it eventually affects almost every major organ system simultaneously. Furthermore, in children it frequently affects the neurological system. This produces many symptoms, including loss of developmental milestones, that progressively affect neurodevelopmental status. Children are likely to become disabled in many areas, including motor, speech, and cognitive functions. For the most part, these children will not be cared for in a hospital, but in a home environment within a community.

This chapter discusses the current state of empirically based knowledge concerning behavioral and psychosocial aspects of HIV/AIDS in children and families, and identifies common weaknesses in current research endeavors. Broad areas for research investigations are suggested. Barriers to conducting research with this population group are explored, and strategies for implementing research with these children and families are discussed.

THE CURRENT STATE OF RESEARCH

Although research abounds concerning many aspects of HIV/AIDS, much of the information to date on psychosocial and behavioral aspects of HIV infection and AIDS in families and children is merely descriptive, derived from anecdotal and clinical observations. Research endeavors, empirically based as well as descriptive, must begin to focus upon this specific population. It is necessary that we begin to develop a solid base of knowledge concerning not only well persons at risk for HIV infection, but also adults and children living in families with maternally transmitted HIV infection.

Current research tends to cluster around certain behavioral and psychosocial variables related to HIV infection in children and families: central nervous system (CNS) involvement in children; attitudes about HIV/AIDS of various groups, including adolescents, women, and different cultural/ethnic groups; identification of risk behaviors and risk-reducing behaviors; psychosocial responses of caretakers of HIV-infected persons; and "prevention" strategies for high-risk groups. The research in these areas has been reviewed in earlier chapters in this book, and therefore is mentioned only briefly here.

Research on CNS Complications

Although studies concerning CNS complications of HIV/AIDS in children comprise a large body of literature, the focus is primarily on the pathophysiology (Belman et al., 1988; Mintz et al., 1989; Falloon et al., 1989; Price et al., 1988), descriptions of neurological and developmental complications (Oleske et al., 1983; Rubinstein, 1983; Rubinstein et al., 1983; Belman et al., 1985; Epstein et al., 1986; Andiman, 1989), and prevalence (Epstein et al., 1986; Ultmann et al., 1987).

Few well-designed, large-scale empirical studies to date have focused on the psychosocial effects of CNS complications on children or families. In addition, existing studies suffer from methodological limitations. For example, natural history studies that follow a cohort of children throughout the spectrum of HIV disease from asymptomatic infection to AIDS proper need to be designed, to help identify the points at which children are most at risk for functional neurological/neuropsychological deficits. Such studies need to include a comparison group of HIV-seronegative children, so that effects of various other potential contributing factors (e.g., prenatal alcohol or drug exposure) may be quantified and separated from effects of HIV infection. In addition, such studies should use a comprehensive assessment battery to measure effects of CNS involvement, including developmental, neurological, neuroradiological, cognitive, and psychiatric measures that are sensitive and specific enough to permit relatively subtle differential diagnoses. Finally, because there are so many con-

founding variables, multivariate analysis of data should be applied to
these studies to deal with the complex context in which CNS complications develop in children.

Research on Attitudes

A second large body of research-based literature concerns the wide
variety of attitudes about HIV/AIDS, including surveys of groups considered "at risk" for infection.

Research to date has surveyed two main groups whose attitudes
may have a significant effect on the nature and incidence of maternally transmitted HIV infection: adolescents (DiClemente et al., 1986; Strunin & Hingson, 1987; Hingson et al., 1990) and women (Hutchinson
& Kurth, 1991; Flaskerud & Thompson, 1991; Rivera Robles et al.,
1990; Flaskerud & Rush, 1989; Abdool Karim et al., 1989; Beaman &
Strader, 1989; Nyamathi & Vasquez, 1989; Baker et al., 1990; Brown
& Rundell, 1990). Respondents to these surveys include African-
Americans, Whites, and Latinos/Latinas; members of low-income
groups; partners of injection drug users; rape victims; and individuals
with sexually transmitted diseases (STDs). Such studies provide data
on attitudes toward sexuality and reproductive decision making,
avoidance of risk, and knowledge about decision making; this information is needed in the development of preventive educational and
other strategies for specific high-risk groups. Again, however, many
of these studies do suffer from methodological weaknesses, especially concerning survey questionnaires and data collection procedures.
Another problem is a lack of focus on the less accessible "high-risk"
population, such as drug-using persons, and on persons who are already HIV-infected.

Research on Risk-Taking
and Risk-Reducing Behaviors

A smaller body of literature is concerned with identification of both
risk-taking and risk-reducing behaviors (Rapkin & Erickson, 1990; Lesnick & Pace, 1990; O'Dowd & McKegney, 1990; Thomas et al., 1989;
Quinn et al., 1988; Harrison et al., 1991; Brown et al., 1989; Rickert,
1989; Bowser, 1989; Sherr et al., 1990; Fullilove et al., 1990;
Rotheram-Borus & Koopman, 1991; Strunin & Hingson, 1987). Again,
various populations are included in these descriptive studies, including minority women and adolescents, college students, patients in STD
clinics, and women drug users. Such studies, like attitude surveys, are

needed to provide the baseline for development of specific interventions to eliminate risk-taking behaviors and to establish risk-reducing behaviors, which would theoretically prevent and eventually eliminate the risk of infection.

Research on Caretakers

Very few studies have focused on responses of caretakers of children with HIV/AIDS (Brown & Powell-Cope, 1991; Marin et al., 1990). There are studies dealing with caretakers of HIV-infected gay men; however, the different concerns and issues of the two infected populations (children/families and gay men) make it difficult to generalize findings from one group to the other. Existing studies concerning caretakers of children with HIV/AIDS have examined psychosocial concerns of caretakers of children in the home environment, and have compared responses of caretakers of hospitalized and nonhospitalized children.

The potential caretaker environments in which children with maternally transmitted HIV infection live are often deprived and chaotic, composed of individuals who are highly stressed and psychologically fragile. Yet clinicians have observed strength and resilience in these families as well. Many additional studies are needed in this area to identify appropriate care strategies for families and children living with HIV/AIDS in the community and home.

Research on Preventive Strategies

A small but growing number of studies deal with strategies designed to prevent the acquisition of HIV among a variety of high- and low-risk populations (Nelson, 1991; Schilling et al., 1991; Jemmott & Jemmott, 1991; Flaskerud & Nyamathi, 1990; Berrier et al., 1991). Educational strategies have been tested for use with adolescents, injection drug users, minority women, and pregnant women. Behaviors encouraged in these educational sessions include use of condoms and sterilization of injection equipment. Preventive interventions are currently seen as the primary means to contain the spread of HIV/AIDS. It is likely, however, that many strategies used to change behaviors are targeted toward middle-class populations (who also need to learn to prevent HIV infection) and not toward other cultural/ethnic or socioeconomic groups. Baseline data on learning in different population groups need to be acquired, and interventions must be developed specifically for all segments of the population. Although intervention studies are desperately needed in this area, they need to be grounded in empirical, cross-cultural research.

PROBLEMS WITH EXISTING RESEARCH

As can be seen from the discussion above, many potential areas for research into the psychosocial dimensions of HIV/AIDS in children and families remain to be studied. Furthermore, many existing studies have methodological problems that confound the interpretation of data. Systematic studies of the experiences of living with maternally transmitted HIV infection are critically needed, so that the major psychosocial issues of HIV/AIDS may be understood. Such studies require the following:

• *Adequate sample size.* Many studies have involved samples that are too small to have any statistical power. Simply put, such studies have little likelihood of detecting differences or change; even if they do find a difference, the sample will be too small to permit the extension of any generalizations about the findings to other groups.

• *Multivariate analytic techniques.* The children and families affected by HIV/AIDS are highly complex. There are many conflicting, confounding variables present in their lives and environments, in addition to HIV infection. Most HIV-infected children come from poor, inner-city backgrounds and have very young parents. The majority of families with HIV/AIDS are African-American or Latino. Most minority children with HIV/AIDS have at least one parent who is an injection drug user. For all these reasons, these families are extremely difficult to reach and do not respond to conventional outreach methods. Drug-addicted mothers, for instance, may avoid services because they fear that their children will be taken from them. Statistical techniques must sort out the true effects of HIV/AIDS from the "white noise" produced by the multitude of factors present in the environments of the families.

• *Comparison groups.* Meaningful comparison groups for families and children with HIV/AIDS must be identified. Again, since we know so little about uninfected families who have the same demographic characteristics as infected families, baseline data should be established so that research findings on families with HIV/AIDS are meaningful. Only after the "norm" can be established and compared with findings related to HIV/AIDS can the true nature of infected families and children be clarified.

• *Longitudinal designs.* Psychosocial variables, as well as physiological variables, change over time in children and families with HIV/AIDS. Studies that track a cohort of such children and families over time, and have several different data collection points, are desperately needed to ascertain the changes that occur in the psychosocial and behavioral aspects of HIV/AIDS.

Although it is relatively simple to identify what current studies lack, it is less simple to overcome barriers to achieving strong, empirical quantitative studies or descriptive qualitative studies. Later sections discuss these barriers in some detail and suggest strategies to surmount the obstacles to developing strong research designs.

SOME AREAS WHERE RESEARCH IS NEEDED

Research is desperately needed in numerous areas, not only to obtain a clear picture of children and families with HIV/AIDS, but, more importantly, to develop and test relevant interventions and care modalities. Proposed areas for research into psychosocial dimensions of children and families with HIV/AIDS can be grouped into five areas: (1) research concerning the family as a whole; (2) research concerning individual family members, including children; (3) research concerning psychosocial/behavioral interventions or strategies to help children and families; (4) research directed to professional caregivers of HIV-infected children and families; and (5) research into health policy issues related to HIV/AIDS. This topical grouping of suggested areas is not meant to be all-inclusive. It is meant to suggest possible questions to the reader, and to stimulate the reader to identify further areas requiring research.

Research Concerning the Family as a Unit

The first type of research views the family as a system or unit. In particular, it examines how HIV infection affects the interactions among family subsystems, and how it affects the family's relationship with other systems, such as the broader community or school. Areas for research might include the following:

1. Identification and testing of care delivery models and intervention protocols that can be used to care for children and families with HIV in the home and community.
2. Effects of HIV/AIDS on family structure and function, including the stressors experienced by families and children, as well as their coping strategies and adaptation.
3. The effects of HIV/AIDS on the family developmental cycle.
4. Differences between functional and dysfunctional HIV/AIDS families, with an examination of family support systems, communication networks, and patterns of closeness and apartness.
5. Comparative cultural, ethnic, and socioeconomic variations in families with HIV/AIDS.

6. Effects on "survivors" of a family with multiple infected members.
7. Effects of multiple care systems on the family.
8. Relationships between professional and other caregivers and a family with HIV/AIDS.

Research Concerning Individual Family Members (Including Children)

The second type of research focuses on family members, and on how HIV/AIDS affects them as *individuals*. Areas for research might include the following:

1. *Long-term psychological effects.* Researchers need to study the psychological sequelae of having HIV infection over time for specific groups—women; heterosexual men who are parents; injection drug users who have families; children at different developmental stages; and adolescents. Studies are also needed of the psychological stages of dealing with HIV/AIDS as a chronic illness, and how such stages compare to those found in persons with other types of chronic illness. Additional research areas include cultural and other influences on reproductive decision making, and issues of secrecy and stigma for the various groups mentioned above.

2. *Disclosure issues.* Research investigators need to understand the effects of disclosure of a family member's HIV status—the testing–counseling situation, partner notification, and motivations for disclosure or nondisclosure to partners.

3. *Family member issues.* A greatly underrepresented area is that of the special needs and concerns of specific family members. Important topics for research include psychological issues of HIV-negative or seroconverted siblings; concerns of noninfected children with an HIV-infected parent; effects of maternally transmitted HIV infection on extended family members; and effects of the family system and individual members on an HIV-infected child's well-being over time.

4. *Children and education.* There are a number of important issues related to HIV-infected children in school—confidentiality, disclosure of HIV status, reaction of peers and teachers, factors that affect the children's ability to learn, social integration of the children, and factors that promote or hinder this integration.

5. *Injection drug use.* Research should be conducted on drug use of family members and HIV/AIDS—interaction effects on psychological functioning, predisposing factors, treatment and return to addiction in infected and noninfected persons, and drug users' concerns and attitudes about HIV infection.

6. *Adolescents.* This population is underresearched. What is the effect of HIV infection on adolescents' attainment of independence, feelings of hope versus despair, thoughts of suicide, and sexual activity?

7. *Risk reduction issues.* Finally, we need more research on health-promoting behaviors in HIV-infected women, injection and other drug users, children and adolescents.

Research Concerning Interventions to Help Families and Children

The third type of research concerns the development and testing of strategies and interventions to care for families and children with HIV/AIDS. Professionals, funding agencies, and families alike place the highest priorities on development of empirically tested care modalities that will improve the care delivered to these families and children. It is important to remember, however, that interventions must be grounded in real baseline data and knowledge. Most existing care delivery models were designed for middle-class White families. HIV/AIDS, and the families most often affected at this time, present great challenges to care delivery. Research needs to document which present treatments are effective; it also needs to provide the baseline data for developing new appropriate treatments. Research into psychosocial components of care needs to address two levels simultaneously if truly effective treatment models are to be developed: (1) the basic aspects of psychological issues in infected families, and (2) the testing of treatments.

Research into interventions might cover the following topics: self-help strategies; care in the home environment, and effects of the home environment on care; discharge planning needs; managed care paradigms; case management paradigms; techniques to teach a variety of self-care strategies to different population groups; and the actual outcomes of these care strategies. Outcomes of care delivery are a specific research interest of many federal and nonfederal funding agencies, and often have a focus on HIV/AIDS. In addition, outcome research, by documenting which interventions work, plays an important role in health policy decisions (particularly those concerning allocation of resources).

Research Concerning Caregivers of Families and Children

The fourth type of research concerns professionals and other persons who deliver care to HIV-infected children and families in a variety of settings. This type of research, while not focused directly on the families, is important, as caregivers are instrumental in determining the quality of care and level of support families receive. Some areas for research directed to caregivers might include burnout and strategies to avoid burnout (see Chapter 14); motivation for working with HIV-infected persons; fears and doubts concerning HIV infection and infected persons and families; and strategies to change negative attitudes into positive responses.

Research into Related Health Policy Issues

Policies developed concerning HIV/AIDS are likely to have a profound impact on the psychosocial functioning of infected families; such policies are therefore included here as an area for research investigation. Some topics that might be researched include ethical and legal issues concerning HIV/AIDS in children and families (see Chapters 16 and 17); policies related to allocation of resources for HIV/AIDS research and treatment; impact of demonstration projects on policy formation; school policies; policies concerning testing and confidentiality of health professionals and family members; mandatory testing of pregnant women and other high risk groups in the population; public financing and systems of care delivery for persons with HIV/AIDS; impact on HIV/AIDS institutions that deliver care to children and families (hospitals, home health agencies); and methods to contain costs related to HIV/AIDS.

As noted earlier, these suggested research areas are not meant to be exhaustive. Myriad topics for research endeavors may present themselves to the reader from each area mentioned above, or may themselves suggest other areas for research not mentioned. Research into the behavioral and psychosocial aspects of HIV infection in families and children is yet in its infancy. However, as medical and basic physiological research concerning HIV/AIDS and treatments (including drugs) rapidly progresses, children and other family members will be surviving for longer and longer periods. With more persons living with the chronic condition, psychosocial dimensions of HIV infection and disease will become increasingly important as the focus of research investigations.

BARRIERS TO CONDUCTING PSYCHOSOCIAL RESEARCH

Although psychosocial research with HIV/AIDS children and families is vital to establishing appropriate care delivery and to improving their quality of life, it presents formidable challenges to the investigator. This section reviews some of the difficulties in conducting research with families and children with HIV/AIDS. The final section looks at some strategies to overcome these barriers and implement research endeavors.

A pair of articles in the *New England Journal of Medicine* on experimental drugs for HIV infection and AIDS suggest that the norm of traditional rigorous scientific research, the three-phase drug trial, is being challenged. New designs are being pioneered in the conduct of HIV-related drug trials. These include the use of nonrandomized trials; rejection of the untreated control group; statistical rather than design control of multiple confounding variables; and flexible entry criteria (Merigan, 1990; Byar et al., 1990). These strategies indicate the dramatic and unique nature of HIV/AIDS in our society, and the measures that must be taken to gain needed data concerning this disease and the persons whom it affects.

Behavioral and psychosocial research concerned with nonmedical aspects of HIV/AIDS is also affected by the nature of the HIV disease process, the treatment protocols, and the current population most affected by HIV/AIDS. In the study of populations of children and families with maternally transmitted HIV infection, certain conditions may present barriers to conducting the research.

The first of these conditions is the limited number of truly HIV-infected children (and the families of such children) currently documented. The numbers of children currently diagnosed as being infected with HIV are relatively small in many locations. If the researcher wishes to study children who are symptomatic, or who are actually diagnosed as having full-blown AIDS by current CDC or other criteria, those numbers become smaller still. Reasons for some of the low numbers include the artifact of poor screening of children; the as yet inadequate diagnostic techniques in some geographic areas (although laboratory techniques, such as polymerase chain reaction or viral culture, for establishing an early diagnosis of HIV infection are rapidly becoming available); the lack of state policy or law mandating screening for pregnant women or neonates; and the fact that some areas of the country are simply not yet affected with maternally transmitted HIV infection.

The relatively small numbers of children reliably diagnosed as having HIV infection must be balanced against the multiple variables affecting children and families with HIV/AIDS. The problem with so many extraneous variables impinging on the families and children is that complex research designs are necessary to control effects of the unwanted variables—for example, poverty. Complex research designs call for very large sample sizes, which in many locations are impossible at the present time. Sample number projections established by power analysis (the traditional mode of establishing sample size) are very difficult to fulfill under current circumstances. A dilemma exists: Is it better to delay the process of stable inquiry until large numbers of children (and families of such children) diagnosed with HIV infection are available across the country, or is it better to conduct studies despite the limitations imposed on research findings by a sample size not large enough for the multiple extraneous variables involved or the complexity of the design?

Many other conditions pose barriers to conducting research on the population currently affected by maternally transmitted HIV infection. These include the following:

• There is a wide variation in the age at diagnosis of HIV infection in children. Children are entering into research protocols as newly diagnosed subjects at different points in their development. Thus, a child's developmental level becomes one factor that might affect the outcome measure chosen to study the effects of HIV/AIDS on the child or the family.

• No true, accurate severity index for children exists at present. It therefore becomes difficult to control for the severity of the condition of children entered into a study. Some children may be sicker than other children in the study, and no reliable basis exists to limit research participation by severity of the condition. Thus, initial level of illness may confound outcome measures.

• There are differences in prognosis based on presenting symptomatology (e.g., *Pneumocystis carinii* pneumonia in children carries a much worse prognosis than does lymphoid interstitial pneumonitis). Again, since the progress of HIV infection seems to be different in children who have different presenting symptoms, this variable may affect outcome measures. Limiting the sample to children with only certain presenting symptoms would again reduce the numbers of children available.

• There are also differences in prognosis based on age at diagnosis (i.e., children diagnosed at under 1 year of age have a worse prognosis than do children diagnosed at over 1 year of age). As with presenting symptomatology, the age at diagnosis may profoundly affect either what the researcher hopes to find in the study or the effects of an experimental treatment.

• Children may be on one or more medical treatment protocols. Medical treatments are often experimental in nature (in fact, some children may simultaneously be in a medical study investigating a treatment protocol). Effects of medical treatments must be controlled for in psychosocial studies, as the observed effects of a psychosocial treatment may actually be attributable to a medical treatment.

• Children may be participating in one or more drug trials. Like the effects of medical treatment protocols, the effects of the drugs used in drug trials may account for any differences observed in a study population. Furthermore, since some drug trials use a placebo, employ different dosages of a medication, and are "blind" (i.e., the researchers for the drug trial are not aware of which subjects receive the placebo or which receive a particular dosage of the drug), it is very difficult for the behavioral or psychosocial researcher to know what is happening to the subjects in his or her study. Since so many persons with HIV/AIDS are involved in drug trials, to exclude everyone who is involved in such a trial would profoundly affect sample size.

• Great variation exists among children's caretakers and home environments. Children are routinely found in homes with biological parent(s), with extended family members (often grandmothers), or with foster parents. Furthermore, over the course of any study, a child's caretaker or home environment may change—a parent may die, or a child's care may become too difficult for a grandmother. Since many families with maternally transmitted HIV infection currently practice informal adoption, it is common for children to be moved to other environments when one family unit becomes unable to care for them. The nature of the home and caretaker will affect many outcome measures related to a child. Finally, if a child is moved to a caretaker or home a distance from the study site, the child may be lost to the study.

• Families with maternally transmitted HIV infection are frequently connected to the drug culture. A biological mother may use injectable or other drugs, or her partner may be a user. In this instance, the effects of intrauterine or breast-feeding exposure to drugs must be differentiated from effects of HIV/AIDS on the child. Furthermore, effects of drug use on a family may greatly affect outcome measures related to the child, family, or other family members. In addition, data collection with groups involved in the drug culture is highly problematic for many reasons.

• Multiple family members may be HIV-infected in addition to the child. Obviously, the biological mother is always infected in mother–child transmission, and other members may be infected as well. This factor may affect many outcome measures and data collection procedures. For example, if a child's biological mother is a respondent in the study, her level of sickness (especially CNS involvement) may profoundly affect her ability to participate, even if the focus is on the sick child and not on the mother herself.

• Although HIV-infected children are beginning to survive for longer periods, many will still die in a few years. This makes conducting longitudinal studies extremely difficult, as many children may die before complete data can be gathered, and thus will be lost to the investigation.

• Children and families often live in extreme poverty. It is very difficult to assess the effects of HIV/AIDS on children and families when all the factors connected with poverty—such as premature birth, malnutrition, inadequate medical and health care, crime, violence, poor education, unemployment, poor housing, and so on—can also affect these families. Many relevant outcome measures, such as developmental level of children, will be affected by living in such profound poverty as well.

• Children and families with HIV/AIDS are often from minority cultural/ethnic backgrounds. These groups have routinely been excluded from research. Thus, it is difficult or impossible to obtain baseline data on uninfected minority families with which to compare the data on infected families.

• Many low-income families with HIV/AIDS do not trust "authorities," and do not respond to "being studied" in a manner similar to that of middle-class population groups. These families have had negative experiences with a variety of authorities, including health professionals. It takes much time to establish a trusting relationship with such families, and a researcher rarely has sufficient time to do so. For families with HIV/AIDS, participating in a research study, especially one that does not directly benefit them or their children, has little importance.

• HIV-infected families face multiple crises every day of their lives, over and above the infection. It is just one more crisis added to an already overwhelming number of crises. How can participation in research fit into such lives?

• Families with HIV/AIDS are involved with multiple, often uncoordinated systems of care. Often, conflicting systems of care and uncoordinated services are chaotic for the family. A behavioral researcher may appear to be just one more burden. When given a choice to participate in a study, it is little wonder that many family members decline.

Every condition mentioned above is a variable routinely found in the population of families and children currently affected with maternally transmitted HIV infection. Not only must the research design inherently deal with these variables; the conduct of the research must incorporate parameters imposed by such variables. The classic epidemiological design employed in drug trials will often be inappropriate for this group and difficult to implement. Creative, more flexible designs must be pioneered to study this unique group of individuals.

IMPLEMENTING RESEARCH WITH FAMILIES AND CHILDREN

The preceding section has dealt with some of the barriers an investigator might encounter when doing research with families and children who are affected with HIV/AIDS. Although such barriers may seem overwhelming, there are many strategies that can assist the investigator in overcoming them. In general, it is necessary to remember several things about these families that can assist the researcher in carrying out a study. First, although the families may be experiencing very adverse conditions, many of them have strengths that make them very resilient. It is important to identify these strengths, as they can facilitate the implementation of research. The investigator should also remember that many families sincerely want to help not only their own children but other HIV-infected children. Their life events may not always enable them to carry out this desire, but the sentiment is there and can help involve the families in research. Finally, families and children with maternally transmitted HIV infection are a population that we need to understand. Research with this group is necessary and important, and vital to delivery of good-quality care. It is well worth any effort necessary to overcome existing barriers in order to carry out research.

Three considerations must be taken into account in planning to develop a research study focusing on the current population of children and families with HIV/AIDS: (1) the appropriate research design for one's geographic location; (2) the logistics of data collection; and (3) gaining the trust of potential study participants.

An investigator must first consider the geographic pattern of HIV infection and its incidence in his or her locale. Although the pattern is changing, and HIV is spreading from urban epicenters to smaller cities, suburban areas, and rural areas, it is still necessary to consider the absolute numbers of individuals (i.e., children) currently affected in a locale before attempting to fulfill certain types of research designs. For example, a traditional experimental design, with several treatment groups and a control group, can only be carried out in geographic locations where there are sufficient numbers of children to participate in the study and yield generalizable findings. A researcher in, say, Montana, may write a perfect research project of this nature, but may be unable to fulfill the design requirements because of the small number of potential subjects in the area. Such settings lend themselves more readily to qualitative designs—for example, designs using case studies, in which much smaller numbers of participants are necessary to obtain important findings. Otherwise, the investigator will need to consider relocating or setting up consortium projects with researchers in areas more heavily affected by maternally transmitted HIV infection.

A second consideration is that of the logistics necessary for collecting the required data. Where will the researcher have to go to obtain data, and is it feasible to collect data at these sites? Often, collecting psychosocial data concerning children and families may require home visits or visits to places within the community. How will the researcher accomplish this—especially if he or she is not of the same background as the families and is not really familiar with them? What if data must be acquired in communities or families involved with the drug culture? What if children and family members are victims of violence? Although none of these factors will preclude data collection in the appropriate environment, some thought must be given as to how data collection may be carried out in the home or community under any potential circumstances.

It might seem that collecting data in the hospital, clinic, or other environment where children or family members come together as a group (e.g., a site where support group meetings are held) would be an easier way to obtain necessary data. Although this is undoubtedly true, data collection in such environments also requires careful consideration and planning. Again, logistics are vitally important to a successful study. Data collection in a clinic or hospital requires detailed planning with clinic staff members, so as not to disrupt the already hectic flow of work. For example, identifying appropriate participants, finding time during the clinic visit to test participants, or even finding space to do the data collection may become a major issue. Researchers will find that they get little cooperation from staff members if they are perceived as nuisances or impediments to delivering care. Although collecting data from families at support groups does not carry the same problems, the investigator will need to worry about possible participants' showing up at such sessions. Since many of these families do not have telephones, it is difficult to ascertain which families will attend any one session, nor is it often possible to remind families of the session in a timely fashion.

A third consideration in developing a study is gaining the trust of family members themselves. It is not likely that families will inherently trust the investigator, nor is there any reason that they should. Establishing a trusting relationship that will allow for carrying out a complex data collection battery will take a long time. Often researchers do not even know how to communicate appropriately with potential participants. The researcher will have to determine whether he or she is the best person to collect data, or whether there are other persons (research assistants, professional staff, or community persons) who might work more easily with the families. The pros and cons of working with these different individuals to collect data must be considered, and compromises must be made when necessary.

CONCLUSION

Many of the barriers we have described to the conduct of research with children and families with HIV/AIDS are not unique to this situation. They have always been present in the conduct of studies with disenfranchised minority groups living in poverty. In the past, the research community tended to ignore these populations and to focus research on population groups that were easier to work with and involved fewer confounding variables. HIV/AIDS has made it impossible to ignore the conduct of research with the populations currently affected. We may find that traditional research designs must often be altered when studying groups affected by maternally transmitted HIV infection.

The HIV/AIDS epidemic, especially in families and children, is challenging many traditional models of practice and research. The nature of the disease, the diagnostic and treatment protocols that are being developed, and the affected populations all make these models not only inappropriate, but unworkable; continuing to use them would therefore be negligent. New models of research must be evolved and pioneered in order to study HIV infection and the population groups it affects. Although scientific rigor should not be compromised, flexible alternatives to traditional research designs and methods must be developed and refined. The research community, both in the biomedical disciplines and the behavioral/psychosocial disciplines, must share this responsibility.

REFERENCES

Abdool Karim, Q., et al. (1989). Sexual behavior and knowledge of AIDS among urban Black mothers. *South African Medical Journal, 80*(7), 340–343.
Andiman, W. A. (1989). Virologic and serologic aspects of human immuno-

deficiency virus infection in infants and children. *Seminars in Perinatology, 13*(1), 16–26.

Baker, T. C., et al. (1990). Rape victims' concerns about possible exposure to HIV infection. *Journal of Interpersonal Violence, 5*(1), 49–60.

Beaman, M. L., & Strader, M. K. (1989). STD patients' knowledge about AIDS and attitudes toward condom use. *Journal of Community Health Nursing, 6*(3), 155–164.

Belman, A., et al. (1985). Neurological complications in infants and children with acquired immune deficiency syndrome. *Annals of Neurology, 18,* 560–566.

Belman, A., et al. (1988). Pediatric acquired immunodeficiency syndrome: Neurologic syndromes. *American Journal of Diseases of Children, 142,* 29–35.

Berrier, J., et al. (1991). HIV/AIDS education in a prenatal clinic: An assessment. *AIDS Education and Prevention, 3*(2): 100–117.

Boland, M. (1989). *Generations in jeopardy: Responding to HIV infection in children, women, and adolescents in New Jersey.* Newark, NJ: New Jersey Department of Health.

Bowser, B. P. (1989). Crack and AIDS: An ethnographic impression. *Journal of the National Medical Association, 81*(5), 538–540.

Brown, G. R., & Rundell, J. R. (1990). Prospective study of psychiatric morbidity in HIV-seropositive women without AIDS. *General Hospital Psychiatry, 12*(1): 30–35.

Brown, L. S., et al. (1989). Female intravenous drug users and perinatal HIV transmission. *New England Journal of Medicine, 320*(22), 1493–1494.

Brown, M. A., & Powell-Cope, G.M. (1991). AIDS family caregiving: Transitions through uncertainty. *Nursing Research, 40*(6), 338–345.

Buehler, J. W., et al. (1989). Reporting of AIDS: Tracking HIV morbidity and mortality. *Journal of the American Medical Association, 262,* 2896–2897.

Byar, D. P., et al. (1990). Design considerations for AIDS trials. *New England Journal of Medicine, 323*(19), 1343–1348.

DiClemente, R., et al. (1986). Adolescents and AIDS: A survey of knowledge, attitudes and beliefs about AIDS in San Francisco. *American Journal of Public Health, 76,* 1443–1445.

Epstein, L., et al. (1988). Neurological and neuropathological features of HIV in children. *Annals of Neurology, 23*(Suppl.), S19–S23.

Epstein, L., et al. (1986). Neurologic manifestations of human immunodeficiency virus in children. *Pediatrics, 78,* 678–687.

Falloon, J., et al. (1989). Human immunodeficiency virus infection in children. *Journal of Pediatrics, 114*(1), 1–30.

Flaskerud, J. H., & Nyamathi, A. M. (1990). Effects of an AIDS education program on the knowledge, attitudes and practices of low income Black and Latina women. *Journal of Community Health, 15*(6), 343–355.

Flaskerud, J. H., & Rush, C. E. (1989). AIDS and traditional health beliefs and practices of Black women. *Nursing Research, 38*(4), 210–215.

Flaskerud, J. H., & Thompson, J. (1991). Beliefs about AIDS, health, and illness in low-income White women. *Nursing Research, 4*(5), 266–271.

Fullilove, M. T., et al. (1990). Black women and AIDS prevention: A view towards understanding the gender rules. *Journal of Sex Research, 27*(1), 47–64.

Gwinn, M., et al. (1991). Prevalence of HIV infection in childbearing women in the Unites States: Surveillance using newborn blood samples. *Journal of the American Medical Association, 265*(13), 1704–1708.

Harrison, D. F., et al. (1991). AIDS knowledge and risk behaviors among culturally diverse women. *AIDS Education and Prevention, 3*(2), 79–89.

Hingson, R., et al. (1990). Acquired immunodeficiency syndrome transmission: Changes in knowledge and behaviors among teenagers, Massachusetts statewide surveys, 1986 to 1988. *Pediatrics, 85*(1), 24–29.

Hutchinson, M., & Kurth, A. (1991). "I need to know that I have a choice . . . ": A study of women, HIV, and reproductive decision-making. *AIDS Patient Care, 5*(1), 17–25.

Jemmott, L. S., & Jemmott, J. B. (1991). Applying the theory of reasoned action to AIDS risk behavior: Condom use among Black women. *Nursing Research, 640*(4), 228–234.

Lesnick, H., & Pace, B. (1990). Knowledge of AIDS risk factors in South Bronx minority college students. *Journal of Acquired Immune Deficiency Syndromes, 3*(2), 173–176.

Marin, B., et al. (1990). Differences between Hispanics and non-Hispanics in willingness to provide AIDS prevention advice. *Hispanic Journal of Behavioral Sciences, 12*(2), 153–164.

Merigan, T. C. (1990). You can teach an old dog new tricks: How AIDS trials are pioneering new strategies. *New England Journal of Medicine, 323*(19), 1341–1343.

Meyer, A., & Weitzman, M. (1991). Pediatric HIV disease: The newest chronic illness of childhood. *Pediatric Clinics of North America, 38*(1), 169–194.

Mintz, M., et al. (1989). Neurological manifestations of acquired immunodeficiency syndrome in children. *International Pediatrics, 4*(2), 161–171.

Neaigus, A., et al. (1990). Effects of outreach intervention on risk reduction among intravenous drug users. *AIDS Education and Prevention, 2*(4), 253–271.

Nelson, E. W. (1991). Sexual self-defense versus the liaison dangerous: A strategy for AIDS prevention in the '90s. *American Journal of Preventive Medicine, 7*(3), 146–149.

Nyamathi, A., & Vasquez, R. (1989). Impact of poverty, homelessness, and drugs on Hispanic women at risk for HIV infection. *Hispanic Journal of Behavioral Sciences, 11*(4), 299–314.

O'Dowd, M. A., & McKegney, F. P. (1990). AIDS patients compared with others seen in psychiatric consultation. *General Hospital Psychiatry, 12*(1), 50–51.

Oleske, J., et al. (1983). Immune deficiency syndrome in children. *Journal of the American Medical Association, 249*(17), 2345–2349.

Price, R., et al. (1988). The brain in AIDS: Central nervous system HIV-1 infection and AIDS dementia complex. *Science, 239,* 586–592.

Quinn, T. C., et al. (1988). Human immunodeficiency virus infection among patients attending clinics for sexually transmitted diseases. *New England Journal of Medicine, 318*(4), 197–203.

Rapkin, A. J., & Erickson, P. I. (1990). Differences in knowledge of and risk factors for AIDS between Hispanic and non-Hispanic women attending an urban family planning clinic. *AIDS Patient Care, 4*(9), 889–899.

Rickert, E. J. (1989). Differing sexual practices of men and women screened for HIV (AIDS) antibody. *Psychological Reports, 64*(1), 323–326.

Rivera Robles, R., et al. (1990). Social relations and empowerment of sexual partners of IV drug users. *Puerto Rico Health Sciences Journal, 9*(1), 99–104.

Rotheram-Borus, M. J., & Koopman, C. (1991). Sexual risk behaviors, AIDS knowledge, and beliefs about AIDS among runaways. *American Journal of Public Health, 81*(2), 208–210.

Rubinstein, A. (1983). Acquired immunodeficiency syndrome in infants. *American Journal of Diseases of Children, 137*(9), 825–827.

Rubinstein, A., et al. (1983). Acquired immunodeficiency with reversed T4/T8 ratios in infants born to promiscuous and drug-addicted mothers. *Journal of the American Medical Association, 249*(17), 2350–2356.

Schilling, R. F., et al. (1991). Building skills of recovering women drug users to reduce heterosexual AIDS transmission. *Public Health Reports, 106*(3), 297–304.

Sherr, L., et al. (1990). Sexual behavior, condom use and prediction in attenders at sexually transmitted disease clinics: Implications for counseling. *Counseling Psychology Quarterly, 3*(4), 343–352.

Strunin, L., & Hingson, R. (1987). Acquired immunodeficiency syndrome and adolescents: Knowledge, beliefs, attitudes, and behaviors. *Pediatrics, 79,* 835–838.

Thomas, S. B., et al. (1989). Knowledge about AIDS and reported risk behaviors among Black college students. *Journal of American College Health, 38*(2), 61–66.

Ultmann, M., et al. (1987). Developmental abnormalities in children with acquired immunodeficiency syndrome (AIDS): A follow-up study. *International Journal of Neurosciences, 32*(3–4), 661–667.

19

· · · · · · · · · · · · · ·

HIV/AIDS and Public Policy

Recent Developments

· · · · · · · · · · · · · ·

David C. Harvey, MSW, LCSW

> We must try harder to understand than explain.
> —*Vaclav Havel in speech to the 1991*
> *World Economic Forum*

Public policy is the means of defining in a rational and authoritative manner the distribution of goods and services according to benefits and costs in society. This book's previous discussion of HIV epidemiology, and of the psychosocial and psychotherapeutic issues of children and families affected by HIV/AIDS, may suggest that policy makers have the necessary information for an equitable allocation of goods and services in the U.S. health care sector according to a cost–benefit analysis. However, the denial, misinformation, and stigma associated with HIV/AIDS, unparalleled in recent American history in connection with any disease, continue to contribute to a political culture in which effective public policy formation in the areas of prevention, research, and treatment remains inadequate. This is evidenced most acutely in the area of prevention and the continuing surge in HIV infection. As of July 1994, 61,000 cases of HIV infection have been reported to the Centers for Disease Control and Prevention (CDC) from the 27 states with mandated HIV reporting (CDC, 1994c).

In 1991, the National Commission on AIDS warned that "in the months to come [the people of the United States] must either engage seriously the issues and needs posed by this deadly disease or face relentless, expanding tragedy in the decades ahead." In 1993, the commission looked back on this warning and commented that "our nation has continued on [its] short-sighted course. Sadly, we must continue to report that America is still doing poorly."

Political science theory helps explain this response to HIV/AIDS in the United States. As Van Horn, Baumer, and Gormley (1989) discuss in their book *Politics and Public Policy,* our large and diverse political system selects some public policy problems to address and others to disregard. The process may be understood by drawing distinctions between politics and policy and their interdependence, as well as by understanding a framework that includes "issue characteristics." In the public health policy arena, HIV/AIDS was initially ignored because of the issue characteristics (such as homosexuality and injection drug use) linked with HIV transmission. Although politicians and policy analysts have still been reluctant to embrace these social issues, there have been some notable public policy achievements. This is not, however, a statement that indicates success in combating this potentially preventable deadly infection, for which there is currently no cure or vaccine. Furthermore, our failure to combat HIV/AIDS is related to our failure to contain and treat drug abuse and drug-resistant tuberculosis, both of which are linked to HIV infection.

This chapter adopts the multisystem approach to HIV/AIDS that this book on psychotherapeutic issues stresses. The chapter reviews the theory of clinicians as policy makers, the need for advocacy to benefit families with HIV/AIDS, and recent developments at the federal level that affect the delivery of a wide array of HIV-related health and mental health services. The present discussion is by no means complete in an era of massive policy reformation now underway on a national scale in the areas of health care, education, and prevention.

At the time of this writing, large-scale health reform at the federal level of government is now in question, following the failure of legislation in the 103rd Congress. How Congress and the administration will resolve issues of providing health care to low-income and uninsured persons will have significant impact on children, youth, and families living with HIV/AIDS. Further analysis of the reform measures now underway by state governments and their impact on HIV/AIDS services will be needed in the coming years.

CLINICIANS AS POLICY MAKERS

Some social policy analysts suggest that public policy is best understood by examining the role of clinicians and other direct service providers as agents of policy delivery. Lipsky (1980), in *Street-Level Bureaucracy,* contends that public policy is best understood not by studying legislatures or high-ranking administrators, but instead by examining policy as made and implemented by "street-level" workers. Lipsky writes, "Too often social analysts offer generalizations about organizational and governmental actions without concretely explaining how individual citizens and workers are affected by the actions" (p. xi). Clinicians can be the implementers and decision makers regarding key public policy questions, such as who receives what services according to cost–benefit analysis. The dilemma often encountered at the federal level of government in public policy development is that this direct role of clinicians, and their knowledge of how federal policy gets implemented, are not well understood. For the clinician, the problem is a failure to understand the significance of the policy delivery role and the power that this role carries in developing, influencing, and implementing federal policy.

HIV/AIDS PUBLIC POLICY, FAMILIES, AND MENTAL HEALTH

More than five out of every six cases of pediatric HIV infection have resulted from mother–infant transmission, and over 40% of children with AIDS have been born to women with a history of injection drug use. The mothers of another 17% of children with AIDS became infected through sexual intercourse with injection drug users (CDC, 1994a). HIV/AIDS is increasingly coming to affect entire families, and disproportionately affects low-income black or Hispanic persons. Most of these families have limited access to health and social services, transportation, and housing. Mental health services often come as a last priority on a continuum of basic needs that includes primary medical care, food, housing, transportation, and income maintenance. However, counseling and psychological services offered in the context of comprehensive, culturally relevant care can significantly relate to the success (or failure) of medical and social interventions with HIV/AIDS, and can thereby prolong life and improve the quality of life (Harvey, Boland, Burr, & Conviser, 1992; U.S. Department of Health and Human Services [DHHS], 1987, 1988).

Since the end of World War II, mental health policy has gone through cyclical patterns of development based on treatment advances, changing public opinion, fiscal conditions, new technologies, and changes in the political landscape (Mechanic, 1991). HIV/AIDS, along with other problems such as deinstitutionalization and homelessness, has helped usher in a new era of mental health policy dialogue. In relation to HIV/AIDS, mental health policy debate has resulted from concerns about (1) the acute psychological stress reaction to being diagnosed with a stigmatized disease; (2) primary and secondary prevention of HIV infection as a mental health intervention; (3) behavioral research aimed at understanding the psychodynamics of injection drug use and sexual behavior; and (4) financing of mental health services for persons with, or affected by, HIV/AIDS. However, the research literature related to mental health policy continues to focus on the needs of persons with severe or chronic mental illness. Mental health policy research has lagged in the HIV/AIDS area. There is a continuing need for research that analyzes the relationship between HIV/AIDS mental health services and improved life expectancy.

The development of mental health services that are culturally sensitive; that are relevant to the particular social and economic circumstances most children, adolescents, and families with HIV/AIDS encounter; and that can be integrated with comprehensive health care and social services is the primary public policy issue of this chapter. Because of the close link needed between mental health services and medical, legal, and social services, public policy related to HIV/AIDS mental health services has often been a part of larger HIV/AIDS policy and financing initiatives.

THE NEED FOR ADVOCACY

For progress to be gained in expanding HIV/AIDS services and preventing HIV infection, the field needs to be engaged in public policy advocacy that employs a range of strategies. Dicker (1990), in *Stepping Stones: Successful Advocacy for Children,* conducts a systemic analysis of effective advocacy, which brings about changes in government policies and practices that result in the improvement of lives of large numbers of children and families. Dicker cites four elements of successful advocacy: (1) Concrete solutions to problems are addressed; (2) various strategies are used over a prolonged period to achieve goals; (3) partners are recruited and found within the government to achieve implementation and reforms; and (4) care providers, parents, and children are enabled to participate and are empowered to make decisions regarding public policy. The analysis includes five in-depth case examples of successful advocacy efforts that combined inside-government and outside-government partnerships, grassroots organizing of constituents and care providers, specific legislative proposals, and other strategies that resulted in significant change and improvement of services within the system.

In the pediatric, adolescent, and family HIV/AIDS community, there has been a paucity of unified and national (in scope) advocacy efforts that utilize the policy delivery role of clinicians, as well as the direct life experiences of children, adolescents, and their families living with HIV/AIDS. By contrast, there has been some success (however controversial) within the grassroots advocacy efforts of the gay community. Community groups such as the AIDS Coalition to Unleash Power (ACT-UP) attempt to make the life experiences of persons living with HIV/AIDS known; together with professional advocates in Washington, D.C., they have enjoyed a measure of success in helping to expedite approval of experimental HIV/AIDS drugs, to enhance funding for HIV/AIDS service programs, and to refocus the HIV/AIDS research programs within the National Institutes of Health (NIH).

National coalitions in Washington, including the Pediatric AIDS Coalition and the National Organizations Responding to AIDS, convene and organize national constituency groups around HIV/AIDS public policy. What differs between HIV/AIDS advocacy efforts for the gay community and for families and children at this point in time is the ability to mobilize and conduct grassroots efforts. These efforts with families and children have been hampered because families with HIV/AIDS are overwhelmed with other problems in daily living, such as housing, food, transportation, day care, and other needs. However, successful advocacy strategies usually involve constituents in a primary role. Advocates for children, adolescents, and families with HIV/AIDS are faced with the difficult challenge of how to ensure accountability to family members who often cannot speak for themselves. One strategy is to rely on the experience of care providers to advocate for their clients. Advocates, however, must continue to search for ways to bring families with HIV/AIDS to Washington to be heard and to convene family councils to ensure that the families are a part of national advocacy campaigns.

A new national organization formed in 1994, the AIDS Policy Center for Children, Youth and Families, has a central mission to convene providers, families and youth living with HIV to participate in the national policy dialogue concerning HIV/AIDS and to fill the gap in addressing the policy concerns of this group.

FEDERAL GOVERNMENT RESPONSE

In response to public policy debate by Congress and efforts within the larger HIV/AIDS advocacy community, the federal government now spends a significant amount of funds on HIV/AIDS. These funds are dispersed through many government agencies. The primary HIV/AIDS mental health service and prevention activities are conducted through the Public Health Service (PHS) within the U.S. Department of Health and Human Services. Within the PHS, the majority of funds are spent through the NIH, the CDC, and the Substance Abuse and Mental Health Services Administration (SAMHSA). NIH funding is primarily for medical and laboratory research; SAMHSA funds research in areas of high-risk behaviors and prevention; CDC funding is for research, surveillance, and prevention implementation.

ADMS Block Grant Program

Under the auspices of the PHS, the Alcohol, Drug Abuse and Mental Health Services (ADMS) Block Grant Program is the major federal program providing financial assistance to states and territories for prevention, treatment, and rehabilitation programs related to mental illness, alcoholism, and drug abuse. Within this program are initiatives to cope with the HIV/AIDS epidemic. In 1981, several separate programs supporting community mental health centers, drug and alcohol treatment programs, and state mental health planning programs were combined under the Public Health Service Act, which was again later amended under the ADMS Amendments Act of 1984. At this time, two set-asides were established under the ADMS Block Grant Program: a 10% set-aside to serve underserved populations, with emphasis on children and adolescents; and a 5% set-aside for women under state substance abuse programs. Given the high correlation between injection drug use and HIV infection among women and children, these programs became the focus for HIV/AIDS prevention efforts and mental health counseling related to substance abuse and HIV/AIDS.

In 1992, with far-reaching ramifications for the delivery of HIV/AIDS mental health and prevention services, Congress passed legislation reorganizing the Alcohol, Drug Abuse and Mental Health Administration (ADAMHA), which administers the ADMS Block Grant Program (U.S. Congress, 1992). This administration was renamed SAMHSA, and now consists of the Center for Substance Abuse Prevention, the Center for Substance Abuse Treatment, and the Center for Mental Health Services. In addition, the National Institute on Alcoholism and Alcohol Abuse, the National Institute of Drug Abuse, and the National Institute of Mental Health are now placed under authority of the NIH. The May 1992 congressional conference report accompanying the legislation states:

> The principal purpose of the reorganization is to fully develop the Federal government's ability to target effectively substance abuse and men-

tal health services to the people most in need, and to translate research in these areas more effectively and more rapidly into the general health care system. (U.S. Congress, 1992)

ADMS Block Grant funds can be used to support community mental health centers and coordination with medical services, as well as research in areas of drug abuse and alcoholism, and HIV/AIDS. Community mental health centers are a major resource for children and families with HIV/AIDS in local communities, because they are publicly financed.

In the congressional conference report (U.S. Congress, 1992), the authors comment that HIV/AIDS has not received the level of attention at ADAMHA that would be expected. A new central office is recommended to administer substance abuse and HIV/AIDS research and services, as well as new requirements regarding categorical grant programs to help treat substance-using pregnant women and their children.

The 10% set-aside for childhood mental health services has been refocused to develop systems of care for children in at least one geographic location in a state. An additional set-aside under the ADMS Block Grant formula to states for 1993 and 1994 increases services to pregnant women and women with dependent children, while specifically commenting that pregnant women and injection drug users must have preferential treatment in admission to treatment programs, and that states are required to provide interim services if a waiting period exists for admission to treatment. A special focus is placed on HIV/AIDS prevention and counseling services and tuberculosis services, and states with more than 10 cases per 100,000 of AIDS must set aside additional funds for HIV early intervention services. A new Children of Substance Abusers Program provides funds for comprehensive services to children and families affected by parental substance abuse, and requires programs to link with existing related programs.

NIH Maternal and Pediatric HIV/AIDS Research

The maternal and pediatric HIV/AIDS research programs conducted by the National Cancer Institute, the National Institute of Allergy and Infectious Disease (NIAID), and the National Institute of Child Health and Development (NICHD) have two basic components: (1) biomedical research in HIV/AIDS in infants, children, pregnant women, and mothers; and (2) therapeutic clinical trials in these same groups. Biomedical research encompasses the study of epidemiology, natural history, diagnosis, and transmission of HIV infection in women and children. Clinical trials research focuses on the development and evaluation of safe and effective therapies that are life-prolonging and that will eventually be life-saving in mothers and children infected by HIV.

The NIH Revitalization Act of 1993 restructured HIV/AIDS programs within the NIH, in the belief that research programs would be enhanced by (1) strengthening the NIH Office of AIDS Research and appointing a full-time director; (2) developing strategic plans across institutes and coordinating research programs; (3) creating an Office of AIDS Research Advisory Council; and (4) granting budget authority to the Office of AIDS Research to allocate funds and to create a discretionary fund.

Biomedical Research

Despite some impressive gains in understanding brought about by maternal and pediatric HIV/AIDS biomedical research, many basic biomedical questions remain unanswered. The epidemiology of HIV infection in pregnant women, infants, and children, and the role of the placenta in viral transmission, are among the areas needing further study. Additional diagnostic technology for earlier detection of HIV in neonates, infants, and children is an area of rapid development, and access to these new technologies will need to be provided. Some of the outcomes of pediatric HIV/AIDS biomedical research may have benefits for our understanding of other areas, including the development of dementia; the development of the immune system and its relationship to the body's ability to cope with disease; and the transmission of viruses from mother to fetus *in utero* (Pediatric AIDS Coalition, 1993).

A recent and important gain in the AIDS research field is the results of a study sponsored by NIH that has shown that the drug zidovudine (ZDV or AZT) used by a carefully selected group of "well" immunocompetent HIV-infected women during the second and third trimester of pregnancy, infused during labor, and administered to the infant during the first six weeks of life reduced the rate of HIV transmission to newborns by two-thirds (CDC, 1994b). This finding has wide-ranging implications for HIV care and prevention for women and children, particularly young women who represented a significant proportion of the initial study participants. Specific legal and policy issues related to informed consent, access to therapy, and care will need to be addressed. The mental health consequences of providing counseling, obtaining informed consent, and offering this new therapy will need to be addressed immediately.

Clinical Trials

Women, particularly women of color, have traditionally experienced obstacles in gaining access to clinical HIV/AIDS drug trials, funded through NIAID and NICHD. Obstacles to participation include the inadequate number of protocols, lack of transportation and day care, lack of education and outreach, cultural issues, and legal barriers, among other needs. Likewise, the lack of uniform access to primary care for children, women, and families with HIV/AIDS has hampered efforts to enroll patients in clinical trials. Although primary and comprehensive HIV/AIDS services should have as one component access to HIV/AIDS therapeutic trials, this is not always the case.

Concern about the vulnerabilities of children and pregnant women as research subjects, as well as specific legal concerns, also initially resulted in these populations being left out of clinical trials. This process has now been reversed, but concerns continue about access to clinical trials and balancing patients' rights to participate versus risks (National Commission on AIDS, 1991).

The Need for Behavioral Research

Another major focus of recent policy debate has been the permissibility of sexual behavior research through the National Institute of Mental Health and other NIH research institutes. Regarded as essential by researchers in evaluating prevention services, maintaining surveillance, and projecting the future epidemiological course of HIV/AIDS, sexual behavior research has been disallowed under various congressional appropriations bills. The arguments for understanding sexual behavior in the context of prevention, adolescent development, drug use, and basic homosexual and heterosexual psychosexual issues have thus far been regarded as inadequate. The relative paucity of information on the behavioral factors related to HIV transmission led the Commission on Behavioral and Social Sciences and Education of the National Research Council to establish an HIV/AIDS Research Committee (Institute of Medicine, National Academy of Sciences, 1988).

Although several limited sexual behavior research studies have been carried out or are in progress, other major proposed studies, especially ones dealing with adolescents, were canceled by the Bush administration and Congress. In 1992, although two sexual behavior studies were forbidden by specific appropriations amendments, the Senate did pass another amendment expressing support for such research. This amendment contained provisions to take research decisions out of the political realm (Youngstrom, 1992), but whether additional research in this area will be supported is uncertain.

Pediatric/Family HIV/AIDS Health Care Program

In 1988 Congress established the Pediatric/Family HIV/AIDS Health Care Program—the main federally sponsored comprehensive health care system for children, adolescents, women, and families—to meet the challenges of preventing the further spread of HIV/AIDS and delivering care to families with HIV/AIDS through the development of collaborative systems of care at the community level. By 1994, 37 direct service sites had been funded in 22 states, the District of Columbia, and Puerto Rico. These projects have become an important component of the health care infrastructure, but do not serve all children and families affected by HIV/AIDS in the United States.

The projects have emphasized prevention within the comprehensive care system in order to reduce mother–infant transmission of HIV, especially among minorities and adolescents. The projects also work at developing effective models of delivering mental health services in the context of prevention and psychosocial interventions through family support groups, family-to-family networks, and individual counseling and case management. Nontraditional approaches to psychosocial interventions have been developed that take into account the particular socioeconomic circumstances of these families. Many of the projects have been successful in conducting outreach and education activities with women, aimed at preventing the further spread of HIV infection. Injection drug use has been directly or indirectly implicated in the infection of a majority of the children and adults served by the projects, underscoring the need for continuing and improved access to drug treatment and mental health services (Harvey et al., 1992).

Ryan White Comprehensive AIDS Resources Emergency Act

The Ryan White Comprehensive AIDS Resources Emergency (CARE) Act of 1990 provides health care and support services to individuals and families affected by HIV/AIDS (U.S. Congress, 1990). Through four discrete titles, which include formula, supplemental, and categorical grants to cities, states, and other eligible agencies and institutions, comprehensive outpatient and ambulatory care is funded for individuals and families. Funds for Title I, the HIV Emergency Relief Grant Program, provides emergency assistance to high-incidence cities throughout the United States. Funds are distributed to cities through formula, noncompetitive grants. Supplemental grants are also awarded to cities through a competitive process. Specific types of services funded include mental health services.

Under Title II of the act, CARE Grants are provided to states through a formula block grant. States have the option to use these funds to (1) establish and operate HIV/AIDS care consortia; (2) provide home- and community-based case services; (3) provide assistance in continuity of health care coverage; and (4) provide treatments that have been determined to prolong life or prevent deterioration of health. Not less than 15% of the total amount of funds awarded to each state is to be used to provide health and support services to infants, children, women, and families with HIV/AIDS. Types of services that may be funded include mental health and developmental services.

Also under Title II is authority to conduct Special Projects of National Significance (SPNS). Funding for this authority cannot exceed 10% of the amount appropriated for Title II. Grants may be made to assess the effectiveness, innovative nature, and replicability of service models. Other special projects include services for low-income individuals; drug abuse and HIV/AIDS treatment; support and respite care; comprehensive services for unserved hemophilia and HIV/AIDS populations; HIV/AIDS health care and support services to individuals and families; rural services; homeless services; and services for incarcerated persons. In fiscal year 1992, the Health Resources Services Administration awarded mental health demonstration grants under the SPNS authority of the Ryan White CARE Act.

Title IIIb of the CARE Act funds early intervention services at community health centers and other entities to provide outreach and counseling services, establish linkages with HIV testing programs, and provide on-going comprehensive health services for low-income persons affected by HIV infection.

Title IV of the Ryan White CARE Act authorizes programs that provide for comprehensive HIV/AIDS care for children, adolescents, pregnant women, and families; it also has a component that enhances access to HIV/AIDS therapeutic trials. In 1993, because of similar program goals, Congress has consolidated funding for the Pediatric/Family HIV/AIDS Health Care Program within Title IV, thereby authorizing and securing the program.

Major prevention initiatives are funded by the CDC in four basic areas of intervention: mass media campaigns; formal presentations of HIV/AIDS information to groups of people; one-to-one interaction with individuals at risk; and intensive group interventions. Operating under some educational restrictions imposed by Congress, the CDC undertook a seemingly massive prevention effort and stimulated private–public partnerships to provide education and prevention services in the mid-1980s; stimulated HIV/AIDS education programs in public schools; and funded local health departments to work with local community-based organizations and drug treatment centers to provide counseling and testing services, as well as other prevention initiatives (CDC, 1990). However, little outcome evaluation has been conducted with these funds to determine whether interventions have been related to changes in behavior (Scheitinger, 1991).

In addition to health promotion initiatives in the media, national HIV/AIDS information campaigns, and adolescent and school health programs, the Perinatal HIV Prevention Projects, started in 1990, are implementing and testing three prevention models for preventing HIV mother–infant transmission (CDC, 1990). These models include the following components: overcoming obstacles to contraception use by women at risk for HIV infection; utilization of family planning services for women with or at risk of HIV infection; evaluating attitudinal factors related to contraceptive use; and encouraging behavioral change to reduce the risk of HIV infection.

In 1993–1994, Congress and the CDC evaluated programs and implemented a course correction to focus planning efforts at the community level rather than channeling them through state agencies. Congressional legislation was considered to foster these changes, and the CDC implemented administrative revisions to its programs. Proposed legislation in the 104th Congress may further change HIV/AIDS and other STD prevention programs. The emphasis on local community control of prevention activities may be further altered.

FUTURE PUBLIC POLICY DEVELOPMENT

Significant public policy questions related to children, adolescents, and families with HIV/AIDS remain to be addressed in the areas of resource allocation, access to comprehensive services and clinical drug trials, behavioral research and prevention initiatives, access to zidovudine therapy for pregnant women with HIV, and the continued development of effective psychosocial and psychotherapeutic interventions that are culturally sensitive and competent. This will require a coordinated federal response incorporating recommendations that have already been developed by experts in the areas of behavior and biomedical research, service system development and financing, and prevention and mental health services. Future HIV/AIDS mental health services research must analyze the link between successful medical interventions and successful psychosocial and mental health interventions. With no vaccine or cure currently available for HIV/AIDS, the provision of mental health and prevention services is the only means of preventing the further spread of the virus and should be a high-priority public policy concern.

With the potential that cases of perinatal HIV infection can be reduced by offering the drug zidovudine to pregnant women with HIV infection, the role of the mental health clinician in assisting the patient with informed consent, outreach, education, and psychosocial support is crucial and should be further considered in public policy development.

REFERENCES

Centers for Disease Control (CDC). (1990). *CDC plan for preventing HIV infection: A blueprint for the 1990s.* Atlanta: Author.

Centers for Disease Control and Prevention (CDC). (1994a, August). *1993 year-end AIDS surveillance report. HIV/AIDS surveillance.* Atlanta: Author.

Centers for Disease Control and Prevention (CDC). (1994b, August 5). *Recommendations of the U.S. Public Health Service Task Force on the use of zidovudine to reduce perinatal transmission of HIV.* Atlanta: Author.

Centers for Disease Control and Prevention (CDC). (1994c). *HIV/AIDS Surveillance Report, 5*(4), 1–12.

Dicker, S. (1990). *Stepping stones: Successful advocacy for children.* New York: Foundation for Child Development.

Harvey, D. C., Boland, M., Burr, C., & Conviser, R. (1992). *Pediatric/family HIV Health Care Demonstration Grant Program: Clients served, 1988–1990.* Newark, NJ: National Pediatric HIV Resource Center.

Institute of Medicine, National Academy of Sciences. (1988). *Confronting AIDS.* Washington: National Academy Press.

Lipsky, M. (1980). *Street-level bureaucracy: Dilemmas of the individual in public services.* New York: Russell Sage Foundation.

Mechanic, D. (1991). Recent developments in mental health: Perspectives and services. *Annual Review of Public Health, 12,* 1–15.

National Commission on AIDS. (1991). *America living with AIDS.* Washington, DC: U.S. Government Printing Office.

National Commission on AIDS. (1993). *AIDS: An expanding tragedy.* Washington, DC: U.S. Government Printing Office.

Pediatric AIDS Coalition. (1993). *1993–1994 legislative agenda.* Washington, DC: Author.

Scheitinger, H. (1991). *Good intentions: A report on federal HIV prevention programs.* Washington, DC: AIDS Action Council.

U.S. Congress. (1990). *Conference report 101-652: Ryan White Comprehensive AIDS Resources Emergency Act of 1990.* Washington, DC: Government Printing Office.

U.S. Congress. (1992). *Conference report 102-522: ADAMHA Reorganization Act of 1992.* Washington, DC: U.S. Government Printing Office.

U.S. Department of Health and Human Services. (1987). *Report of the Surgeon General's workshop on children with HIV infection and their families.* Washington, DC: U.S. Government Printing Office.

U.S. Department of Health and Human Services. (1988). *Report of the Secretary's work group on pediatric HIV infection and disease.* Washington, DC: U.S. Government Printing Office.

Van Horn, C., Baumer, D., & Gormley, W. (1989). *Politics and public policy.* Washington, DC: Congressional Quarterly Press.

Youngstrom, N. (1992, August). Bush vetoes bill supporting research on sexual behavior. *APA Monitor, 23*(8), 40.

Index